Get Through

MRCP Part I: BOFs

Get Through
MRCP Part I: BOFs

Osama S M Amin MRCPI MRCPS(Glasg)
Department of Neurology, Baghdad Teaching Hospital, Baghdad, Iraq

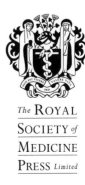

The ROYAL
SOCIETY *of*
MEDICINE
PRESS *Limited*

Published by the Royal Society of Medicine Press Ltd
1 Wimpole Street, London W1G 0AE, UK
Tel: +44 (0)20 7290 2921
Fax: +44 (0)20 7290 2929
E-mail: publishing@rsmpress.co.uk

British Library Cataloguing in Publication Data
A catalogue record for this book is available from the British Library

ISBN: 978-1-85315-823-0

Distribution in Europe and Rest of the World:
Marston Book Services Ltd
PO Box 269
Abingdon
Oxon OX14 4YN, UK
Tel: +44 (0)1235 465500
Fax: +44 (0)1235 465555
Email: direct.order@marston.co.uk

Distribution in USA and Canada:
Royal Society of Medicine Press Ltd
c/o BookMasters Inc
30 Amberwood Parkway
Ashland, OH 44805, USA
Tel: +1 800 247 6553/ +1 800 266 5564
Fax: +1 410 281 6883
Email: order@bookmasters.com

Distribution in Australia and New Zealand:
Elsevier Australia
3052 Smidmore Street
Marrickville NSW 2204, Australia
Tel: +61 2 9517 8999
Fax: +61 2 9517 2249
Email: service@elsevier.com.au

Typeset by Techset Composition Limited, Salisbury, UK
Printed in the UK by Bell & Bain Ltd, Glasgow

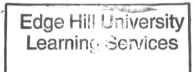

Contents

Foreword

The London MRCP exam began in 1859, so this book arrives one year short of its 150th anniversary. Yet the relevance of the MRCP lies in its place in a two-and-a-half millennium tradition of Hippocratic medicine.

What distinguishes the Hippocratic tradition? I would suggest it has three characteristics. First, it is a scientific tradition, based on observation and evidence, not on authority–when traditions are old it is easy to forget their radical foundations. Second, any tradition that is based on scientific evidence must cope with change–we must be prepared to go where new evidence leads. Progress means change, and quite possibly the science of medicine has made more progress in the last 150 years than in the two-and-a-half millennia before. Candidates sitting the exam now and their counterparts in 1859 would no doubt both be equally surprised, and discomforted, to have their question papers exchanged!

Finally, however, Hippocratic medicine is not just a science, and certainly not just a job. It is a vocation and a profession. From the Hippocratic tradition we have the driving imperative to act only in the patients' best interest, and to seek to never bring them harm. It is this tradition that makes those who share it colleagues, at a deep level, with physicians from other nations and other times.

Any profession must function within specific times and cultures, and medicine is no exception. Postgraduate medical training in the UK is going through a time of turbulent change. But I am glad to say that this book contains no questions about MMC or how to write a good CV. The job may go through good times or bad, but the vocation remains constant. There will always be patients who need intelligent and caring treatment from their physicians. In this Osama Amin serves stunningly well as a role model. If I were working at the Baghdad Teaching Hospital in Iraq, would I be concerning myself with writing medical textbooks? We can be thankful for such an example. For the real accolade for this book is not just that it will help you to pass an exam, but that it will help you to treat patients.

David Misselbrook
Dean, Royal Society of Medicine

Preface

'How do I get started?' 'Which books should I read?' 'Which are the best self-assessment books?' 'How much time do I need for preparation?' These are the usual questions asked by the MRCP candidates. Rumours about the MRCP examination spread like a fire, conveying many wrong ideas and unhelpful 'tips'.

Any type of examination, medical or non-medical, requires preparation. With careful reading, an appropriate duration of study and proper self-assessment, the candidate can safely secure a pass in this examination.

How do I get started? The answer is simple; start by reading *accredited textbooks*, chapter by chapter to build up a wealth of knowledge. An efficient physician should be familiar with the well-known medicine textbooks and their contents.

Which medical books should be read? The market is full of well-accredited textbooks. I would suggest starting with *Davidson's Principles and Practice of Medicine*; it is simple, compact and covers many important aspects and themes of the examination. You should then extend your horizon by reading specialist textbooks.

How much time do I need for preparation? No one can answer this question for you; you are the only one who can judge your starting point and estimate the time needed to assimilate the necessary knowledge base. However, no less than 6 months would suffice for this purpose. The best tip is to take your time and there will be no need to rush.

Which are the best self-assessment books? This is an embarrassing question! The market is full of these books and the number is rising. Self-assessment books should be tackled only after reading textbooks. The idea is to self-assess, i.e. test your level of knowledge. Do not start your MRCP preparation journey by doing this step first. Do as many best of five (BOF) books as you can, identify your weak points and try to fill these gaps.

My examination is tomorrow! There is no need to panic. On the day before examination, for your own self-esteem, skim quickly over BOF questions.

What will happen on the day of examination? Reach the place of the examination at least 1 hour before the expected start time, and bring a grade 2B pencil and a rubber with you (some examination centres supply candidates with these). Each candidate has a dedicated seat labelled with his/her name (and sometimes code number). The MRCP UK Part 1 examination has two papers, 100 BOF questions in each, and each paper lasts 3 hours with a 1 hour break between. The candidate should choose the best possible answer from the five stems.

Verify your name, code number and examination number on the front page of each paper. Paper 1 is usually easier than paper 2. Read individual questions carefully and mark the answer sheet with your choice; if you face any difficult question, skip these and return to them at the end.

According to the MRCP examination regulations, the composition of the papers is as follows:

Specialty	Number of questions*
Cardiology	15
Clinical haematology and oncology	15
Clinical pharmacology, therapeutics and toxicology	20
Clinical sciences**	25
Dermatology	8
Endocrinology	15
Gastroenterology	15
Neurology	15
Ophthalmology	4
Psychiatry	8
Renal medicine	15
Respiratory medicine	15
Rheumatology	15
Tropical medicine, infectious and sexually transmitted diseases	15

*This should be taken as an indication of the likely number of questions; the actual number may vary by two.
**Clinical sciences comprise:

Cell, molecular and membrane biology	2
Clinical anatomy	3
Clinical biochemistry and metabolism	4
Clinical physiology	4
Genetics	3
Immunology	4
Statistics, epidemiology, and evidence-based medicine	5

Adapted with permission from *MRCP (UK) Regulations and Information for Candidates, 2008 edition*. MRCP (UK) Central Office, Royal Colleges of Physicians of the United Kingdom, London, UK. Copyright 2008. All rights reserved.

The examination may include pre-test questions (trial questions that are used for research purposes, and these do not count towards the candidate's final score).

In writing this book, I have tried to cover the examination syllabus and its most important themes, and to provide a rapid review of most of the subjects that can be encountered.

Good luck!

Osama Amin

List of abbreviations

ABPI	ankle:brachial blood pressure index
ACE	angiotensin-converting enzyme
ADH	antidiuretic hormone
AIDS	acquired immune deficiency syndrome
AIP	acute intermittent porphyria
ALT	alanine aminotransferase
ANA	antinuclear antibody
ANCA	antineutrophil cytoplasm antibody
ARDS	acute respiratory distress syndrome
ARMD	age-related macular degeneration
ASD	atrial septal defect
AST	aspartate transaminase
CABG	coronary artery bypass graft
CLI	critical limb ischaemia
CLL	chronic lymphocytic leukaemia
CML	chronic myeloid leukaemia
CMV	cytomegalovirus
CNS	central nervous system
COPD	chronic obstructive pulmonary disease
CPAP	continuous positive airway pressure
CRP	C-reactive protein
CSF	cerebrospinal fluid
DIC	disseminated intravascular coagulation
DIP	distal interphalangeal
DL_{CO}	carbon monoxide diffusion in the lung
DVT	deep vein thrombosis
ECT	electroconvulsive therapy
EEG	electroencephalogram
EIA	enzyme-linked immunoassay
EMG	electromyography
EPO	erythropoietin
ERCP	endoscopic retrograde cholangiopancreatography
FAP	familial adenomatous polyposis
FEV1	forced expiratory volume in 1 second
FiO_2	fractional concentration of oxygen in inspired gas
FVC	forced vital capacity
G6PD	glucose-6-phosphate deficiency
GBM	glomerular basement membrane
GFR	glomerular filtration rate
GIT	gastrointestinal tract
HAART	highly active antiretroviral therapy
hCG	human chorionic gonadotrophin
HDL	high density lipoprotein
IDL	intermediate density lipoprotein
INO	internuclear ophthalmoplegia
INR	international normalized ratio
ITP	idiopathic thrombocytopenic purpura
JVP	jugular venous pressure

LDH	lactate dehydrogenase
LDL	low density lipoprotein
LV	left ventricle
MCV	mean corpuscular volume
MDR	multidrug resistant
MEN	multiple endocrine neoplasia
MGUS	monoclonal gammopathy of undetermined significance
MODY	maturity onset diabetes of the young
MRI	magnetic resonance imaging
NSAID	non-steroid anti-inflammatory drug
PAN	polyarteritis nodosa
PCI	percutaneous coronary intervention
PCR	polymerase chain reaction
PCV	packed cell volume
PEM	protein energy malnutrition
PIP	proximal interphalangeal
PPI	proton pump inhibitor
PTH	parathyroid hormone
RBC	red blood cell
RIBA	recombinant immunoblot assay
RTA	renal tubular acidosis
SBP	spontaneous bacterial peritonitis
SIADH	syndrome of inappropriate ADH secretion
SLE	systemic lupus erythematosus
TB	tuberculosis
TIA	transient ischaemic attack
TIPPS	transjugular intrahepatic portosystemic stent shunt
TSH	thyroid stimulating hormone
TTP	thrombotic thrombocytopenic purpura
UTI	urinary tract infection
VLDL	very low density lipoprotein
VSD	ventricular septal defect
vWD	von Willebrand disease
vWF	von Willebrand factor
WPW	Wolff–Parkinson–White

Recommended reading

Abrahamson M, Aronson M (eds). *ACP Diabetes Care Guide, A Team-Based Practice Manual and Self-Assessment Program*. Philadelphia: American College of Physicians, 2007.

Andreoli T, Carpenter C, Griggs R, Benjamin I. *Andreoli and Carpenter's Cecil's Essentials of Medicine*, 7th edn. Philadelphia: Elsevier, 2007.

Boon NA, Colledge NR, Walker BR (eds). *Davidson's Principles and Practice of Medicine*, 20th edn. Philadelphia: Elsevier, 2006.

Fauci AS, Braunwald E, Kasper DL *et al.* (eds). *Harrison's Principles of Internal Medicine*, 17th ed. New York: McGraw-Hill, 2008.

Goldman L, Ausiello D (eds). *Cecil Textbook of Medicine*, 22nd edn. Philadelphia: Elsevier, 2003.

Kanski J. *Clinical Ophthalmology: A Systematic Approach*, 6th edn. Philadelphia: Elsevier, 2007.

Klippel J, Crofford A, Stone J, Weyand C (eds). *Primer on the Rheumatic Diseases*, 12th edn. Georgia: Arthritis Foundation, 2001.

Larsen P, Kronenberg H, Melmed S, Polonsky K (eds). *William's Textbook of Endocrinology*, 10th edn. Philadelphia: Elsevier, 2003.

Ropper A, Brown R. *Adams and Victor's Principles of Neurology*, 8th edn. New York: McGraw-Hill, 2005.

Warrel D, Cox T, Firth J, Benze E (eds). *Oxford Textbook of Medicine*, 4th edn. New York: Oxford University Press, 2003.

Dedicated to
My Mother, Ghareeba
My Wife, Sarah
My Patients

Acknowledgements

I would like to sincerely thank my patients; their real clinical scenarios were taken to formulate the book's questions. Special thanks go to Sarah Burrows and Sarah Vasey at RSM Press for their kind cooperation during the writing of this work. I am extremely grateful to the RSM Press; without its kind help, this book would not have been published.

I'm also indebted to Lucy Gardner, the copy-editor who has done excellent work, and the following for their contribution: Hannah Wessely, Nora Naughton, Aileen Castell and Mandy Sancto.

I intend to donate my royalty to support the educational activities of the RSM.

1. Cardiology: Questions

1) A 65-year-old retired forest ranger comes for his monthly check-up visit. He sustained an anterior wall myocardial infarction 4 months ago for which he takes aspirin, metoprolol and simvastatin. His blood pressure is 135/80 mmHg. The serum lipid profile that was done 2 days ago showed an LDL-cholesterol of 93 mg/dl. What would you do next?

   a. Add enalapril
   b. Increase the dose of simvastatin
   c. Stop metoprolol
   d. Repeat his lipid profile
   e. Give omeprazole

2) A 70-year-old man with calcific aortic stenosis presents with exertional breathlessness over the past few months. His echocardiography reveals an ejection fraction of 54%, left ventricular hypertrophy and moderate aortic stenosis. He denies chest pain or syncope, but admits to having frequent palpitations associated with light-headedness. What is the best action to take?

   a. Frequent follow-up
   b. Aortic valve replacement
   c. 24-hour Holter monitoring
   d. Prescribe nifedipine
   e. Start a thiazide

3) A 21-year-old woman presents with recurrent attacks of palpitations and presyncope. She denies taking drugs and there is no family history of note. Resting 12-lead ECG shows a short PR interval and slurring of the upstroke of the R wave. Which is the best treatment?

   a. Procainamide
   b. Digoxin
   c. Radiofrequency catheter ablation
   d. Implantable cardioverter–defibrillator
   e. Percutaneous coronary intervention

4) A 7-year-old girl has had recurrent chest infections and her notes indicate a cardiac murmur. Auscultation reveals a continuous machinery murmur at the left subclavicular area. Cardiac catheterization shows patent ductus arteriosus. What is the next best step?

   a. Observe
   b. Heart–lung transplantation
   c. Permanent pacemaker
   d. Endovascular occlusion of the ductus
   e. Infective endocarditis prophylaxis

5) A 43-year-old man with dilated cardiomyopathy complains that he takes many medications daily and is not feeling well. He is dyspnoeic while shaving, toileting and dressing, and is a little short of breath at rest. His regimen includes carvedilol, lisinopril and furosemide. His ECG reveals infrequent multifocal ventricular ectopics. Which one of the following medications should be added to improve this man's chances of survival?

a. Digoxin
b. Fluvastatin
c. Spironolactone
d. Amiodarone
e. Hydralazine

6) A 17-year-old athlete presents with recurrent palpitations at rest. He has a jerky pulse with a double apical impulse. There is a systolic ejection murmur in the aortic area with a mitral regurgitation at the apex. You are considering a diagnosis of hypertrophic cardiomyopathy. Which one of the following would decrease the loudness of the aortic area murmur?

a. Strain phase of Valsalva manoeuvre
b. Standing
c. Post-extrasystolic beat
d. Inspiration
e. Squatting

7) A 45-year-old man has permanent atrial fibrillation for which he takes daily digoxin and aspirin. His ventricular rate is still rapid and you are considering adding another medication to slow it down. Which one of the following medications does *not* increase the serum digoxin level?

a. Amiodarone
b. Quinidine
c. Propafenone
d. Flecainide
e. Metoprolol

8) A 41-year-old woman presents with a 1-hour history of crushing substernal chest pain. She smokes two packets of cigarettes a day and has poorly controlled Type 2 diabetes mellitus. There is a strong family history of premature coronary artery disease. Her 12-lead ECG shows ST segment elevation in leads V2–V4. Which one of the following is not an absolute contraindication to receiving thrombolytic therapy for this ST segment elevation myocardial infarction?

a. Aortic dissection
b. Intracranial Berry's aneurysm
c. Active internal bleeding
d. Current menstruation
e. Brain tumour

9) A 62-year-old man who is a heavy smoker presents with a 6-hour history of central chest pain that had started when he was watching TV. He has long-standing hypertension for which he takes daily lisinopril. His ECG shows non-specific ST–T changes. His serum cardiac troponin T level is slightly raised. Chest X-ray is unremarkable. What is the diagnosis?

a. Unstable angina
b. Full thickness myocardial infarction
c. Acute pericarditis
d. Diffuse oesophageal spasm
e. Type A aortic dissection

10) A 68-year-old man develops sudden haemodynamic collapse and shortness of breath four days after sustaining an anterior wall myocardial infarction. Cardiac catheterization shows a step-up in oxygen saturation from the right atrium to the right ventricle, and a large v wave in the pulmonary capillary trace. What has developed in this patient?

a. Papillary muscle rupture
b. Ventricular septum rupture
c. Left ventricular free wall rupture
d. Ruptured sinus of Valsalva
e. Ruptured mitral valve chordae

11) A 14-year-old man with post-ductal coarctation of the aorta has a systolic ejection murmur at the aortic area as well as a murmur at the left upper back. What is the likely cause of the precordial murmur?

a. The site of coarctation
b. The presence of collaterals
c. Associated bicuspid aortic valve
d. Associated pulmonary stenosis
e. An innocent flow murmur

12) A 43-year-old woman with long-standing rheumatic mitral regurgitation presents for a check-up. She denies any symptoms. She is a librarian who lives alone in a two-story house and who shops daily. Which one of the following indicates the need for mitral valve surgery in this woman?

a. Presence of thumping beats
b. Ejection fraction of 40%
c. Left ventricular end-systolic volume 40 ml
d. Left ventricular end-diastolic volume 60 ml
e. Presence of apical thrill

13) A 54-year-old woman with ischaemic heart disease in the form of chronic stable angina, Canadian functional class I, is about to undergo non-cardiac surgery. Which one of the following procedures does *not* carry a high risk for perioperative vascular events?

a. Emergency operation
b. Aortic aneurysm surgery
c. Cataract extraction
d. Prolonged operation with major fluid shift
e. Vascular surgery of lower limbs

14) A 69-year-old man with long-standing, poorly controlled hypertension presents with severe tearing central chest pain radiating to the back. Chest X-ray shows a widened upper mediastinum. His ECG reveals 4-mm ST segment elevation in leads II, III and aVF. What is the cause of his abnormal ECG?

a. Dissection of the left main coronary artery
b. Cardiac tamponade
c. Involvement of the right coronary artery ostium
d. Aortic rupture into the left pleural space
e. Coronary artery spasm

15) A 50-year-old man has a blood pressure of 160/105 mmHg, which is repeatedly confirmed to be high. He has migraine without aura for which he takes sumatriptan during pain episodes. Which is the best antihypertensive medication for this patient to be given initially?

a. Ramipril
b. Propranolol
c. Hydrochlorothiazide
d. Losartan
e. Alpha methyldopa

16) A 67-year-old man who is a heavy smoker presents with calf pain upon exercise. He reports feeling this pain when walking about 50 metres on the flat level and that it goes away during rest. His peripheral pulses are feeble and his feet are cold. Neurological examination of the lower limbs is unremarkable as is his lumbar spine X-ray film. The ankle:brachial blood pressure index indicates the presence of peripheral vascular disease if it is:

a. <3
b. >2
c. <0.9
d. >0.5
e. 1

17) A 72-year-old man presents with abdominal pain that is suggestive of peptic ulceration. You have detected a palpable pulsating mass in the epigastrium. A trial of lansoprazole has produced a dramatic symptomatic relief. Abdominal ultrasonography reveals dilated abdominal aorta. You advised repeat of this investigation at regular intervals. Elective aneurysmal repair is warranted when the rate of aortic dilatation exceeds:

a. 2 cm/6 months
b. 0.5 cm/12 months
c. 5 mm/6 months
d. 10 mm/3 months
e. 1.5 cm/4 months

18) A 28-year-old man attends A&E, after having an upper respiratory tract infection, with central chest pain that worsens when lying down, swallowing and deep breathing. He is reasonably well and healthy and he does not take drugs. His 12-lead ECG shows widespread ST segment elevation. The pain is partially responsive to indometacin. You are reluctant to prescribe prednisolone because:

a. It is ineffective
b. High doses are needed
c. It increases the risk of developing relapsing/recurrent inflammation
d. It is contraindicated
e. Long-term treatment is mandated

19) A 62-year-old man with a diagnosis of chronic stable angina still has chest pain upon exertion. His current medications are optimal doses of atenolol, diltiazem, isosorbide dinitrate and aspirin. He insists that he is compliant with his medications and there has been no significant change in his daily activities. What is the next best step?

a. Arrange for coronary angiography
b. Refer for coronary artery bypass grafting
c. Add fluvastatin
d. Start heparin infusion
e. Add enalapril

20) A 23-year-old university student presents to A&E with a 1-hour history of rapid palpitation. Apart from dizziness, she reports no other symptoms. Her blood pressure is 110/50 mmHg. A 12-lead ECG is consistent with supraventricular tachycardia. Vagal manoeuvres fail to abort this tachyarrhythmia. What medication should you give?

a. Oral adenosine
b. Intravenous adenosine bolus
c. Slow intravenous adenosine over 30 minutes
d. Subcutaneous adenosine pump
e. Sublingual adenosine

21) A 49-year-old man with long-standing hypertension comes to see you after developing gradual breathlessness on exertion. His blood pressure is 150/100 mmHg with grade II hypertensive retinal changes but no raised JVP. Examination reveals S4 with clear lung bases. His echocardiography shows concentric left ventricular hypertrophy and an ejection fraction of 60%. What is the cause of his exertional dyspnoea?

a. Restrictive cardiomyopathy
b. Congestive heart failure
c. Pericardial constriction
d. Diastolic dysfunction
e. Drug-induced pulmonary fibrosis

22) A 54-year-old man with chronic stable angina presents to A&E with a 1-hour history of crushing central chest pain that is not responsive to rest and sublingual nitroglycerin. He has raised JVP, hypotension and clear lung bases. His ECG shows ST segment elevation in some leads, with raised cardiac markers. Which coronary artery is likely to be the cause?

a. Left main stem
b. Left anterior descending
c. Left circumference
d. Right coronary
e. Combined right coronary and left anterior descending

23) A 68-year-old man with long-standing hypertension presents to A&E with his son, complaining of prolonged and severe, tearing chest pain. His blood pressure is 70/30 mmHg. Chest X-ray shows a widened upper mediastinum. All of the following can result in this low blood pressure, except:

a. Involvement of the aortic valve
b. Rupture into the pericardium
c. Rupture into the mediastinum
d. Left anterior descending artery occlusion
e. Rupture into the pleural space

24) A 32-year-old man has a 3-hour history of rapid and pounding heart beats. After reviewing his 12-lead ECG, you are considering a diagnosis of atrial flutter with 2:1 conduction. How can you confirm your clinical suspicion?

a. Give an infusion of lidocaine
b. Start oral metoprolol
c. Give a bolus of adenosine
d. Wait and see
e. Apply a nitroglycerin skin patch

25) A 36-year-old man with chronic lone atrial fibrillation complains of feeling dizzy and unwell for 2 days. He has noticed that he becomes dizzy during exertion and when he walks in the garden. He smokes 2–3 cigarettes a day and drinks beer at weekends. His ECG reveals rapid atrial fibrillation and his blood pressure is 110/70 mmHg. Which of the following medications would control the ventricular rate during exercise?

   a. Digoxin
   b. Amiodarone
   c. Atenolol
   d. Clonidine
   e. Procainamide

26) A 57-year-old man is about to undergo exercise ECG testing for exertional chest pain that appears to be ischaemic. His resting 12-lead ECG is consistent with marked left ventricular hypertrophy. The next best step is:

   a. Delay the exercise ECG testing for 1 month
   b. Shorten the duration of the Bruce protocol
   c. Start ramipril before the test
   d. Arrange for myocardial perfusion imaging
   e. Do coronary intervention before the test

27) A 66-year-old man develops two generalized tonic–clonic seizures one day after admission to the coronary care unit because of anterior wall myocardial infarction and short-lived, successfully terminated, ventricular fibrillation. You are considering a diagnosis of drug induced seizures. Which one of the following medications could be responsible for this man's seizures?

   a. Metoprolol
   b. Lidocaine
   c. Captopril
   d. Morphine
   e. Aspirin

28) A 37-year-old woman presents with prostration and fever. On examination you note a skin rash, splenomegaly, palpable tender nodules on the finger pulps and cardiac murmurs. Which one of the following carries the highest risk for developing infective endocarditis?

   a. Patent ductus arteriosus
   b. Aortic coarctation
   c. Previous infective endocarditis
   d. Hypertrophic cardiomyopathy
   e. Mitral valve prolapse with cusp thickening

29) A 35-year-old male vagrant, intravenous drug abuser presents to A&E with shortness of breath and high fever. He has a pansystolic murmur down the left lower sternal border that increases on inspiration. Previously he has been seen by many doctors in the outpatient clinic for his fever, but no improvement has been observed. His blood culture is repeatedly negative. What is the cause of this negative blood culture?

a. *Candida* infection
b. *Brucella* infection
c. Prior antibiotic therapy
d. *HACEK* group infection
e. *Staphylococcus albus* infection

30) A 33-year-old writer with a 2-year history of congestive heart failure presents to A&E with rapid onset of severe shortness of breath and cough. He admits to being non-compliant with his medications lately. His chest X-ray reveals bilateral perihilar shadows in a bat-wing distribution. You start high-flow oxygen and furosemide. What medication should be given next?

a. Oral ramipril
b. Intravenous nesiritide
c. Oral digoxin
d. Intravenous amiodarone drip
e. Oral carvedilol

31) A 21-year-old male university student desperate for help, visits you for advice. He says that his two older brothers died suddenly when they were young. His ECG shows right bundle branch block and ST segment elevation in leads V1 and V2. This prompts coronary angiography, which is normal. What is this young man's diagnosis?

a. Romano–Ward syndrome
b. Wolff–Parkinson–White syndrome
c. Brugada's syndrome
d. Jervell–Lange–Nielsen syndrome
e. Mark–Thomas syndrome

32) A 54-year-old diabetic man has pain in his forefeet at night. He experiences pain in both calves whenever he walks about 40 metres on the flat that is relieved within 5 minutes of rest. Examination reveals ulcers on the toes. Ankle blood pressure is 40 mmHg. What is this man's diagnosis?

a. Intermittent claudication
b. Intermittent pseudoclaudication
c. Critical limb ischaemia
d. Cholesterol atheroembolic disease
e. Small vessel vasculitis

33) A 51-year-old man after being brought to A&E with cardiovascular collapse, underwent successful cardioversion. He takes daily amiodarone to prevent episodes of supraventricular tachycardia. His wife states that their GP has recently introduced a medication. Attempts to call the GP and to verify the medication have not been successful. All of the following medications might have been added, except:

a. Chlorpromazine
b. Cisapride
c. Terfinadine
d. Imipramine
e. Ciprofloxacin

34) A 66-year-old man is to undergo surgical repair of his type B aortic dissection. He is taking chlorthalidone and ramipril for long-standing hypertension, and metformine for Type 2 diabetes. Examination reveals a cold, pulseless paralyzed left leg. What is the indication for surgical intervention in type B aortic dissection in this man?

a. Associated diabetes
b. The duration of hypertension
c. Presence of acute limb ischaemia
d. Patient's age
e. Hypertension per se

35) A 10-year-old boy presents with rapid atrial fibrillation and central cyanosis. Echocardiography shows atrialization of the right ventricle. His mother has bipolar disorder and she took lithium salt during her pregnancy. What is the cause of cyanosis in this boy?

a. Associated large pulmonary arteriovenous malformation
b. Development of Eisenmenger's syndrome
c. Coexistent congenital methaemogloblinaemia
d. Right to left shunt through the patent foramen ovale
e. Severe secondary polycythaemia

36) A 61-year-old man while still receiving chemotherapy for his small cell lung cancer, presents with tachycardia, hypotension and raised JVP. His cardiac silhouette is globular, and his echocardiography is consistent with a large pericardial effusion. Which one of the following can be seen on examination of his JVP?

a. Cannon waves
b. Fixed elevation of the JVP
c. Blunted y descent
d. Irregular filling
e. Negative hepatojugular reflux

37) A 22-year-old woman survived an out-of-hospital cardiac death through prompt resuscitation, and is worried because she thinks that this will happen again. Her ECG, echocardiography and coronary angiogram are all normal. She is not on any medications and she takes no illicit drugs. Her family history is unremarkable. What is the best option to prevent this cardiac death from recurring?

a. Amiodarone
b. Bi-ventricular pacing
c. VVI pacing
d. Implantable cardioverter–defibrillator
e. Radiofrequency catheter ablation

38) A 29-year-old woman presents with progressive impairment in her exercise tolerance, and cough. Examination reveals an apical mid-diastolic murmur, and her chest X-ray shows straightening of the left heart border. Her past medical history is unremarkable, as is her family history. Which one of the following indicates non-eligibility to undergo mitral balloon valvuloplasty for rheumatic mitral stenosis?

a. The presence of trivial regurgitation
b. No valvular cusp calcification
c. The presence of left atrial thrombus
d. Sinus rhythm
e. Patient's age

39) A recent ECG for a 63-year-old man with diabetes is consistent with left axis deviation, but there are no voltage criteria for left ventricular hypertrophy. Echocardiography confirms the latter observation. This can be explained by:

a. Posterior wall myocardial infarction
b. Right bundle branch block
c. Limb lead reversal
d. Left anterior hemiblock
e. Mirror image dextrocardia

40) A 67-year-old man has chronic atrial fibrillation. You are considering starting him on anticoagulation with warfarin because he has a very high risk of thromboembolic phenomena. Which one of the following would incur such a very high risk?

a. Diabetes
b. Left ventricular dysfunction
c. Hypertension
d. Transient ischaemic attacks
e. Mitral regurgitation

41) A 19-year-old man with rapid palpitations and dizziness is brought to A&E by his older sister. He is otherwise healthy with no chronic illnesses. He denies any illicit drug ingestion. A 12-lead ECG reveals wide QRS complex tachycardia. Which one of the following is suggestive of supraventricular tachycardia with aberrant conduction rather than ventricular tachycardia?

a. Fusion beats
b. Extreme left axis deviation
c. Very wide QRS complexes
d. History of ischaemic heart disease
e. Rate slowing with intravenous adenosine

42) A 54-year-old man with essential hypertension comes for a scheduled weekly visit because of high uncontrolled blood pressure. His blood pressure is 160/105 mmHg. He takes daily atenolol, enalapril and hydrochlorothiazide. What is the most common cause of his refractory hypertension?

a. Renal artery stenosis
b. Phaeochromocytoma
c. Subclinical hyperthyroidism
d. Exogenous steroid ingestion
e. Non-compliance

43) A 36-year-old man with NYHA functional class III idiopathic dilated cardiomyopathy visits the cardiology outpatient clinic for a check-up. There is a trace of leg oedema with clear lung bases. An echocardiography that was done 1 week ago revealed global poor contractility and an ejection fraction of 42%. He receives daily digoxin, captopril and furosemide. You are considering adding a beta-blocker to his regimen. Which one of the following beta-blockers would you choose?

a. Sotalol
b. Bisprolol
c. Atenolol
d. Propranolol
e. Esmolol

44) A systolic click is detected in a 22-year-old woman during a routine pre-employment examination. She is otherwise healthy, enjoys an independent life and lives in an apartment with her boyfriend. All of the following are potential causes for a systolic click except:

a. Floppy mitral valve
b. Valvular aortic stenosis
c. Prosthetic valve
d. Tricuspid valvular stenosis
e. Pulmonary valvular stenosis

45) A 12-year-old girl has recurrent attacks of torsades de pointes ventricular tachycardia because of Romano–Ward syndrome. Which one of the following should be avoided?

a. Beta-blockers
b. Intravenous isoprenaline
c. Left stellate ganglion ablation
d. Cardiac pacing
e. Intravenous magnesium

46) A 57-year-old man has been admitted to the coronary care unit with anterioseptal myocardial infarction. Five days later he reports the same prolonged central crushing chest pain. You consider this may be due to a re-infarction. Which one of the following enzymes would be helpful in consolidating your clinical impression?

a. Troponin T
b. Troponin I
c. ALT
d. MB isozyme of creatine kinase
e. AST

47) A 54-year-old man has NYHA functional class II congestive heart failure. His condition rapidly deteriorates in his condition within a few days. His JVP is raised and there are prominent pitting leg oedema and bibasal rales. All of the following can result in his cardiac decompensation except:

a. Pulmonary thromboembolism
b. Tachyarrhythmia
c. Bradycardia
d. Polycythemia
e. Chest infection

48) A 33-year-old man with rheumatic mitral regurgitation presents with a 3-week history of fever, lassitude, weight loss and pallor. Serial blood cultures isolate viridans *streptococci*. His transthoracic echocardiography fails to demonstrate any vegetation. What is next best step?

a. Repeat blood cultures
b. Repeat transthoracic echocardiography after 3 days
c. Do transoesophageal echocardiography
d. Liver function testing
e. Coagulation studies

49) A 30-year-old woman presents with progressive exertional breath-lessness. She was told that she has a pansystolic murmur when she was a child. Examination reveals central cyanosis and clubbing. What is the likely cause of this woman's current presentation?

   a. Tricuspid atresia
   b. Eisenmenger's syndrome
   c. Infective endocarditis
   d. Secundum atrial septal defect
   e. Tetralogy of Fallot

50) A 32-year-old refugee from Africa presents with marked ascites, raised JVP with prominent x descent, pitting leg oedema and loud S_3. Chest films show clear lung fields and a normal heart size, but there are flecks of calcification within the cardiac silhouette. What is the likely cause of his presentation?

   a. Previous tuberculous infection
   b. Mediastinal irradiation
   c. Drug-induced
   d. HIV infection
   e. Parasitic infestation

51) A 41-year-old man comes for his annual check-up. He denies any symptoms, and neither smokes nor drinks alcohol. His past medical history is unremarkable and there is no family history of note. Examination is unremarkable and his body mass index is 22 kg/m². However, his 12-lead ECG reveals the presence of wide-spread low voltage QRS complexes. Which one of the following is the likely explanation for his abnormal ECG?

   a. Emphysema
   b. Obesity
   c. Hypothyroidism
   d. Incorrect standardization
   e. Hypopituitarism

52) A 74-year-old man with multiple pathologies is seen to have absent P wave on ECG monitoring while being managed in the intensive care unit. His 12 lead ECG confirms this observation. Which one of the following is *not* a potential cause of this finding?

   a. Atrial fibrillation
   b. Hyperkalaemia
   c. Nodal rhythm
   d. SA block
   e. Brugada's syndrome

53) A 24-year-old man was found to have a bigeminal rhythm during a routine pre-employment assessment. Apart from the occasional dropped beat, he reports feeling fine. He denies taking drugs and there is no family history of the same complaint. Which one of the following is the likely cause of this cardiac rhythm?

a. Atrial flutter with alternating 4:1 and 2:1 conduction
b. Mobitz type II second-degree AV block with 3:2 conduction
c. Alternating ventricular premature complexes
d. Alternating atrial extrasystoles
e. Alternating nodal ectopics

54) A 50-year-old man is referred by his GP for further assessment. The GP states that the patient has an irregularly irregular right radial pulse and he is unable to define its origin and cause. Which one of the following is *not* implicated as a potential cause of this physical finding?

a. Marked respiratory sinus arrhythmia
b. Multiple multifocal ventricular premature complexes
c. Paroxysmal atrial tachycardia with variable block
d. Wandering atrial pacemaker
e. Atrial flutter with 4:1 conduction

55) A 12-year-old child comes with his mother to the cardiology out-patient clinic because of recurrent short-lived palpitations at rest that terminate spontaneously after a few minutes. His mother has been told that her child has atrialization of his right ventricle. A 12-lead ECG reveals a short PR interval and negative QRS complex in lead V_1. What is the likely cause of these palpitations?

a. Atrial fibrillation
b. Wolff–Parkinson–White syndrome type B
c. Anomalous left coronary artery
d. Romano–Ward syndrome
e. Wolff–Parkinson–White syndrome type A

56) A 2-month-old infant is referred for management of cyanosis and failure to thrive. Echocardiography suggests tricuspid atresia. Which one of the following ECG findings would be consistent with the echo result?

a. Right ventricular hypertrophy
b. Right bundle branch block
c. Left axis deviation
d. Short PR interval
e. P-congenitale

57) A 22-year-old healthy-looking athlete requests a cardiac examination. He is seeking help after reading an article published on the internet about hypertrophic cardiomyopathy. Which one of the following is consistent with this form of heart disease?

a. Family history must be present
b. Aortic area murmur that is non-audible in the neck
c. Mitral stenosis murmur
d. Bisferiens pulse
e. Favourable response to digoxin

58) A 65-year-old man with features of pulmonary oedema presents to A&E. He is dyspnoeic with hypoxaemia. Chest X-ray confirms your clinical impression of pulmonary oedema, but the cardiac size looks normal. Which one of the following might be responsible for this?

a. Mitral regurgitation
b. Constrictive pericarditis
c. Combined aortic stenosis and reflux
d. Chagas' disease
e. Keshan's cardiomyopathy

59) A 15-year-old male patient with ventricular septal defect presents to A&E in a dyspnoeic state. After careful examination the SHO suggests the development of Eisenmenger's syndrome. You re-examine the patient and find something that points away from the SHO's diagnosis. What have you found?

a. Clubbing
b. Central cyanosis
c. Soft P_2
d. Single S_2
e. Graham–Steell murmur

60) A general practitioner is in a dilemma over a case he has referred to you. He says that the referred 31-year-old man has no myocardial infarction or ischaemic heart disease, but his 12-lead-ECG shows many Q waves. Which one of the following is *not* responsible for this man's ECG Q wave?

a. Hyperkalaemia
b. Hypertrophic cardiomyopathy
c. Wolff–Parkinson–White syndrome
d. Limb lead reversal
e. True posterior wall myocardial infarction

Cardiology: Answers

1) a.
Secondary prophylaxis programmes for patients with established coronary artery disease should always include (if no contraindication or intolerance) aspirin, a β-blocker, an ACE inhibitor and a statin. This man's LDL-cholesterol is within the target of <100 mg/dl which does not necessitate dose escalation for simvastatin. Although his blood pressure is well-controlled, an ACE inhibitor should be added. ACE inhibitors have been shown to counteract ventricular remodelling, prevent the onset of overt heart failure and reduce hospitalization. By taking daily aspirin, this man is at risk of NSAID-induced peptic ulceration; omeprazole is a reasonable medication to add, but top priority for maximum cardiovascular protection is an ACE inhibitor. Repeating his lipid profile after 3–4 months is part of his follow-up, but there is no need to check it again within 2 days.

2) b.
Symptomatic aortic stenosis calls for aortic valve surgery irrespective of its severity. This surgery is the cornerstone in the treatment of symptomatic patients fit for surgery. The presence of exertional symptoms, like dyspnoea, indicates that this patient is at risk of sudden death (patients succumb rapidly once the disease becomes symptomatic). Aortic valve replacement offers the best therapeutic intervention, while aortic balloon valvuloplasty has good results in children and can be used as a palliative measure in individuals unfit for surgery. Nifedipine has been shown to delay the need for surgery in aortic regurgitation, not stenosis. A diuretic may improve his pulmonary congestion because of diastolic dysfunction, but at this point valvular surgery is the most important step. The patient's palpitations might well be due to ventricular dysrhythmia (especially VT) and Holter monitoring is a good option to consider.

3) c.
Radiofrequency catheter ablation offers the best cure rate for symptomatic patients with troublesome WPW syndrome and avoids long-term treatment with antiarrhythmics. Asymptomatic patients have an excellent prognosis and need reassurance only. Digoxin and verapamil are contraindicated because they increase the conduction velocity in the accessory pathway. The most common arrhythmia in WPW syndrome is AV nodal re-entrant tachycardia. Atrial fibrillation is uncommon but can degenerate rapidly to ventricular fibrillation.

4) d.
Generally speaking, patients with patent ductus arteriosus should have their ductus occluded. This will eliminate any risk of infective endocarditis. The occlusion can be achieved via a thoracotomy approach or using endovascular techniques. Certain patients with complex cardiac anomalies may need to maintain an 'open' ductus to allow circulation

between the right and left sides of the heart. Note that, although small lesions may be totally asymptomatic, they still confer a risk of infective endocarditis. All patients with an open ductus need infective endocarditis prophylaxis. The presence of a persistent shunt post-surgery does not eliminate the risk of infective endocarditis.

5) c.
This patient has stage III heart failure of NYHA functional class IV. Improving his survival is an important part of the overall management plan. Adding an aldosterone antagonist, like spironolactone, in severe congestive heart failure has been shown to decrease mortality. Combined hydralazine/isosorbide dinitrate can be used in those who cannot take ACE inhibitors (because of intolerance or contraindication) and has the same mortality benefit. Digoxin has been shown to reduce hospitalization but has no impact on mortality. Amiodarone can be used to suppress serious arrhythmias, but does not influence mortality rate. Statins have a mortality benefit in ischaemic heart disease.

6) e.
Squatting (which increases the left ventricle cavity size) and isometric hand exercise (which increases the afterload) decrease the loudness of the ejection systolic murmur heard at the aortic area. The first three options increase the loudness, while inspiration increases the loudness of right-sided cardiac lesions.

7) e.
Metoprolol does not affect the serum digoxin level but it may increase that of lidocaine. Digoxin interactions should always be kept in mind as this medication is commonly used with other cardiac medications and toxicity can ensue rapidly. Amiodarone potentiates the effects of digoxin, ciclosporin and warfarin.

8) d.
Menstruation is neither an absolute nor a relative contraindication to receiving thrombolytic therapy. Pregnancy is an absolute contraindication, as is the presence of acute pericarditis and past intracranial haemorrhage. Bleeding diathesis, proliferative diabetic retinopathy and prolonged cardiopulmonary resuscitation are relative contraindications.

9) a.
Questions giving a brief patient scenario are extremely common in the MRCP examination. This man has ischaemic chest pain with a slightly raised cardiac marker and inconclusive ECG; only unstable angina fits the few clues given.

10) b.
The first three options are mechanical complications of acute myocardial infarction, which usually appear 3–5 days after the acute ischaemic event.

Thrombolytic therapy appears to hasten their appearance but does not consistently increase their incidence. The cardiac catheterization study reflects oxygenated blood being shunted from the left to the right ventricle. Note that both VSD and ruptured papillary muscles produce a large v wave in the pulmonary capillary trace. Echocardiography is an excellent investigation for a rapid diagnosis.

11) c.
Bicuspid aortic valve is commonly seen in coarctation patients. The coarctation murmur is heard at the left upper back while that of the enlarged collaterals is best heard around the scapulae.

12) b.
Symptomatic patients should undergo surgery irrespective of disease severity. Asymptomatic patients should be operated upon in the presence of any one of the following: asymptomatic LV dysfunction, atrial fibrillation, evidence of pulmonary hypertension and progressive LV dilatation (LV end-systolic volume >45 ml and LV end-diastolic volume >70 ml). A thrill is a sign of severity, but does not justify surgery per se. Thumping beats might well be due to ectopics.

13) c.
All options except the third are high-risk procedures (>5%) for perioperative vascular events (death, myocardial infarction and congestive heart failure). Low-risk (<1%) procedures are endoscopic procedures, breast biopsy and cataract extraction.

14) c.
The overall picture is of type A aortic dissection that has progressed proximally to involve and occlude the ostium of the right coronary artery, resulting in inferior wall myocardial infarction. Note that patients with this type of myocardial infarction should *not* receive thrombolytic therapy – a 'trap' that has been used in past examinations.

15) b.
A beta-blocker would tackle the hypertension as well as being a good option for migraine prophylaxis. Co-morbidities should always be taken into account when treating hypertension.

16) c.
The ankle:brachial blood pressure index (ABPI) indicates the presence of peripheral vascular disease if it is <0.9. Some symptomatic patients may have an ABPI in the range of 0.9–1.2. Patients such as the man described here (i.e. those who report calf pain on exercising who have a risk factor(s) for peripheral vascular disease and a normal neurological examination of the lower limbs) should have their ABPI measured whilst exercising; if it is falls below 0.9, it indicates peripheral vascular disease.

17) c.

Asymptomatic abdominal aortic aneurysms should be repaired if their maximum diameter exceeds 5.5 cm or their rate of expansion exceeds 0.5 cm/6 months. The presence of symptoms or complications, like abdominal pain, impending rupture and downstream embolization, calls for surgery regardless of the aneurysm size. Note that this patient's abdominal pain was due to peptic ulcer, not the aneurysm itself, which was detected incidentally.

18) c.

Acute viral/idiopathic pericarditis responds well to NSAIDs. Severe cases or those who respond partially to NSAIDs may benefit from adding a glucocorticoid, usually prednisolone. However, prednisolone increases the incidence of relapsing/recurrent acute pericarditis. Steroids suppress symptoms but do not accelerate cure.

19) a.

This patient's chronic stable angina is not responding to optimal medical treatment. He is a candidate for coronary angiography with possible intervention. The anatomy and status of the coronary vasculature need to be defined, as this will guide the physician as to what to do next, i.e. percutaneous coronary intervention (PCI) or coronary artery bypass grafting (CABG). Jumping to CABG would be unreasonable. Although a statin and an ACE inhibitor should be prescribed as part of his secondary prophylaxis, neither is the next best step at this time. Nothing in the patient's history points towards a possible unstable angina and therefore there is no justification for starting heparin infusion.

20) b.

Adenosine is not available as an oral preparation. It has a very short half-life and has to be given via the intravenous route as a bolus. Three boluses, of 3, 6 and 12 mg, can be given at 2-minute intervals if no response occurs initially. It is well-tolerated; however, some patients may experience short-lived distressing flushing, chest tightness and even chest pain. It can result in bronchospasm and therefore is best avoided in asthmatic patients. The action of adenosine is potentiated by dipyridamole and antagonized by xanthenes (like theophylline).

21) d.

Diastolic heart failure impedes the filling of the ventricles, which in this patient has resulted from hypertension-induced LVH. The left ventricular filling pressures rise, especially with exertion, producing pulmonary congestion and dyspnoea. The JVP is normal.

22) d.

Right ventricular infarction can result in hypotension and raised JVP, with clear lung bases. On ECG, occlusion of the right coronary artery would be expected to show ST segment elevation in the inferior leads (II, III, aVF) and/or right chest leads.

23) d.
Dissecting aortic aneurysm type A has several complications, all of which can lead to cardiovascular collapse. Acute aortic regurgitation, cardiac tamponade, rupture into the mediastinum or pleural space, and occlusion of the ostium of the right coronary artery resulting in right ventricular infarction are the causes to look for.

24) c.
Supraventricular tachycardia can be easily confused with atrial flutter with 2:1 conduction, and even with a sinus tachycardia. Giving a bolus of intravenous adenosine would help settle this issue by transiently increasing the AV conduction block and revealing the typical 'saw-tooth' pattern of atrial flutter. The same approach will terminate the supraventricular tachycardia in a substantial number of patients.

25) c.
Beta-blockers are the medications of choice to control ventricular rate, especially in young active people whose ventricular rate increases on exercise or exertion. Clonidine has no antiarrhythmic action.

26) d.
Exercise ECG is of virtually no value if the resting ECG is highly abnormal; abnormal 12-lead resting ECG (like the changes induced by digoxin or LVH) would definitely interfere with the interpretation of the exercise testing and result in a false-positive test (e.g. wrongly suggesting ischaemic heart disease by showing ST segment depression). If the resting ECG is abnormal, or the patient can not undergo a formal exercise test, a stress imaging method should be substituted, like dobutamine echocardiography or dipyridamole myocardial perfusion imaging.

27) b.
Intravenous lidocaine, by virtue of its CNS effects, can result in seizures that are usually generalized. Pethidine (meperidine) can lower the seizure threshold and enhances lidocaine toxicity.

28) c.
High-risk groups for infective endocarditis are those with a history of infective endocarditis; a prosthetic valve; complex cyanotic congenital heart disease; and a surgically constructed systemic–pulmonary shunt. Intermediate-risk patients are those with most acquired valvular and congenital heart lesions, as well as mitral valve prolapse with significant regurgitation.

29) c.
This man's infective endocarditis has involved the tricuspid valve, causing regurgitation. He has been seen by many doctors who may well have prescribed antibiotics for his fever. The doses of these antibiotics will certainly have been suboptimal for his infection, but they may have been

sufficient to sterilize his blood culture. The most common cause (90%) of culture-negative endocarditis is prior antibiotic exposure. Other causes (10%) are infection with a fastidious organism like the HACEK group, or with an organism that requires a special culture medium, like fungi and brucella. Do not forget non-infective causes like Libman–Sack's endocarditis or thrombotic (marantic) endocarditis.

30) b.
This is a difficult question with many reasonable answers. Intravenous infusion of a B-type natriuretic peptide has been shown to be beneficial in the management of acute pulmonary oedema due to acute LV failure. The treatment of acute pulmonary oedema in general involves high-flow, high concentration oxygen, morphine, loop diuretics, intravenous nitroglycerin and inotropics. The addition of nesiritide further improves management. It can be used in decompensated heart failure with dyspnoea at rest or minimal exertion. Hypotension and elevation in serum creatinine are its commonest side effects.

31) c.
This young man demonstrates the full-fledged Brugada's syndrome, a defect in sodium channel function, resulting in the typical ECG changes mentioned and possibly leading to torsades de pointes ventricular tachycardia or sudden death, without prolonging the QT interval (unlike options in Romano–Ward syndrome and Jervell–Lange–Nielsen syndrome). The inclusion of Mark Thomas syndrome in the options is a distraction as there is no such syndrome, and the picture is inconsistent with WPW syndrome.

32) c.
Critical limb ischaemia (CLI) is defined as the presence of pain at rest (mainly at night) in the forefoot that usually requires opiates and/or the presence of ischaemic ulceration and tissue loss, with an ankle blood pressure of <50 mmHg. This patient has features of intermittent claudication, but these are overshadowed by the CLI. Intermittent pseudoclaudication is neurogenic in origin due to spinal stenosis.

33) e.
The history given is short and inconclusive. However, you can guess that there is a grave arrhythmia which has necessitated cardioversion in A&E. Giving a new medication in addition to amiodarone (which prolongs the QT interval) might well have further prolonged this interval, resulting in torsades de pointes ventricular tachycardia. Questions such as this which give a short, confusing scenario are commonly seen in the MRCP examination.

34) c.
Type B aortic dissection is usually treated medically with an intravenous beta-blocker. The presence of actual or impending rupture, or the

presence of complications (like the acute limb ischaemia in this patient, or gut or renal involvement) call for emergency surgical intervention.

35) d.
Epstein's anomaly, in which the tricuspid valve is dysplastic and displaced downward, resulting in atrialization of the right ventricle and tricuspid regurgitation, causes central cyanosis through a right to left shunt via a patent foramen ovale or associated ASD. WPW syndrome can be associated, especially type B. Lithium exposure in utero has been defined as an aetiological factor for Epstein's anomaly.

36) c.
In cardiac tamponade, there is a prominent x descent and a blunted y descent, while in constrictive pericarditis there are prominent x and y descents. Pulsus paradoxus is more consistent with cardiac tamponade, while Kussmaul's sign is more consistent with constrictive pericarditis.

37) d.
The indications for the use of an implantable cardioverter–defibrillator are gradually increasing. Failed cardiac death in the absence of myocardial infarction or any reversible cause, a history of myocardial infarction with an ejection fraction of <35% and sustained VT, as well as certain high risk groups (arrhythmogenic right ventricular dysplasia, congenital long QT syndromes and hypertrophic cardiomyopathy) are the usual indications that feature in the MRCP examination. Biventricular pacing, termed re-synchronization therapy, is used in congestive heart failure with a prolonged QRS complex; this has been shown to improve symptoms.

38) c.
The presence of a favourable valve anatomy is an important predictor of successful valvuloplasty. The presence of any of the following would cancel out any benefit obtained from this intervention: heavy calcification of the mitral valve apparatus, significant (+++ or ++++) mitral regurgitation, left atrial thrombus and atrial fibrillation. Age per se does not influence the clinical decision.

39) d.
'Hemiblocks' do not broaden the QRS complex; instead, they alter the mean QRS axis, resulting in left axis deviation in left anterior hemiblock, and right axis deviation in left posterior hemiblock. Options a–c result in a tall R wave in lead V_1. Mirror image dextrocardia is one of the causes of a tall R wave in lead V_1 which might wrongly suggest right ventricular dominance and right axis deviation.

40) d.
Apart from option transient ischaemic attacks (TIAs), none of the other options alone confers a very high or even high risk of thromboembolic events. Very high-risk (12%/year) patients are those who have a history of

ischaemic stroke or TIAs. High-risk (6.5%/year) groups should have two or more risk factors plus an age >65 years. Risk factors for thromboembolic events in patients with atrial fibrillation are a history of ischaemic stroke or TIAs, mitral valve disease, heart failure, diabetes, hypertension and age >65 years. Echocardiographic evidence of LV dysfunction (which might be asymptomatic) and mitral valve annulus calcification are additional risk factors.

41) e.
The presence of fusion beats, capture beats and AV dissociation is pathognomonic for ventricular tachycardia in the appropriate setting. Ventricular tachycardia does not slow upon applying vagal manoeuvres or intravenous adenosine. If you are still unsure, treat as VT.

42) e.
The most common cause of refractory hypertension is non-compliance with medications, and the next is an inadequate drug regimen/dosage. Unrecognized secondary causes or the development of complications (such as renal failure and renal artery stenosis) are uncommon in clinical practice.

43) b.
Only three beta-blockers have been studied extensively and have been shown to reduce mortality in congestive heart failure: carvedilol, metoprolol and bisprolol. Each of these should be given in small escalated doses as they may precipitate acute on chronic heart failure. When appropriately prescribed, they produce symptomatic improvement, increase the ejection fraction, reduce hospitalization rate and most importantly, decrease the mortality rate.

44) d.
Mitral and tricuspid valvular stenoses produce opening snaps (in early diastole). Systolic clicks are brief, high intensity sounds that occur in early or mid-systole. When lost in stenotic valves, they indicate severe valvular thickening and/or calcification. A lost systolic click in a prosthetic valve occurs when the valve is obstructed by thrombus or vegetation.

45) b.
Episodes of torsades de pointes VT usually respond favourably to intravenous magnesium. Bradycardia-associated cases are managed with pacemaker insertion or intravenous isoprenaline. The latter should be avoided in congenital cases, as there is already an increased sympathetic tone which can easily be augmented further by the isoprenaline infusion. Prevention of recurrence in congenital syndromes can be achieved by left stellate ganglion ablation or long-term treatment with beta-blockers.

46) d.
Cardiac troponins are the most sensitive cardiac markers, starting to rise after 4–6 hours but remaining elevated for up to 2 weeks; therefore they are of no value in this patient. The MB isozyme of creatine kinase starts to rise after 4–6 hours and returns to normal within 2–3 days, so it is a useful marker in this patient who experiences a re-infarction on day 5. ALT is marker for liver disease. AST starts to rise later, peaks within 2–3 days and returns to normal within 4–5 days; however, it is neither sensitive nor specific for the cardiac myocyte.

47) d.
Many patients with heart failure will have a decompensation at some point during the course of their illness. This may result from non-compliance with medication, sudden change in the regimen, adding a counterproductive medication(s), brady- and tachy-arrhythmia, chest infection (actually any cause of fever), occult pulmonary thromboembolism, anaemia and hyperthyroidism. The cause should be identified and removed if possible.

48) c.
Infective endocarditis is highly likely in this at-risk patient. The question does not mention treatment, and instead addresses the diagnostic approach for infective endocarditis. The blood culture is positive for a 'typical' organism and there is no need to repeat it. Transthoracic echocardiography has a sensitivity of 65% for detecting vegetations; this figure rises to 95% with the transoesophageal approach.

49) b.
The pansystolic murmur in childhood may well represent VSD which has progressed over time to Eisenmenger's syndrome, resulting in pulmonary hypertension, clubbing and central cyanosis. The initial murmur does not fit the other options, and tetralogy of Fallot is cyanotic early in life.

50) a.
The overall picture points toward constrictive pericarditis. Given the patient's ethnic origin, TB infection seems the likely culprit. There is nothing in the history to suggest a possible malignancy treated by irradiation. Chagas disease is seen in South America and can cause congestive heart failure and heart block. The drug history is negative. HIV infection per se does not constrict the pericardium.

51) d.
The commonest cause of low-voltage ECG is the so-called incorrect standardization (the ECG machine is wrongly calibrated). This patient's clinical scenario is totally benign, and the other options are highly unlikely.

52) e.
Brugada's syndrome is one of the causes of sudden cardiac death and its ECG features are right bundle branch block and ST segment elevation in leads V_1–V_2. The first four options are causes of absent P wave.

53) c.
Bigeminal rhythm is common in cardiology practice, and alternating ventricular premature complexes are the commonest culprit. All the other options are true causes of this abnormal rhythm, but are uncommon in clinical practice.

54) e.
Atrial flutter with 4:1 conduction results in a slow regular ventricular rate; note the high-grade AV block. Do not forget atrial fibrillation as a cause of the irregularly irregular rhythm in this patient (this together with multiple multifocal ventricular and/or atrial ectopics are the commonest causes).

55) b.
This patient has Ebstein's anomaly. This cardiac malformation is associated with WPW syndrome, usually type B (note the ECG finding of below baseline negative QRS complex in lead V_1). Type A has above baseline lead V_1 QRS complex. WPW syndrome may result in AV nodal re-entrant tachycardia that may well be responsible for this child's short-lived palpitations.

56) c.
The majority of congenital heart anomalies have right ventricular dominance and right axis deviation; tricuspid atresia is an exception in that it has *left* axis deviation and *left* ventricular dominance. P-congenitale is due to right atrial hypertrophy and dilatation, resulting from pulmonary stenosis.

57) b.
The aortic area murmur is maximum at the left lower sternum and does not radiate to the carotids. It should be differentiated from that of aortic stenosis which is maximal at the aortic area and usually radiates to the carotids. A family history may be present and a family history of sudden death should always be looked for. A mitral regurgitant murmur is commonly heard, and hypertrophic cardiomyopathy is an important differential diagnosis in any patient with combined aortic stenosis and mitral regurgitation. A bisferiens pulse indicates combined aortic valve disease with predominant regurgitation. Digoxin is contraindicated, as are vasodilators.

58) b.
There are both cardiac and non-cardiac causes of pulmonary oedema with normal size heart: mitral stenosis (especially when early and when

complicated by atrial fibrillation); acute myocardial infarction; chronic constrictive pericarditis; emphysema (patients have a long thin heart shadow that might appear completely normal in cardiac diseases); non-cardiogenic pulmonary oedema, neurogenic pulmonary oedema, toxic inhalation, and aspiration. Note that Keshan cardiomyopathy is a form of dilated cardiomyopathy due to selenium deficiency. The other options result in cardiac dilatation.

59) c.
The pulmonary component of the second heart sound is prominently loud (it may be palpable as well) in Eisenmenger's syndrome. Clubbing is a late feature. Advanced cases have features of right-sided heart failure. The Graham–Steell murmur is the pulmonary regurgitant one.

60) e.
True posterior wall myocardial infarction is a cause of a tall R wave in lead V_1; it does not produce a Q wave in that lead. Limb lead reversal and high lead placement are common causes of 'Q waves' in clinical practice; mirror image dextrocardia is a rare one. Hypertrophic cardiomyopathy and WPW syndrome can result in a pseudo-infarction pattern; this is especially seen in the former when there can be a prominent septal Q wave. Other causes of Q waves are cardiac contusion, amyloid heart disease, myocarditis and left bundle branch block. Hyperkalaemia may prolong the QRS complex and even produce the so-called sine wave, but it may induce a transient Q wave.

2. Respiratory medicine: Questions

1) A 65-year-old factory worker presents with chronic cough, exertional dyspnoea and hyperinflated chest. The JVP is not raised and there is no cyanosis. He is a life-long heavy smoker. Chest X-ray shows diffuse hyperlucent lung zones, flat diaphragms and a narrow heart. Which of the following is the most effective option to prolong his life?

   a. Inhaled glucocorticoid
   b. Oral prednisolone
   c. Advise smoking cessation
   d. Refer for heart–lung transplantation
   e. Pneumococcal vaccination

2) A 22-year-old woman seeks help for repeated chest infections and pleurisy. She has had a daily cough productive of copious putrid sputum for the past 4 years. Her notes reveal a severe attack of childhood whooping cough. What is the current diagnosis?

   a. Allergic bronchopulmonary aspergillosis
   b. Church–Strauss vasculitis
   c. Chronic persistent asthma
   d. Bronchiectasis
   e. Retained foreign body

3) A 68-year-old man, who is confused and irritable, is brought to A&E by his sons. He has a 2-week history of increasing cough, diffuse bone pain and prostration. He is an ex-smoker after 40 years of heavy cigarette smoking. Chest X-ray shows a left hilar mass with an irregular border. Serum potassium is 3.0 mEq/L, blood urea is 10 mg/dl and serum calcium is 12.0 mg/dl. What is the likely diagnosis?

   a. Small cell lung cancer
   b. Squamous cell cancer of the lung
   c. Colonic secondary tumour
   d. Old healed tuberculosis
   e. Old calcified hamartoma

4) An 8-year-old boy has mild intermittent asthma which has worsened lately because of an upper respiratory tract infection. He takes daily inhaled terbutaline. Chest X-ray shows prominent bronchovascular markings. His PEFR is <60% of his previous best value. What should be done?

a. Add co-amoxiclav
b. Increase the dose of his inhaled β2-agonist
c. Increase the frequency of the inhaled β2-agonist
d. Start oral prednisolone
e. Give slow-release theophylline

5) A 32-year-old farmer presents with flu-like symptoms 8 hours after going into his barn. He experiences these symptoms every time he goes into the barn. Which one of the following would cast a doubt upon the diagnosis of farmer's lung?

a. Low grade fever
b. Eosinophil count 1×10^9/L
c. Low DL_{CO}
d. Bilateral interstitial shadowing in mid and upper lung zones
e. FEV_1/FVC ratio of 80%

6) A 33-year-old woman has a 4-month history of exertional dyspnoea, chest pain and syncope. She denies being on any medication or taking illicit drugs. Her family history is unremarkable. Examination reveals central cyanosis, clear lung fields and pulmonary and tricuspid refluxes. The mean pulmonary artery pressure is 40 mmHg with a normal sized left atrium. What is your preliminary diagnosis?

a. Primary pulmonary hypertension
b. Bronchiectasis
c. Chronic obstructive airway disease
d. Progressive massive fibrosis
e. Mitral stenosis

7) A 51-year-old man presents with tachypnoea and dyspnoea, one week after undergoing left-sided total knee replacement. Chest examination is unremarkable as is the plain chest X-ray. Pulse oximetry is 85%. What is your diagnosis?

a. Hyperventilation syndrome
b. Tension pneumothorax
c. Pulmonary thromboembolism
d. Lung aspiration
e. *Mycoplasma* pneumonia

8) A 65-year-old woman presents with dyspnoea on exertion and a dry irritative cough. Examination shows clubbing, cyanosis and bibasal crackles. Which one of the following is *not* consistent with your provisional diagnosis of idiopathic pulmonary fibrosis?

a. Raised ESR
b. Positive serum rheumatoid factor
c. Raised hemidiaphragms
d. Upper zone interstitial infiltrates on chest X-ray
e. Low K_{CO}

9) A 40-year-old black man presents with dry cough and arthralgia. Examination reveals tender raised nodules on both shins with low-grade fever. Chest X-ray reveals bilateral hilar enlargement. Biopsy of the cervical lymph node shows non-caseating granuloma. Which one of the following is an indication for treatment with prednisolone in this patient?

a. Stage I of the disease
b. Normal ECG
c. Bilateral facial palsy
d. Serum calcium of 9 mg/dl
e. No ocular complaints

10) A 66-year-old ex-smoker presents with chest tightness. Plain chest X-ray indicates large left-sided pleural effusion, aspiration of which reveals many malignant-looking cells. Which one of the following is a contraindication to surgical treatment in non-small cell lung cancer?

a. Serum calcium of 13 mg/dl
b. Pleural effusion
c. Tender distal forearms
d. Fixed raised JVP
e. Haemoglobin of 10 g/dl

11) A 55-year-old man with COPD presents to A&E with a 2-hour history of increased shortness of breath associated with pleuritic chest pain. His blood pressure is 70/40 mmHg with a rapid pulse rate. Chest X-ray shows a 10% right-sided pneumothorax. What is the best treatment for the time being?

a. Wait and see
b. Repeated aspiration
c. Chest tube underwater seal apparatus
d. Referral for chest surgery
e. Controlled oxygen

12) A 43-year-old man presents with fever, prostration, weight loss and night sweats. His cough is productive of scanty, whitish sputum with streaks of blood. Despite complying with his anti-TB medications, his sputum is still positive for acid-fast bacilli 5 months after starting therapy. Which one of the following is *not* a predictor of infection with a multidrug resistant (MDR) TB strain?

a. Exposure to MDR TB patient
b. Eastern European origin
c. Previous non-compliance with medications
d. HIV infection
e. Diabetes

13) A patient is admitted to the intensive care unit with severe pneumonia. He had been reasonably well and healthy prior to his chest infection. Which one of the following is a predictor of high mortality in pneumonia?

a. Age > 30 years
b. High abbreviated mental status examination score
c. Negative blood culture
d. Serum albumin 25 g/L
e. White cell count 5 x 10^9/L

14) A 21-year-old woman with asthma presents with severe shortness of breath, tachypnoea and wheezes. Conventional treatment in A&E failed to produce any improvement. Which one of the following should be kept in mind?

a. Development of pneumothorax
b. Foreign body inhalation
c. Smoke inhalation
d. Suboptimal treatment
e. Nebulization-induced bronchospasm

15) A 65-year-old man with COPD has rapid progression of his exertional dyspnoea. He is asking whether adding prednisolone to his daily medications would benefit him. Which of the following is *not* an indication for the use of oral glucocorticoids in patients with COPD?

a. During exacerbations
b. Failure of bronchodilator therapy
c. Patient is already taking glucocorticoids
d. Previous clinical response to glucocorticoids
e. Emphysema-predominant disease

16) A 54-year-old man presents with progressive chest tightness. Examination shows stony dullness and diminished breath sounds over the left lower hemithorax. Which one of the following causes of transudative pleural effusion can also result in exudative pleural effusion?

a. Congestive heart failure
b. Liver cirrhosis
c. Pulmonary infarction
d. Nephrotic syndrome
e. Uraemia

17) A 55-year-old police officer presents with increasing chest tightness, cough and increased sputum production 5 days after an apparently benign episode of flu. He has moderate COPD for which he takes daily regular inhaled terbutalin. Examination reveals global confusion, cyanosis, warm extremities and chest hyperinflation. Blood gas analysis shows PaO$_2$ 50 mmHg, PaCO$_2$ 70 mmHg and blood pH 7.2. What is the best treatment for this patient?

a. Non-invasive ventilation
b. Oral prednisolone
c. Controlled oxygen therapy
d. Endotracheal intubation with mechanical ventilation
e. Intravenous doxapram

18) A 32-year-old farmer with a 15-year-history of asthma consults you because of a deterioration in his asthma control. He has a daily productive cough with copious putrid sputum and recurrent pleuritic chest pain; the latter responds well to oral antibiotics. The development of which of the following should be considered in this patient?

a. Farmer's lung
b. Occupational asthma
c. Allergic bronchopulmonary aspergillosis
d. Bilateral pneumothoraces
e. Post-primary pulmonary tuberculosis

19) A 17-year-old girl presents with fever, headache, chest tightness, ear pain and dry cough. She has had mild flu for 5 days. Examination reveals bullous erythematous lesion on her eardrums. Chest examination is unremarkable. Chest X-ray reveals bilateral patchy infiltrates and hilar lymph node enlargement. What is the likely diagnosis?

a. Legionnaire's disease
b. *Mycoplasma pneumoniae* infection
c. *Staphylococcus aureus* lung abscess
d. Lymphangitis carcinomatosa
e. Pulmonary aspiration

20) A 21-year-old man presents with a 4-week history of fever, night sweats and prostration. He has daily cough and haemoptysis. Chest examination reveals biapical crepitations which become more prominent post-tussively. Which one of the following does *not* increase the risk of developing pulmonary tuberculosis?

a. Silicosis
b. Uraemia
c. Type I diabetes
d. Asbestosis
e. Gastrectomy

21) A 66-year-old heavy smoker presents with increasing cough and lassitude. Sputum examination shows many malignant-looking cells. Blood film reveals anaemia with a leucoerythroblastic blood picture. The diagnosis is a small cell lung cancer. How would you treat this patient?

a. Chemotherapy
b. Radiotherapy
c. Chemotherapy and radiotherapy
d. Hospice care
e. Surgical removal of the tumour

22) A 49-year-old woman is referred to the chest clinic because of progressive dyspnoea on exertion and dry cough. Her chest X-ray reveals bilateral upper zone fibrosis. Which of the following could *not* be responsible for this X-ray appearance?

a. Ankylosing spondylitis
b. Silicosis
c. Old healed tuberculosis
d. Chronic hypersensitivity pneumonitis
e. Asbestosis

23) A 60-year-old man has had reduced exercise tolerance for 8 months. He worked in the manufacture of fireproof insulating materials for 40 years. Plain chest X-ray reveals calcified diaphragmatic plaques and bilateral lower zones fibrosis with shaggy heart borders. Which of the following statements is true regarding the treatment of this illness?

a. There is no specific treatment
b. Use high-dose oral prednisolone
c. A trial of cyclophosphamide for 2 months is worthwhile
d. Weekly methotrexate is a useful adjunctive
e. Monthly nebulized pentamidine

24) A 27-year-old man has a chronic illness for which he has taken daily medication for the past few months. Which one of the following does *not* cause pulmonary eosinophilia?

a. Bromocriptine
b. Sulasalazine
c. Chlorpromazine
d. Gold
e. Imipramine

25) A 51-year-old man presents with fever, breathlessness and cough. Chest X-ray reveals bilateral diffuse perihilar shadows with air bronchogram. Bronchoalveolar lavage confirms the diagnosis of alveolar proteinosis. Which one of the following statements is correct regarding the treatment of this patient?

a. Usually responds to ciclosporin
b. May respond to GM-CSF
c. Does not respond to whole lung lavage
d. May be treated with oestrogen ablation therapy
e. Responds dramatically to smoke cessation

26) A 24-year-old woman visits A&E with severe dyspnoea and tachypnoea. She gave birth to a full-term baby last week. Her right ankle is swollen and her calf is tender. Which one of the following virtually excludes a diagnosis of massive pulmonary thromboembolism?

a. Normal chest X-ray
b. 100 mmHg PaO_2
c. 85% SaO_2
d. Right ventricular dilatation
e. T wave inversion in V_1–V_4

27) A 30-year-old office clerk presents with fever, one week after being successfully treated for a pneumonic illness. He is due to have a chest X-ray. Which one of the following is *not* a potential cause of his fever?

a. Empyema thoracis
b. Deep venous thrombosis
c. Lung abscess
d. Drug-fever
e. Erythema gyratum repens

28) A 54-year-old man with congestive heart failure attends the cardiology clinic for a scheduled follow-up visit. A chest X-ray that was done 1 week ago revealed moderate right-sided pleural effusion for which he has received furosemide. The effusion has decreased dramatically and today's pleural fluid analysis reveals a protein level of 35 g/L. What is the cause of this pleural fluid protein level?

a. Tuberculous infection
b. Complicated parapneumonic effusion
c. Pseudo-exudative effusion
d. Pulmonary thromboembolism
e. Malignant effusion

29) A 35-year-old airline pilot consults you regarding his chest problem. He had a small left-sided pneumothorax 7 months ago which was managed by observation alone. What is your advice?

a. Surgical obliteration of the pleural spaces
b. Repeating the chest X-ray
c. Nicotine replacement therapy
d. Chest tube underwater seal
e. Frequent follow-up

30) A 68-year-old man is referred to the thoracic surgeon because of a cavitory mass on plain chest X-ray. Which one of the following is *not* a cause of this lung lesion?

a. Squamous cell cancer of the lung
b. Wegener's granulomatosis
c. Pulmonary infarction
d. Legionnaire's disease
e. Long-term amiodarone therapy

31) A 32-year-old woman presents with progressive breathlessness. A further evaluation confirms the diagnosis of lymphangioleiomyomatosis. Which one of the following risks is carried by this lung disease?

a. Recurrent pneumothoraces
b. Bleeding tendency
c. Bronchospasm
d. Pulmonary–bronchial arterial shunt
e. Pulmonary tuberculosis

32) A 43-year-old woman presents with a new pulmonary infarction. This is the fourth one within 10 months despite the patient being compliant with once-daily 5 mg warfarin. Her current INR is 3.5. What action should you should take?

a. Increase the dose of warfarin
b. Split the daily warfarin into two doses
c. Inferior vena cava filter
d. Add daily clopidogrel
e. Add daily aspirin

33) A 30-year-old woman with exertional breathlessness is diagnosed with primary pulmonary hypertension after undergoing invasive investigations. Which one of the following medications is *not* used in the medical treatment of this woman?

a. Inhaled nitrous oxide
b. Prostacyclin infusion
c. Prostacyclin nebulization
d. Warfarin
e. Endothelin infusion

34) A 60-year-old heavy smoker presents with a 3-day history of hoarse voice. He is afebrile and denies flu symptoms. Which one of the following investigations would you choose to explore his voice change?

a. Complete blood count
b. Chest CT scan
c. Rhinoscopy
d. Oesophagoscopy
e. Flow–volume loop

35) A 20-year-old woman comes to A&E complaining that she can not breathe. Her chest examination is unremarkable, as is her chest X-ray. Her SaO$_2$ is 97%. Which one of the following statements is inconsistent with psychogenic hyperventilation?

a. Inability to take a deep breath
b. Erratic breathing at rest
c. Inability to cope with spirometry
d. PaO$_2$ 7.5 kPa
e. Frequent sighing at rest

36) A 35-year-old obese man consults you with his wife. She says that her husband snores all night and in all sleeping positions. He admits to having excessive daytime sleepiness. Full night polysomnography is highly suggestive of obstructive sleep apnoea. Which one the following would *not* be part of your management plan for this patient?

a. Weight reduction
b. Avoidance of alcohol in the evening
c. Doxapram
d. CPAP
e. Mandibular advancement device

37) A 21-year-old university student presents with a few days' history of headache, chest tightness and dry cough. His plain chest X-ray is suggestive of pneumonic illness. Cold agglutinin titre is high. He received oral doxycyclin for 2 days, after which he developed retrosternal chest pain. What would you do?

a. Repeat chest X-ray
b. ECG
c. *Legionella* urinary antigen
d. Blood culture
e. Sputum immunofluorescence study

38) A 9-year-old girl is brought to see you by her parents with severe shortness of breath. She has had moderate intermittent asthma from the age of 4 years. She is severely dyspnoeic but her chest examination is unremarkable. Chest X-ray shows bilateral hyperlucent lung zones. She is confused and uncooperative with the examination. What is the best action to be taken?

a. Nebulized β2-agonists
b. Intravenous aminophylline
c. Oral prednisolone
d. Mechanical ventilation
e. Chest tube insertion

39) A 67-year-old man presents with dyspnoea. His chest X-ray reveals small 1–3-mm rounded shadows all over both lung fields. Which one of the following does *not* produce a similar X-ray picture?

a. Sarcoidosis
b. Secondary malignancy
c. Pneumoconiosis
d. Tuberculosis
e. Systemic lupus erythematosus

40) A 20-year-old man presents with a prolonged episode of flu. There is skin tuberculin conversion and a primary complex is noted on the plain chest X-ray. Which one of the following features is a hypersensitivity reaction in patients with primary pulmonary tuberculosis?

a. Hilar enlargement
b. Cough
c. Pericarditis
d. Meningitis
e. Dactylitis

41) A 47-year-old woman with acute lymphoblastic leukaemia develops fever, malaise, headache, breathlessness and cough with bloody sputum near the end of her remission induction therapeutic regimen. The chest X-ray shows pneumonic consolidation with areas of cavitations. One-week treatment with piperacillin and gentamicin fails to produce any improvement. What would you suggest?

a. Increasing the dose of piperacillin
b. Using amphotericin B
c. Adding metronidazole
d. Monotherapy with ceftriaxone
e. GM-CSF

42) A 71-year old man is given a diagnosis of small cell lung cancer following tissue sampling after having a slowly resolving pneumonia. Which one of the following would cast doubt upon this diagnosis?

a. Haemoptysis
b. Weight loss
c. Clubbing
d. Lung collapse
e. Low threshold bone fracture

43) A 40-year-old man presents with a 4-week history of fever, cough and haemoptysis. His occupation involves quarrying and stone dressing. Old chest X-rays reveal egg-shell calcification within an enlarged hilar shadow. What is the likely cause of the current presentation?

a. Asbestosis
b. Pleural mesothelioma
c. Bronchoalveolar carcinoma
d. Post-primary tuberculosis
e. Exacerbation of COPD

44) A 40-year-old woman presents with fever, lassitude, dry cough and dyspnoea. Her chest X-ray reveals bilateral lung parenchymal shadows, mostly in the periphery and upper zones. She has shown an excellent response to prednisolone. What is the likely diagnosis?

a. Rheumatoid lung
b. Wegener's granulomatosis
c. Chronic eosinophilic pneumonia
d. Drug-induced pulmonary fibrosis
e. Cardiogenic pulmonary oedema

45) A 46-year-old woman presents with cough and dyspnoea. Her current X-ray reveals an opacity in the chest and the lateral view localizes the opacity to the anterior mediastinum. Which one of the following does *not* impart an anterior mediastinal shadow?

a. Lymphoma
b. Retrosternal goitre
c. Foregut duplication
d. Dermoid cyst
e. Pericardial cyst

46) A 70-year-old man presents with pain down his left arm and increased cough. His left eyelid is drooped and there is dullness in the left apical lung zone. The small muscles of the left hand are wasted. The patient is a life-long heavy smoker. What is the likely diagnosis?

a. Old healed tuberculosis
b. Pancoast's tumour
c. Cervical rib
d. Carcinoid tumour
e. Sarcoidosis

47) A 34-year-old with an abnormal chest X-ray is referred to the chest clinic. The radiologist insists that the left hemidiaphragm is raised. Which one of the following is *not* a cause of this radiological abnormality?

a. Left-sided pulmonary infarction
b. Severe pleuritic chest pain
c. Left recurrent laryngeal nerve palsy
d. Large volume of gastric gas
e. Left lung lobectomy

48) A 39-year-old man presents with weight loss, cough and breathlessness with lung collapse. Tissue sampling of a lung mass confirms lung cancer. He has never smoked. Which one of the following is *not* a recognized risk factor for the development of lung cancer?

a. Chromium
b. Asbestos
c. Radon
d. Thallium
e. Passive smoking

49) A 33-year-old homosexual man presents with fever, cough and prostration. His sputum is positive for acid-fast bacilli. Which one of the following antituberculous medications is contraindicated in a patient with AIDS?

a. Isoniazid
b. Thiacetazone
c. Rifabutin
d. Ethionamide
e. Cycloserine

50) A 50-year-old man with septicaemia develops severe shortness of breath, cough and irritability. Which one of the following is inconsistent with the diagnosis of adult respiratory distress syndrome?

a. PaO_2/FiO_2 150 mmHg
b. Reduced lung compliance
c. Bilateral interstitial infiltrate
d. Bilateral alveolar infiltrate
e. Pulmonary artery capillary tracing of 25 mmHg

Respiratory medicine: Answers

1) c.
Apart from cessation of smoking (completely and permanently) and long-term domiciliary oxygen therapy (LTOT), no intervention has been shown to affect survival and disease outcome in COPD patients. All patients should be advised about the benefits of cessation of smoking and encouraged to enrol in a smoke cessation group (if motivated). Proper advice, nicotine replacement therapy and use of bupropion have been shown to improve the rate of quitting. The patient has no features suggestive of cor pulmonale, and referring him for heart–lung transplantation is not justified at this time.

2) d.
This young woman demonstrates a full picture of bronchiectasis. Childhood measles and whooping cough are risk factors for future development of bronchiectasis. Recurrent pneumonia and pleurisy are well characterized complications, and secondary 'AA' amyloidosis puts the patient at risk of nephrotic syndrome.

3) a.
The history and imaging point towards a primary lung cancer; nothing is suggestive of an abdominal pathology. The low blood urea and serum potassium may well be due to SIADH, and the hypercalcaemia with diffuse bone pain is likely to represent diffuse bony metastasis. These features would fit small cell lung cancer. Hypercalcaemia due to PTH-related peptide secretion in squamous cell cancer is rare and this type of lung cancer does not produce SIADH–this is the 'trick' option. The patient's confusion could be due to brain secondaries, SIADH (hyponatraemia) or hypercalcaemia, or a combination of these.

4) d.
This boy is having an exacerbation and his lung functions have worsened following a recent viral upper respiratory tract infection. Rescue courses of glucocorticoids may be needed at any stage of the disease and at any time. Rapid control is important, and a step down of the daily oral steroid dosage (when symptoms are controlled) is better than a step up (when no control is achieved). This boy's PEFR is much reduced and neither increasing the dose nor escalating the frequency of inhaled β_2-agonsits would efficiently improve his PEFR.

5) b.
Farmer's lung, a form of hypersensitivity pneumonitis, is due to exposure to organic dust containing *Micropolyspora faenae* and *Aspergillus fumigatus*. The constellation of fever, dyspnoea, malaise and headache with no wheezes that occurs 6–8 hours post-exposure is highly suggestive of this

diagnosis. Eosinophilia is not seen with farmer's lung as it is an immune complex type III (and type IV to a lesser extent) disease. During the acute event, there is hypoxia with normo- or hypo-capnia, and the DL_{CO} is low with normal or increased FEV_1/FVC, as farmer's lung is an interstitial disease.

6) a.
The normal lung examination with pulmonary hypertension and right-sided heart signs should prompt a search for primary pulmonary hypertension or thromboembolic pulmonary hypertension. An occult mitral stenosis may have a similar presentation, but the normal left atrial size rules out this option.

7) c.
This patient has undergone surgery that carries a high risk for pulmonary thromboembolism. The normal chest examination and the 'apparently' normal chest X-ray with hypoxaemia in a dyspnoeic and tachypnoeic patient who is at risk of thromboembolic phenomena, are highly suggestive of this diagnosis. The patient should be treated with heparin while undergoing confirmatory investigation.

8) d.
Idiopathic pulmonary fibrosis targets the elderly. The ESR and serum LDH are commonly raised, and antinuclear and rheumatoid factor are positive in up to 50% of cases (and therefore are unhelpful in screening for underlying connective tissue diseases). The pathology dominates in the lower zones bilaterally, with lung shrinkage and raised hemidiaphragms. Isolated upper zone opacities virtually exclude the diagnosis.

9) c.
The overall picture is suggestive of acute sarcoidosis, which has an excellent prognosis. Indications for treatment in sarcoidosis are vital organ involvement (neurological, heart, eye), hypercalcaemia and/or hypercalciuria, lupus pernio, rapidly progressive stage II/III and stage IV disease. Bilateral facial weakness may well represent neurosarcoidosis (it is also seen in the uveoparotid fever variant).

10) d.
Contraindications to surgical treatment in non-small cell lung cancer are M_1, T_4 and N_3, i.e. presence of metastatic disease, involvement of mediastinal structures (great vessels, oesophagus, recurrent laryngeal nerve) and contralateral hilar lymph node involvement, respectively. This man's fixed raised JVP reflects superior vena cava involvement. Hypercalcaemia could be due to metastatic disease, or secondary to the secretion of PTH-related peptide; the information given is not biased to either of these. Anaemia of chronic diseases is common, and therefore not a contraindication per se to surgery unless it is secondary to bone marrow infiltration (note the question mentions a leucoerythroblastic blood picture). Pleural effusion could be due to post-obstructive infection

with pleurisy, or to malignant infiltration (the latter is a contraindication to surgery). Hypertrophic pulmonary osteoarthropathy (HPOA) is a paraneoplastic picture that does not reflect a locally advanced or metastatic disease.

11) c.

This man's pneumothorax should be assumed to be in tension because of the haemodynamic collapse, regardless of its size and absence of chest X-ray features of tension. Besides, this pneumothorax is secondary to underlying lung disease, resulting in rapid deterioration. These features call for immediate intervention in the form of insertion of a chest tube underwater seal apparatus.

12) e.

Type 1 diabetes per se increases the risk of developing TB, but does not confer an increased risk of acquiring or developing an MDR strain.

13) d.

Predictors of high mortality in pneumonia are age >60 years, presence of confusion, respiratory rate >30/minute, systolic blood pressure <90 mmHg, diastolic blood pressure <60 mmHg, presence of co-morbidities, involvement of two or more lobes on chest X-ray, white cell count $<4 \times 10^9$/L or $>20 \times 10^9$/L, PaO_2 <8 kPa, blood urea >7 mmol/L, positive blood culture and low serum albumin.

14) a.

The development of uni- or bi-lateral pneumothorax is a well-known but often underestimated complication of acute asthmatic attacks. All patients should be asked specifically about sudden pleuritic chest pain and should undergo a chest X-ray. The presence of thick tenacious bronchial secretions may produce lobar collapse and resistance to conventional therapy. None of the clues in the question point to any of the other options.

15) e.

The first four options are the usual indications. Emphysema-predominant disease per se does not influence the use of these medications. Low-dose inhaled steroids should not be used routinely; they should be considered in those with severe disease and frequent exacerbations that require hospitalization. They do not affect the rate of annual fall in the FEV_1.

16) c.

Pulmonary infarction usually results in exudative pleural effusion, which is usually serous or blood stained with red cells and eosinophils; rarely the effusion is truly transudative. The patient may have risk factors for venous thrombosis and lung parenchymal evidence of pulmonary infarction may be seen.

17) d.

This patient is unfortunate in that the episode of flu has exacerbated his COPD, which appears to have been well-controlled and compensated. Rapid deterioration has ensued and has resulted in a highly acidic blood pH. The patient is confused and cyanosed. As the question does not mention any severe co-morbidity or poor life-expectancy, intravenous doxapram in the first place is not warranted. Non-invasive ventilation would be an excellent first step if his blood pH was 7.35–7.25. However, the clinical picture mandates endotracheal intubation and mechanical ventilation. CPAP may be used in the recovery phase and when weaning the patient from the ventilator. Oral prednisolone and controlled oxygen therapy are used in clinical practice as part of the management plan, but they are not the best option when life-saving treatment is required, as in this case.

18) c.

The development of bronchiectasis with worsening of symptoms in a patient with long-term asthma should always prompt a search for allergic bronchopulmonary aspergillosis. Worsening of symptoms may well be due to occupational asthma or farmer's lung, but neither of these would explain the copious putrid sputum and recurrent pneumonia.

19) b.

The picture is consistent with a pneumonic illness secondary to a preceding upper respiratory tract infection. The clues to *Mycoplasma pneumoniae* are the bullous myringitis and the X-ray findings (note the hilar enlargement). It usually targets young people during autumn and has 3–4 yearly cycles.

20) d.

Silicosis, but not asbestosis, confers an increased risk of developing pulmonary TB. Other risk factors are HIV infection, malignancy, immune compromised states, malabsorption and jenuno-ileal bypass. The disease tends mainly to affect the following groups: children, especially first-generation children of immigrants from highly endemic areas; those who have close contact with smear-positive pulmonary TB patients; and individuals who had a primary infection less than 1 year ago.

21) a.

Small cell lung cancer is staged into limited (treated with a combination of radiotherapy and chemotherapy) and extensive (treated with chemotherapy alone). A limited cancer is limited to a hemi-chest and within the field of radiotherapy. This patient's blood picture indicates bone marrow irritation, which may well represent bone marrow secondary tumour infiltration, suggesting this patient has an extensive disease.

22) e.
The pulmonary parenchymal fibrosis of asbestosis, idiopathic pulmonary fibrosis, pulmonary fibrosis associated with connective tissue diseases and drug-induced pulmonary fibrosis predominates in the lower lung zones.

23) a.
There is no specific treatment for asbestosis. Immune suppressive therapy has no value. Nebulized pentamidine is a prophylactic regimen used to prevent *Pneumocystis carinii* pneumonia in HIV-infected patients.

24) a.
Bromocriptine and methysergide can cause pleural fibrosis and effusion. In addition to the other options, causes of pulmonary eosinophilia are nitrofurantoin, aspirin, phenytoin, bleomycin, naproxen and nalidixic acid.

25) b.
Whole lung lavage with large volumes of normal saline is both diagnostic and therapeutic. Spontaneous remission is seen in up to 30% of cases. The disease may respond to GM-CSF. A dramatic response to smoke cessation may be seen in histiocytosis-X of the lung. Oestrogen ablation therapy is of doubtful value in pulmonary lymphangioleiomyomatosis.

26) b.
The normal PaO_2 virtually excludes massive pulmonary thromboembolism in the appropriate clinical setting. There is usually hypoxaemia with normo- or hypo-capnia. CT pulmonary angiography is the investigation of choice. The chest X-ray is usually 'normal looking' at first glance; however, subtle changes are common, like a focal area of oligaemia or a prominent pulmonary artery.

27) e.
Persistent or recurrent fever in patients with pneumonia should prompt a search for complications; empyema should rank highest. Development of lung abscess, canula-associated superficial thrombophlebitis, metastatic abscesses, drug fever, infective endocarditis and local extension to produce pericarditis are the usual causes. Failure of medical therapy should be kept in mind. Erythema gyratum repens is a skin paraneoplastic manifestation of lung cancer (and to a lesser extent, breast and oesophageal cancers).

28) c.
Furosemide has drawn the pleural fluid, leaving its protein content behind (the latter needs time to be absorbed), thus creating a pseudo-exudate. Venous thrombosis and pulmonary infarction may occur in patients with congestive heart failure, but a pseudo-exudate is more likely in view of the diuretic therapy and the rapid reduction in the fluid volume. The history is not indicative of tuberculous infection. No clues are given to

suggest an underlying malignancy. The lack of a preceding history of pneumonic illness rules out a parapneumonic effusion.

29) a.

Any pneumothorax, regardless of its size and whether it is unilateral or bilateral, in high-risk persons (like pilots and divers) calls for obliteration of the pleural spaces, as the recurrence rate is very high and will interfere with the individual's occupation.

30) e.

The most common causes of cavitory lung lesions are lung abscesses (usually due to *Staphylococcus aureus*) and cavitory lung cancer (usually squamous). Amiodarone can result in an idiopathic pulmonary fibrosis-like picture (non-eosinophilic alveolitis) and pleural disease. Infective causes of multiple lung abscesses are *Staphylococcus aureus*, *Klebsiella*, tuberculosis and, rarely, Legionnaire's disease.

31) a.

This grave pulmonary disease results in widespread thin-walled cysts throughout the lung fields. Besides chylous pleural effusions and haemoptysis, recurrent pneumothoraces are common and complicate an already gloomy picture. Death usually occurs within 10 years. Lung transplantation offers the only hope. Oestrogen ablation therapy is still controversial. Pulmonary lymphangioleiomyomatosis does not confer an increased risk of TB, and enlargement of bronchial arteries is seen in bronchiectasis. The disease does not affect haemostasis and the dyspnoea is not due to bronchospasm.

32) c.

The question does not address the cause of the embolic phenomenon, but highlights the recurrent lung events despite adequate anticoagulation; the patient has failure of anticoagulation. The best action is to place an inferior vena cava filter. This therapy is also indicated when anticoagulation is contraindicated or is difficult to achieve.

33) e.

The prognosis of this pulmonary vascular disease was gloomy before the introduction of inhaled or intravenous prostacyclin (iloprost, epoprostenol). Warfarin has been shown to improve the prognosis of severe cases. Continuous prostacyclin infusion produces symptomatic improvement and prolongs survival. Endothelin is the most potent vasoconstrictor in the body and therefore has no place in the management of this patient.

34) b.

The occurrence of sudden hoarseness in a life-long heavy smoker should always prompt a search for underlying lung cancer with recurrent laryngeal nerve involvement. The patient should be referred for ENT examination; meanwhile, arranging for a chest CT scan/bronchoscopy is a reasonable approach.

35) d.
A PaO_2 of 7.5 kPa indicates hypoxaemia, which should cast a strong doubt on the diagnosis of psychogenic hyperventilation. In addition to the other options, inconsistent spirometry manoeuvres, easy induction of symptoms during submaximal hyperventilation and a resting end-tidal CO_2 of <4.5% are other features of psychogenic hyperventilation.

36) c.
In some patients weight reduction and avoidance of alcohol in the evening is all that is required. CPAP keeps the upper airways open during sleep by creating a local pressure that is higher than the atmospheric one. However, up to 50% of patient cannot tolerate this form of therapy. Mandibular advancement devices are effective in selected patients. Uvuolplasty is not very effective in the majority of patients. Resistant cases may call for tracheostomy, but this should be the last resort. Intravenous doxapram has no place in the management of obstructive sleep apnoea.

37) b.
The short scenario is consistent with *Mycoplasma* pneumonia. The development of retrosternal chest pain may well indicate the development of pericarditis. An ECG is an easy way of confirming or refuting this clinical suspicion.

38) d.
The 'silent' chest and the confusion place this girl in the life-threatening category of asthma. Mechanical ventilation should be started immediately.

39) e.
Miliary shadowing is not seen with SLE. In addition to the other options, histoplasmosis may also show miliary shadowing.

40) e.
The hypersensitivity reactions seen in primary TB are dactylitis, phlyctenular conjunctivitis and erythema nodosum. Lymph node enlargement is usually seen in the hilar group and is usually unilateral; the mediastinal and paratracheal groups may also be affected.

41) b.
Patients with prolonged neutropenia and severe suppurative pneumonic illness that is not responsive to conventional antibiotics should be treated for invasive pulmonary aspergillosis. Amphotericin B (with flucytosine) is the recommended regimen.

42) c.
Clubbing is suggestive of non-small cell lung cancer. SIADH, ectopic ACTH and Lambert–Eaton myasthenic syndrome are paraneoplastic manifestations of small cell lung cancer.

43) d.
The patient's occupation puts him at risk of silicosis; the chest X-ray film is consistent with silicosis. Such patients have an increased risk of developing pulmonary tuberculosis, which is the likely cause in this patient.

44) c.
The history itself is inconclusive, but the X-ray findings of photographic negative image of pulmonary oedema together with the dramatic response to steroids put chronic eosinophilic pneumonia at the top of list of differential diagnoses.

45) c.
Foregut duplication, paravertebral abscesses, neurogenic tumours and oesophageal lesions are posterior mediastinal masses. Other causes of anterior mediastinal masses are thymic tumours, germ cell tumours, Morgagni hiatus hernia and aortic aneurysms.

46) b.
The history points to a Pancoast tumour of the lung. The left-sided Horner's syndrome, T_1 wasting of the small muscles of the hand and the neuropathic pain are all consistent with the diagnosis in this heavy smoker.

47) c.
Phrenic nerve palsy, but not recurrent laryngeal nerve palsy, is a cause of a raised hemidiaphragm. Other causes are subphrenic abscess, large masses in the liver, eventration of the diaphragm, and any cause of volume loss in one lung such as pulmonary fibrosis.

48) d.
Cigarette smoking is responsible for about 90% of all cases of lung cancer, making it the most preventable aetiological factor for this disease. Around 5% of lung cancers occur in passive smokers, and another 5% are associated with exposure to environmental radon. Environmental or occupational exposure to chromium, asbestos, cadmium and beryllium is a rare cause of this cancer.

49) b.
Thiacetazone is a bacteriostatic medication that should *not* be used in *HIV*-positive patients. In those taking protease inhibitors, rifabutin should be used instead of rifampicin.

50) e.
Adult respiratory distress syndrome has an acute picture, with severe hypoxaemia (PaO_2/FiO_2 <200 mmHg), bilateral interstitial and/or alveolar infiltrates and a pulmonary artery capillary pressure of <15 mmHg. This patient's elevated PCWP points towards left-sided heart failure.

3. Renal medicine: Questions

1) A 12-year-old boy is referred to the nephrology clinic for further evaluation because of periorbital puffiness and bilateral pitting leg oedema. He has been given a diagnosis of minimal change nephropathy and is about to receive treatment for it. Which one of the following, when present at the time of diagnosis, should cast doubt upon the diagnosis?

   a. Selective proteinuria
   b. Impaired renal function
   c. Normal blood pressure
   d. Hypercholesterolaemia
   e. Bland urinary sediment

2) A 54-year-old man who has had Type 2 diabetes mellitus for 6 years attends for a check-up. He has not seen a doctor for 5 years and is unaware that his diabetes places him at risk of developing renal disease. His urine is negative on albumin dipstick testing. What would you do next?

   a. Repeat the albumin stick testing after 6 months
   b. Spot urine testing for albumin:creatinine ratio
   c. Send for renal ultrasound
   d. Urine culture and sensitivity
   e. 24-hour collection of urine for protein

3) A 32-year-old woman presents with rising blood urea and creatinine over a 3-week period. Her urinary sediment is active and her blood pressure is high. Serum complement levels are low. Which one of the following causes of glomerulopathy does *not* lower serum complement levels?

   a. Infective endocarditis
   b. Post-streptococcal glomerulonephritis
   c. Microscopic polyangiitis
   d. Systemic lupus erythematosus
   e. Cholesterol atheroembolic disease

4) A 66-year-old man with ischaemic heart disease and recurrent TIA presents with refractory hypertension. He is compliant with his daily antihypertensive medications which are prescribed in optimal doses. You detect a right-sided renal bruit. Which one of the following is consistent with right renal artery stenosis?

   a. Right kidney smaller than the left by 3 cm
   b. Left kidney smaller than the right by 4 cm
   c. Right kidney size more than 16 cm
   d. Dilated right renal pelvis
   e. Bright right kidney pyramids

5) A 32-year-old woman forms recurrent renal stones. Her stones are of calcium oxalate type. You suspect idiopathic hypercalciuria. Which medication would you prescribe?

a. Furosemide
b. Penicillamine
c. Captopril
d. Hydrochlorothiazide
e. Allopurinol

6) A 54-year-old woman with a chronic headache syndrome presents with nausea, vomiting, abdominal pain and muscle twitching. Her blood urea and serum creatinine are high and she is to undergo dialysis. The intravenous urogram shows approximation of both mid-ureters. Which one of the following medications could be the cause of this disease?

a. Paracetamol
b. Phenacetin
c. Methysergide
d. Diclofenac
e. Oxycodone

7) A 69-year-old man who is a heavy smoker has left loin pain and a palpable loin mass with haematuria. Renal ultrasound shows a large complex mass in the upper left kidney pole. His haemoglobin is 18 g/dl. What is the cause of this haemoglobin value?

a. Paraneoplastic manifestation
b. Haemoconcentration
c. Syndrome of inappropriate ADH secretion
d. Bone marrow irritation by cancer cells
e. Polycythemia vera

8) A 65-year-old man presents with a few months' history of urinary hesitancy, frequency and recurrent cystitis. Pelvic ultrasound examination shows bladder outlet obstruction by an enlarged prostate of 37 cm^3. How should his prostatism be treated?

a. Use finasteride
b. Give prazosin
c. Wait and see
d. Low dose daily trimethoprim
e. Bilateral orchidectomy

9) A 65-year-old man presents with recurrent painless haematuria. Cystoscopy reveals a small suspicious area, biopsy of which shows the presence of superficial transitional cell bladder cancer. What is the treatment?

a. Intravenous mitomycin-C
b. Cystectomy
c. Transurethral resection of the tumour
d. Deep X-ray therapy
e. Frequent follow-up

10) A 34-year-old man with chronic renal failure comes for a scheduled follow-up. He is taking multiple medications, one of which is intravenous erythropoietin (EPO) given twice a week. His current packed cell volume is 45%. Which one of the following is a reasonable next step?

a. Increase the frequency of EPO
b. Increase the dose of EPO
c. Decrease the frequency of EPO
d. Stop EPO transiently
e. Add oral folate and iron

11) A 33-year-old police officer develops repeated vomiting, muscle twitching and confusion after sustaining a bullet injury in the left thigh with prolonged shock. His blood urea is 100 mg/dl with hyperkalaemia. What is your best action?

a. Dialysis
b. Forced diuresis
c. Oral calcium resonium
d. Nebulized salbutamol
e. Sodium bicarbonate infusion

12) A 48-year-old woman has chronic arthritis of her knees, for which she takes daily phenacetin for the past 3 years. Her renal function is impaired. She has persistent microscopic haematuria on follow-up visits. Which one of the following complications may have occurred?

a. Hydronephrosis
b. Renal artery stenosis
c. Transitional cell cancer of the renal pelvis
d. Polycystic kidney
e. Clear renal cell cancer

13) A 22-year-old male has recurrent renal colic and macroscopic hae-maturia because of multiple renal stones. You suspect cystinuria as a cause. Which investigation would you choose to consolidate your suspicion?

a. Serum oxalate
b. 24-hour urinary calcium
c. Serum uric acid
d. Chromatographic analysis of stone
e. Faecal amino acid chromatography

14) A 47-year-old man with generalized oedema visits the nephrologist. His 24-hour urinary protein is 7 g. He is obese, a heroin addict and is HIV-positive. What type of nephrotic syndrome is he likely to have?

a. Minimal change disease
b. Membranous nephropathy
c. Goodpasture's syndrome
d. Focal segmental glomerulosclerosis
e. Diabetic nephropathy

15) A 22-year-old man is brought to the casualty unit with deep acidotic breathing following a severe crushing injury. His urine myoglobin is very high. You suspect myoglobinuria. Which one of the following laboratory findings would you *not* expect to find in this patient?

a. Hypekalaemia
b. Hyperuricaemia
c. Hypercalcaemia
d. Raised blood urea nitrogen
e. Hyperphosphataemia

16) A 43-year-old woman presents with hiccough, bone pain, pallor and nausea. Her blood urea is 200 mg/dl and serum potassium is 5.7 mEq/L. Abdominal ultrasound shows enlarged kidneys. Which one of the following conditions could be responsible for this uraemia with large kidneys?

a. Chronic glomerulonephritis
b. Reflux nephropathy
c. Retroperitoneal fibrosis
d. HIV infection
e. Analgesic nephropathy

17) A 45-year-old woman presents with hypokalaemia and increased 24-hour urinary potassium. Renal tubular acidosis is suspected. Her renal ultrasound reveals many medullary crystals. Which type of renal tubular acidosis is she likely to have?

a. Type I
b. Type II
c. Type III
d. Type IV
e. Type V

18) A 31-year-old man is referred to you after having a positive dipstick test for protein in a routine pre-employment examination. His clinical examination is totally unremarkable, as is the laboratory testing. Which one of the following could be responsible for his abnormal urine testing?

a. Cold exposure
b. Minimal change disease
c. Congestive heart failure
d. Chronic constrictive pericarditis
e. Mesangiocapillary glomerulonephritis

19) A 54-year-old woman with diabetic nephropathy has undergone renal transplantation. This is her fifth postoperative day and her urine output is <30 ml/hour. Which one of the following is *not* a potential cause of this prolonged post-transplant oliguria?

a. Acute tubular necrosis
b. Arterial anastomotic stenosis
c. Hyperacute rejection
d. Ciclosporin toxicity
e. Ureteral lymphocele

20) A 17-year-old female patient with chronic renal failure due to reflux nephropathy has reached a disease stage that requires renal replacement therapy. You are considering the use of continuous ambulatory peritoneal dialysis. Which one of the following side effects is *not* encountered with this form of dialysis?

a. Peritonitis
b. Development of abdominal wall hernias
c. Amino acids overload
d. Hyperglycaemia
e. Basal atelectasis

21) A 46-year-old man who has multiple chronic illnesses has been recently diagnosed with uraemia. He is concerned about the hazards of taking his current medications that may be imposed by his kidney condition. All of the following medications need major dose reduction in this patient except:

a. Digoxin
b. Vancomycin
c. Ethambutol
d. Tolbutamide
e. Cimetidine

22) A 53-year-old man with ischaemic heart disease needs coronary angiography, but his cardiologist is concerned about the development of contrast nephropathy because he is at risk of this condition. Which one of the following does *not* confer an increased risk of contrast nephropathy?

a. Multiple myeloma
b. Diabetes mellitus
c. Infants
d. Renal artery stenosis
e. Elderly age

23) A 39-year-old patient with membranous nephropathy has non-selective proteinuria. He asks for an explanation of 'non-selective'. Loss of which one of the following substances in urine marks the proteinuria as being non-selective?

a. Albumin
b. Transferrin
c. IgG
d. C_4 complement
e. Thyroid hormone-binding globulin

24) A 10-year-old boy has been recently diagnosed as having renal tubular acidosis type II due to Fanconi's syndrome. All of the following can be seen in this syndrome, except:

a. Positive urinary sugar testing
b. Hyperuricaemia
c. Hypokalaemia
d. Hypophosphataemia
e. Tubular proteinuria

25) A 26-year-old patient with multiple chronic illnesses has heavy crystaluria. He takes many daily medications and is concerned about this new urinary finding. Which of the following medications *cannot* result in this abnormal urine test?

a. Indinavir
b. Aciclovir
c. Acetazolamide
d. Sulphonamides
e. Prednisolone

26) A 54-year-old man presents with hypovolaemic shock following massive peptic ulcer-related upper GIT bleeding. His blood urea is 155 mg/dl with hyperkalaemia. Which one of the following is inconsistent with pre-renal failure?

a. Urine:plasma osmolality >1.1
b. Urinary sodium >20 mEq/L
c. Urinary osmolality >500 mosmol/L
d. Urine:plasma creatinine concentration > 20
e. Fractional sodium excretion <1

27) A 43-year-old uraemic patient is on regular haemodialysis. He complains that many features of the disease have not improved after many sessions of haemodialysis. Which one of the following is usually improved by dialysis?

a. Encephalopathy
b. Anaemia
c. Pericarditis
d. Osteodystrophy
e. Peripheral neuropathy

28) A 54-year-old man presents with resistant hypertension, fluid retention and renal impairment. His 24-hour urinary urine is 5 g with active urinary sediment. You suspect this nephrotic/nephritic picture is due to mesangiocapillary glomerulonephritis. All of the following can result in a secondary form of this glomerulopathy, except:

a. Hepatitis B infection
b. Lung cancer
c. Hepatitis C infection
d. Partial lipodystrophy
e. Type II cryoglobulinaemia

29) A 37-year-old man presents with seizures following a renal transplant 1 month ago. He has had a mild upper respiratory tract infection for which his GP prescribed clarithromycin 1 week ago. What is the likely cause of these seizures?

a. Steroid-induced psychosis
b. Acute graft rejection
c. Ciclosporin toxicity
d. Toxoplasma brain abscess
e. CMV encephalitis

30) A 34-year-old man presents with recurrent macroscopic haematuria and hypertension. Abdominal ultrasound suggests polycystic kidneys. All of the following are extra-renal manifestations of this disease, except:

a. Mitral regurgitation
b. Biscuspid aortic valve
c. Divarication of recti
d. Hepatic cysts
e. Brain Berry's aneurysm

31) A 49-year-old woman developed progressive renal impairment with eosinophilia and eosinophiluria a few days after starting a medication prescribed by her GP. Her daily urine output is nearly maintained. Which one of the following *cannot* be implicated as a cause of this non-oliguric acute interstitial nephritis?

a. Allopurinol
b. Rifampicin
c. Warfarin
d. Mefenamic acid
e. Meticillin

32) A 30-year-old man is referred to you for further evaluation of his hypertension and leg oedema. Investigations disclose a nephritic/nephrotic picture with a positive test for C_3 nephritic factor. His physique demonstrates partial lipodystrophy. Which one of the following would fit his clinical picture?

a. Membranous nephropathy
b. Post-streptococcal glomerulonephritis
c. Mesangiocapillary glomerulonephritis type I
d. IgA nephropathy
e. Mesangiocapillary glomerulonephritis type II

33) A 16-year-old boy presents with progressive renal impairment. He has a positive family history. You are considering a diagnosis of Alport's syndrome. Which one of the following would suggest an alternative diagnosis?

a. Progressive thickening of the glomerular basement membrane
b. Bilateral anterior lenticonus
c. Sensorineural deafness
d. X-linked pattern of inheritance
e. Macrothrombocytopenia

34) A 56-year-old man presents with loss of renal function, proteinuria and haematuria a few days following successful coronary artery stenting. He has blue toes and livedo reticularis over the ankles. What has developed in this man?

a. Contrast nephropathy
b. Polyarteritis nodosa
c. Cholesterol atheroembolic disease
d. Malignant hypertension
e. Microscopic polyangiitis

35) A 27-year-old man is being considered for renal transplantation because of small contracted kidneys. Which one of the following medications is *not* usually given to increase the graft survival?

a. Tacrolimus
b. Rapamycin
c. Mycophenolate mofetil
d. Thioguanine
e. Prednisolone

36) A 39-year-old uraemic man has persistent fatigue and low exercise tolerance despite regular dialysis. His bone disease is responsive to vitamin D metabolite and phosphate binders. He has anaemia which is partially responsive to erythropoietin injections. All of the following are possible causes of this erythropoietin treatment failure, except:

a. Aluminium toxicity
b. Iron deficiency
c. Active inflammation
d. Malignancy
e. Hypocalcaemia

37) A 47-year-old patient presents with fatigue, muscle cramps, drowsiness and hiccough. His breathing is deep and he has a sallow colouration of skin and urea frost. Which one of the following is the most common cause of chronic renal failure in the West?

a. Hypertension
b. Chronic tubulointerstitial disease
c. Inherited nephropathy
d. Diabetes mellitus
e. Unknown cause

38) A 50-year-old woman presents with progressive renal impairment over just 3 weeks. Her urine is positive for blood and protein. Her kidneys are normal in size on ultrasound examination. What is the likely diagnosis?

a. Vesicoureteric reflux
b. Congenital renal dysgenesis
c. Rapidly progressive glomerulonephritis
d. Membranous nephropathy
e. Repetitive renal trauma

39) A 43-year-old man who has had severe upper GIT bleeding develops a progressive rise in blood urea and serum creatinine. The laboratory findings are consistent with pre-renal failure except that the fractional sodium excretion is >1. How would you explain this latter finding?

a. Established acute tubular necrosis
b. Obstructive uropathy
c. Prolonged shock
d. Concomitant furosemide therapy
e. Laboratory error

40) A 43-year-old woman presents with features of urinary tract obstruction, raised ESR and C-reactive protein, and medial deviation of the mid-ureters on intravenous urography. Which one of the following is the commonest cause of retroperitoneal fibrosis?

a. Proctolol
b. Malignant infiltration
c. Radiation
d. Blood seepage from aortic aneurysm
e. Idiopathic

41) A 14-year-old boy with bilateral loin heaviness after drinking a large volume of water was found to have gross bilateral hydronephrosis with normal-sized ureters. No stones were found. Which diagnosis in this boy is the commonest cause of pelviureteric junction obstruction?

a. Malignant involvement
b. Radiolucent stones
c. Ureteric wall muscular hyperplasia
d. Idiopathic
e. Aberrant renal artery

42) A 43-year-old woman with idiopathic membranous nephropathy presents with haemoptysis 5 days after having gross haematuria with impaired renal function. Which one of the following could explain this presentation?

a. Lower limb DVT with pulmonary infarction
b. Real artery occlusion and DVT
c. Renal vein thrombosis and pulmonary embolism
d. Acute pyelonephritis and pulmonary TB
e. Malignant hypertension and chest trauma

43) A 36-year-old woman with SLE presents with proteinuria. Which one of the following would be suggestive of a glomerular origin for the proteinuria?

a. β_2-microglobulin in urine
b. Dysmorphic RBCs in urine
c. Eosinophils in urine
d. Xanthine crystals in urine
e. Oxalate crystals in urine

44) A 23-year-old man presents with progressive drowsiness and rising blood pressure. His bloods reveal progressive loss of renal function. Ultrasound examination fails to discover any site of urinary tract obstruction. What is the best action?

a. Give dopamine infusion
b. Perform a renal biopsy
c. Repeat blood urea nitrogen
d. Test urine for protein
e. Blood culture

45) A 72-year-old man develops deep, sighing breathing and drowsiness with hypertension within 12 hours of an apparently benign aortic root angiography for aneurysmal formation. What is the likely diagnosis?

a. Cholesterol atheroembolic disease
b. Pulmonary embolism
c. Contrast nephropathy
d. Bilateral renal artery occlusion
e. Septic shock

46) A 54-year-old man is about to have his glomerular filtration rate (GFR) measured using creatinine clearance. He has Type 2 diabetes with positive testing for microalbuminuria. He takes daily amlodipine for high blood pressure and a statin for raised LDL cholesterol. Which one of the following is true regarding the creatinine clearance method of measuring the GFR?

a. It is a difficult method to perform
b. It is inaccurate
c. It overestimates the GFR in poor renal function
d. It is not affected by medications
e. It requires a spot random urine sample

47) A 55-year-old heavy smoker develops loin pain and haematuria. He has weight loss, fever and raised ESR. On abdominal ultrasound a mass is seen at the right upper kidney pole, which appears to be malignant, as well as four target lesions in the liver. What is the next step?

a. Proceed with nephrectomy
b. Bone marrow examination
c. Lumbar puncture
d. Brain MRI
e. Chest X-ray

48) A 29-year-old man has a high serum phosphate. He has been diagnosed with chronic renal failure. Which one of the following does *not* produce hyperphosphataemia?

a. Acute renal failure
b. Rhabdomyolysis
c. Tumour lysis syndrome
d. Massive haemolysis
e. Haemodialysis

49) A 22-year-old university student consults you about his current health. He denies any symptoms, and takes no medications or illicit drugs. He does not smoke, but drinks alcohol occasionally. Three of his first-degree relatives have adult polycystic kidney disease. He wants to know if he has this disease. Which one of the following tests would you choose to screen for this disease in this young man?

a. Regular blood pressure measurement
b. Annual urine for microscopic haematuria
c. Abdominal CT scan at 3-year intervals
d. Abdominal ultrasound
e. Intravenous urogram

50) A 28-year-old patient with severe inflammatory bowel disease on prolonged parenteral nutrition develops a low serum phosphate. Which one of the following is *not* caused by prolonged or severe hypophosphataemia?

a. Cardiac arrhythmia
b. Hypercoagulable state
c. Seizures
d. Rhabdomyolysis
e. Hypoventilation

51) A 36-year-old patient is referred to you because of acidosis. His serum electrolytes are Na^+ 135 mEq/L, K^+ 3.0 mEq/L, HCO_3^- 15 mEq/L, and Cl^- 110 mEq/L. Which one of the following cannot be responsible for this patient's acidosis?

a. Renal tubular acidosis type I
b. Acetazolamide therapy
c. Ureterosigmoidostomy
d. Methanol poisoning
e. Chronic diarrhoea

52) A 44-year-old woman develops profound lactic acidosis following a suicide attempt using a drug. Which one of the following could be a cause of lactic acidosis type B?

a. Septic shock
b. Methanol poisoning
c. Cyanide poisoning
d. Respiratory failure
e. Severe anaemia

53) A 12-year-old boy has muscle weakness and cardiac arrhythmia because of hypokalaemia. He denies any bowel symptoms. His toxicology screen was negative for laxatives and diuretics. Which one of the following inherited syndromes does *not* cause hypokalaemia?

a. Bartter's syndrome
b. Liddle's syndrome
c. Fanconi's syndrome
d. Gitelman's syndrome
e. Alport's syndrome

54) A 70-year-old man with Type 2 diabetes on chlorpropamide presents with confusion. His serum glucose is 145 mg/dl, serum sodium 122 mEq/l, blood urea 10 mg/dl and plasma osmolality 262 mosmol/kg. Which one of the following urinary osmolalities would suggest an alternative cause for this man's new presentation?

a. 140 mosmol/kg
b. 435 mosmol/kg
c. 450 mosmol/kg
d. 490 mosmol/kg
e. 500 mosmol/kg

55) A 45-year-old man has polyuria. Serum potassium, calcium and glucose are normal. He denies excessive drinking of water. Toxicology screen is negative for diuretics. A water deprivation test reveals the following: plasma osmolality 305 mosmol/kg and urinary osmolality 210 mosmol/kg at the start of test. After 8 hours, urinary osmolality is 240 mosmol/kg, and is raised to 260 mosmol/kg after vasopressin injection. Which one of the following is *not* a potential cause of this man's illness?

a. Cystinosis
b. Demeclocyclin
c. Hypocalcaemia
d. Lithium
e. Mercury poisoning

56) A 52-year-old man presents with renal colic. Plain abdominal X-ray reveals a single small stone in the right kidney pelvis, an observation confirmed by renal ultrasound. The patient passes the stone in urine after 2 days. Which one of the following investigations is *not* required at this time?

a. Serum calcium
b. Chemical analysis of the stone
c. 24-Hour urine for calcium
d. Serum electrolytes
e. Blood urea

57) A 32-year-old woman presents with burning micturition and urinary frequency. Her urine examination shows many pus cells. She improves after a course of ciprofloxacin, but returns to you 2 weeks later with the same complaints. Why do her symptoms recur?

a. Wrong initial diagnosis
b. Bacterial resistance
c. Factitious illness
d. Re-infection
e. Urethral syndrome

58) A 14-year-old boy has been diagnosed clinically with minimal change disease because of generalized oedema and nephrotic range proteinuria. After 6 months of prednisolone, his urine is still heavily proteinuric with generalized oedema. He is compliant with his medications. How would you respond?

a. Increase the dose of prednisolone
b. Add cyclophosphamide
c. Do renal biopsy
d. Extend the treatment to 1 year
e. Replace prednisolone with ciclosporin

59) A 23-year-old recently married woman presents with dysuria and suprapubic discomfort. She is afebrile with no loin pain. Her past medical history is unremarkable. How would you treat her empirically?

a. Intravenous ciprofloxacin
b. Oral rifampicin
c. Oral co-amoxiclav
d. Intramuscular gentamicin
e. Oral vancomycin

60) A 55-year-old man presents with gross haematuria. He has recurrent urinary bladder stones. Rapid bedside ultrasound examination fails to demonstrate any stone, but there is a fungating bladder mass. What type of bladder cancer is likely?

a. Transitional cell cancer
b. Clear cell cancer
c. Squamous cell cancer
d. Leiomyosarcoma
e. Bladder lymphoma

Renal medicine: Answers

1) b.

Minimal change disease is the commonest cause of nephrotic syndrome in children. The disease has an excellent prognosis. The proteinuria is highly selective, with normal blood pressure, renal function and bland urinary sediment. Hypoalbuminaemia and dyslipidaemia are seen in nephrotic syndromes regardless of the aetiology. If renal function is impaired, the blood pressure is high, urinary sediment is active or the proteinuria is non-selective, the diagnosis should be reviewed. NSAID therapy, HLA-DR7 and atopy are associated with minimal change disease. The disease has a normal appearance on light microscopy and there are no immune deposits.

2) b.

Testing a spot random urinary sample for the albumin:creatinine ratio (ACR) is the screening method of choice for microalbuminuria when the dipstick albumin test is negative. Normal values are <2.5 mg/mmol in men and <3.5 mg/mmol in women. The test is rapid, convenient, cheap and accurate. If the test is positive, 24-hour urine testing for protein and creatinine (to co-measure the GFR) should be done, and if this is positive, should be reconfirmed twice within a 3–6-month period. The microalbuminuric range for albumin excretion is 30–300 mg/day; higher values are frank albuminuria. Persistent microalbuminuria in diabetic patients is a sign of incipient nephropathy and confers an increased risk of atherosclerosis and cardiovascular events. Screening should begin at the time of diagnosis in Type 2 diabetes, and then annually if negative.

3) c.

Microscopic polyangiitis, Wegener's granulomatosis, polyarteritis nodosa, Goodpasture's syndrome and IgA nephropathy do not produce hypocomplementaemia. Shunt nephritis, cryoglobulinaemia and type II mesangiocapillary glomerulonephritis also lower serum complement level. Hypocomplementaemia is a marker of disease activity in SLE.

4) a.

Atherosclerotic renal artery stenosis is unilateral in 50% of cases. Ischaemic atrophy of the affected kidney occurs and the detection of asymmetric kidney size is a useful clue to the diagnosis, but it is insensitive and unfortunately is a late sign. Bright pyramids indicate medullary crystallization, calcinosis or stone formation. Renal artery stenosis should be suspected if the hypertension is severe, of recent onset or difficult to control, and there is asymmetric kidney size with evidence of vascular disease elsewhere (ischaemic heart disease, stroke and peripheral vascular disease). Renal artery angiography is the gold standard in the diagnosis of renal artery stenosis; however, MRA is becoming the screening investigation of choice.

5) d.

Thiazide diuretics decrease the urinary calcium excretion; furosemide has the opposite effect. Penicillamine and captopril are used in cystine stones of cystinuria. Allopurinol is a useful adjunct in calcium oxalate stone treatment, even in the absence of hyperuricaemia. All patients should be encouraged to increase their fluid intake. Alkalization of urine is useful in uric acid and cystine stones, while urinary acidification is helpful in struvite stones. Low dietary oxalate, a calcium-rich diet (calcium binds oxalate to form insoluble salts) is helpful in reducing urinary oxalate execretion in urine. Sodium intake should be restricted, while that of protein should be moderated.

6) c.

Methysergide and proctolol can result in retroperitoneal fibrosis. This woman probably has migraine headaches for which she takes daily methysergide. Approximation of the mid-third of both ureters is the clue to this conclusion. She has developed obstructive uropathy and uraemic syndrome. Note that retroperitoneal fibrosis is one of the causes of hydronephrosis with normal-sized kidneys; other causes are severe dehydration and acute obstruction. The phrasing of the question may misdirect you towards analgesic nephropathy.

7) a.

Paraneoplastic erythropoietin secretion is rarely seen ($<5\%$ of cases) in renal cell cancer. Anaemia is more common. The triad of loin mass, loin pain and haematuria is a useful indicator of the disease, but it is a late constellation and is seen in only 15% of cases. Bone marrow irritation by cancer cells would produce a leucoerythroblastic blood picture. The tumour may also secrete renin, gonadotrophins and PTH; these may be useful tumour markers.

8) b.

Benign prostatic hypertrophy is a common cause of bladder outlet obstruction. A prostate size of <40 cm^3 would probably respond to α-blocking agents like prazosin; this rapidly relaxes the bladder neck and improves the obstruction and urinary flow in up to 70% of cases. A patient with a prostate size >40 cm^3 should be given a 5α-reductase inhibitor like finasteride; this slowly shrinks the enlarged gland with gradual improvement in symptoms. Surgical intervention may take the form of transurethral resection, laser therapy or open prostatectomy. Thermotherapy has been shown to be an effective mode of treatment. Low-dose trimethoprim is useful in preventing recurrent UTI in those with prostatism, but prazosin is the better option in this man as it will relax the bladder neck and improve his urine output. Androgen ablation therapy is useful in advanced prostate cancer.

9) c.

Superficial bladder tumours, even when large or multiple, can be treated by endoscopic resection. Intravesical chemotherapy with mitomycin-C or epirubicin is useful in treating multiple tumours or to prevent recurrence after endoscopic resection. All patients should be educated about regular cystoscopy. If there is a recurrence, it can be treated by diathermy. Very rarely, removal of the bladder is contemplated.

10) d.

The target PCV in uraemic patients given EPO injections is 30–36%; higher values are associated with increased risk of hypertension and thrombosis of surgical shunts. Transient withholding of EPO injections is a good option for the time being; they can be re-introduced once the PCV is within its target value and adjusted to keep the target value stable. The injections usually raise blood pressure and modification of antihypertensive therapy is usually required.

11) a.

The patient has prominent uraemic symptoms and dialysis is the only option left. Nebulized β_2-agonists and intravenous sodium bicarbonate are useful adjuncts in the management of hyperkalaemia, but they should not be used on their own to treat this patient's uraemia.

12) c.

Analgesic nephropathy results from long-term ingestion of any NSAID. There is prominent tubulointerstitial atrophy and fibrosis with papillary necrosis. Ten per cent of all patients have hypotension due to salt-losing nephropathy; hypertension occurs in at least 60% of cases. Recurrent UTI is very common. Sloughing of necrotic papillae may result in renal colic, urinary tract obstruction and even acute renal failure. Painless haematuria should prompt the search for urothelial cancer, especially of the renal pelvis.

13) d.

Chromatographic analysis of the renal stones or urinary cystine level can be used to diagnose cystinuria. Cystinuria results from a tubular defect in the reabsorption of di-basic amino acids. However, only the excessive excretion of cystine is clinically significant because it leads to the formation of renal cystine stones. All patients should increase their fluid intake; alkalization of urine and penicillamine (which binds cysteine, forming insoluble complex) or captopril are useful in the treatment. These stones are semi-opaque.

14) d.

Although membranous nephropathy is the commonest cause of nephrotic syndrome in adults, this patient demonstrates three risk factors for focal segmental glomerulosclerosis: obesity, heroin misuse and HIV infection. In some patients, the glomerular scarring is due to vasculitis, haemolytic uraemic syndrome or cholesterol atheroembolic disease.

15) c.

Acute rhabdomyolysis results in the release of intracellular contents, causing hyperkalaemia, hyperuricaemia and hyperphosphataemia. The serum calcium initially falls but gradually normalizes, and rebound hypercalcaemia may even be seen later. This patient's temporal profile indicates an early course and hypocalcaemia would be expected.

16) d.

Chronic renal failure with enlarged kidney size is seen in diabetic nephropathy, HIV nephropathy, polycystic kidneys, hydronephrosis (except in retroperitoneal fibrosis, where the hydronephrosis is encased within a thick fibrous envelop), amyloidosis, acromegaly, compensatory hypertrophy in a single kidney and in some cases of hepatic cirrhosis.

17) a.

Type I (distal) renal tubular acidosis (RTA) results in a normal anion gap metabolic acidosis. In type I, there is hypercalciuria and hyperphosphaturia. Long-standing cases show osteomalacia, nephrocalcinosis and renal stone formation. The nephrocalcinosis rules out proximal type II RTA.

18) a.

The normal examination essentially rules out the last four options. In otherwise normal individuals, positive albumin dipstick testing might result from exposure to extremes of temperature, heavy exercise, mild or asymptomatic UTI and, do not forget, orthostatic proteinuria.

19) c.

Acute, but not hyperacute, rejection could be the cause. The causes mentioned in the question should always be kept in mind in this clinical setting. The commonest causes are acute rejection and acute tubular necrosis (due to prolonged ischaemic injury during the operation). Ureteric obstruction by a haematoma or lymphocele is rare and can be ruled out by ultrasound examination. Ciclosporin toxicity can be ruled out simply by measuring its serum level. Septic shock should always be considered if the scenario is suggestive.

20) c.

Peritonitis is usually due to *Staphylococcus albus*; Gram-negative infections should raise the suspicion of visceral perforation. Protein and amino acid *depletion* is common in long-term cases. Hyperglycaemia may occur if the fluid is hypertonic, with secondary hypertriglyceridaemia and obesity. Due to tension in the abdominal wall, abdominal wall hernias may occur. This form of dialysis is reasonable for any patient who is unsuitable for haemodialysis: patients with diabetes, cardiovascular instability, inadequate vascular access, heparin contraindication, geographical remoteness, religious reason (Jehovah's Witness) and children. Pulmonary basal atelectasis and reactionary pleural effusion might be seen.

21) d.
Dose reduction is not usually required for digitoxin, hydralazine, prazosin, prednisolone, azathioprine, heparin, doxycyclin, tolbutamide and glibenclamide. Major dose reduction is needed for cimetidine, digoxin, vancomycin, penicillin-G, ampicillin, ticarcillin, aminoglycosides, sulphonamides and ethambutol.

22) d.
Renal artery stenosis per se does not impose an increased risk of contrast nephropathy. The usual risk factors are pre-existent renal impairment, diabetes mellitus (especially if treated with metformin), multiple myeloma, infant, the elderly and the use of high osmolar contrast materials. The most important step in the management is prevention; proper hydration and avoidance of nephrotoxic medications are the cornerstone steps. If there is any doubt, use low osmolar contrast material, although it is best to avoid the procedure all together in patients who are already at high risk.

23) c.
Selective proteinuria is characterized by loss of albumin and/or transferrin in urine. The loss of IgG in urine, measured by the ratio of albumin to IgG in urine, marks the proteinuria as being non-selective. Highly selective proteinuria predicts a favourable response to corticosteroids. Prolonged loss of transferrin in urine results in iron-resistant iron-deficiency anaemia.

24) b.
Fanconi's syndrome is characterized by generalized proximal tubular defect. There will be glycosuria in the presence of normal serum glucose, hypophosphataemia (which results in rickets in the long-term), aminoaciduria (clinically insignificant), hypokalaemia and hypouricaemia. Tubular proteinuria is characterized by predominant loss of β_2-microglobulin in urine.

25) e.
Prednisolone does not precipitate in urine and it decreases the urinary calcium excretion. Other causes of heavy crystaluria are high-dose vitamin C therapy, nitrofurantoin and ethylene glycol poisoning.

26) b.
The differentiation of pre-renal from intrinsic causes of renal failure is important, not only for the treatment plan, but also for prognostic purposes. Pre-renal failure causes avid reabsorption of sodium and water, resulting in a low urinary concentration of this cation (fractional sodium excretion of < 1 and urinary sodium concentration of < 10 mEq/L) and concentrated urine. Note that the kidneys in hepatorenal syndrome of cirrhotic patients reabsorb sodium avidly in a way similar to that seen in prerenal failure, although the renal failure in the former is due to intrinsic renal abnormality. There are many exceptions that will be discussed in

other questions. Established acute tubular necrosis results in the following values: urine sodium >20 mEq/L, fractional sodium excretion >1, urinary osmolality <400 mosmol/L, urine:plasma osmolality 0.9–1.05 and urine:plasma creatinine concentration <15.

27) a.

Some features of uraemic syndromes are unfortunately resistant to or, at best, only partially responsive to haemodialysis: severe peripheral or autonomic neuropathy, pericarditis, pruritis, arteriosclerosis, osteodystrophy and anaemia.

28) b.

Mesangiocapillary glomerulonephritis type I is associated with bacterial infections, hepatitis B and C infections, and cryoglobulinaemia. It is the commonest form of glomerulopathy to be associated with infective endocarditis. Type II disease has been linked to partial lipodystrophy and C_3 nephritic factor. Lung cancer is associated with membranous nephropathy.

29) c.

The duration of immune suppression is too short to cause brain toxoplasma or CMV infection; besides, the question contains no clues pointing to these conditions. The recent introduction of an enzyme inhibitor to the regimen containing seizure-inducing (in toxic levels) medication explains the clinical deterioration. Acute rejection may results in acute renal failure, but the picture would be different. Steroid-induced psychosis is not an epileptogenic condition.

30) b.

Adult polycystic kidney disease is commonly associated with mitral and aortic regurgitations; these are usually mild. Colonic diverticulae and abdominal wall herniae are well-characterized associations. Hepatic cysts are seen in one-third of cases but hepatic dysfunction is extremely uncommon. Berry's aneurysm is seen in 10% of cases, a figure that rises to 20% if there is a positive family history of subarachnoid haemorrhage. Renal replacement therapy is needed in only 50% of cases.

31) c.

Warfarin has not been shown to produce acute interstitial nephritis. In this renal disorder, the renal parenchyma is intensely infiltrated with polymorphonuclear cells and lymphocytes; eosinophils are common, especially in drug-induced causes. Eosinophilia is seen in one-third of cases, while eosinophiluria occurs in 70%. Most patients are not oliguric, but the picture can be dramatic; a rapidly progressive glomerulonephritis-like picture.

32) e.
In type II mesangiocapillary glomerulonephritis, the mesangial cells interpose between the glomerular basement membrane and the endothelium, and an immunofluorescence study will reveal intramembranous dense immune deposits. Hypocomplementaemia is common. In type I disease, the immune deposits are subendothelial.

33) a.
Alport's syndrome is usually an X-linked recessive disease due to a mutation in the *COL4A5* gene encoding the alpha subunit of type IV collagen. It ranks second to adult polycystic kidney disease in the list of inherited causes of chronic renal failure. The hallmark of the disease is progressive *degeneration* of the glomerular basement membrane. Type IV collagen is seen in the cochlea and the ocular tissue. Bilateral sensorineural deafness and ocular abnormalities (bilateral anterior lenticonus and macular degeneration) are seen. The disease does not recur in the transplant tissue; however, antiglomerular basement membrane disease can develop in the renal graft, but only a small minority develop graft destruction.

34) c.
Cholesterol atheroembolic disease occurs days to weeks after an invasive vascular procedure (e.g. angiography, stenting). To a lesser extent, the disease occurs spontaneously, especially in those taking warfarin. The kidney function progressively deteriorates, with signs in the lower limbs (toe gangrene and livedo reticularis). Hypertension is common, and complement levels are usually reduced. The picture may resemble polyarteritis nodosa. There is no specific treatment. Contrast nephropathy occurs *within* 24 hours of using an intravenous contrast medium.

35) d.
Azathioprine, not thioguanine, is used. A common regimen is to combine prednisolone, azathioprine and ciclosporin. The 3-year graft survival is usually 80%. This immune suppression increases the risk of skin and lymphoreticular malignancies. Do not forget ciclosporin toxicity in the MRCP examination.

36) e.
The anaemia of chronic renal failure usually responds to erythropoietin injections; the target PCV is 30–36%. Failure of haemoglobin to rise might result from the first four options.

37) d.
Diabetes mellitus accounts for up to 40% of cases of uraemia in the West; hypertension ranks second (70% of cases when both causes are combined). Five to 20% of uraemia cases have no detectable cause. Inherited and congenital causes make a 5% contribution.

38) c.
This short scenario fits the definition of rapidly progressive glomerulonephritis. The usual causes are systemic vasculitis, SLE, Goodpasture's syndrome and severe IgA nephropathy. Renal function is lost over a matter of days to few weeks, with active urinary sediment. Obstructive causes are never implicated, and kidney size should be normal or increased. Together with renal biopsy, testing of ANA, ANCAs, anti-GBM antibodies and complement levels is required to define the underlying disease. Aggressive immune suppression is needed, usually with prednisolone and cyclophosphamide. Dialysis may be indicated in the appropriate clinical setting.

39) d.
The avid sodium retention in pre-renal failure lowers the urinary sodium content, with a fractional excretion of < 1; however, pre-existent renal disease, or concomitant diuretic therapy, impairs retention and raises this figure. This should always be kept in mind in cases of clear-cut pre-renal failure. Acute tubular necrosis renders the tubules inefficient at reabsorbing the tubular fluid sodium, resulting in elevated urinary sodium. Acute hepatorenal syndrome in advanced cirrhosis has a fractional sodium excretion of < 1 despite it being an intrinsic renal disease. These confusing numbers are commonly encountered in the MRCP examination.

40) e.
The majority of cases of retroperitoneal fibrosis are idiopathic; however, excluding secondary causes is mandatory. The idiopathic variety responds favourably to corticosteroids; medical treatment failure calls for surgical intervention for relief and exclusion of malignancy.

41) d.
Idiopathic hydronephrosis results from functional obstruction of the pelviureteric junction; electron microscopy fails to show any abnormality. The disease is bilateral in 50% of cases. It is rarely asymptomatic. Surgical treatment (pyeloplasty) is usually effective.

42) c.
Only renal vein thrombosis with pulmonary embolism explains all the manifestations mentioned in the question. This is one of the causes of renal disease and haemoptysis. Other causes are Legionnaire's disease, anti-GBM disease and Wegener's granulomatosis.

43) b.
$\beta2$-Microglobulin comes predominantly from the renal tubules. Dysmorphic RBCs in urine (seen on contrast-phase microscopy) indicate a glomerular origin of urinary tract bleeding. If proteinuria coexists, a nephritic picture is highly likely.

44) b.

This unexplained acute renal failure calls for renal biopsy. Other indications for renal biopsy are nephrotic syndrome in adults, atypical nephrotic syndrome in children, chronic renal failure with normal-sized kidneys and isolated haematuria with dysmorphic RBCs. The procedure is contraindicated in bleeding tendency, severe uncontrolled hypertension and small kidney size (<60% of the predicted size). The presence of a single kidney is a relative contraindication, except in renal grafts.

45) c.

Contrast nephropathy occurs within 24 hours of using an intravenous contrast material for imaging studies. Atheroembolic disease occurs after a few days to few weeks. There are no clues to renal artery occlusion or septic shock. Pulmonary thromboembolism results in rapid shallow (not sighing) breathing, and the interval in this case is too short for a thrombosis to establish itself and to embolize.

46) c.

Creatinine clearance (CrCl) is a relatively simple method of measuring the GFR. Measurement of serum creatinine and 24-hour urinary creatinine is all that is required to calculate the CrCl; no injected substances are needed.

$$\text{CrCl (ml/min)} = \frac{\text{24-Hour urinary creatinine}}{\text{Serum creatinine}} \times \frac{1000}{1400}$$

The drawbacks are that it depends on accurate urine collection, many medications interfere with tubular creatinine excretion (e.g. trimethoprim and cimetidine) and it tends to exaggerate the GFR in poor kidney function (because of a compensatory increase in tubular creatinine excretion in the hypertrophied nephrons).

47) a.

This man has metastatic renal cancer. Even in metastatic disease, nephrectomy should be done if possible, as it has been shown to improve the systemic symptoms of the tumour and may even regress metastatic deposits. Renal cell cancers (usually adenocarcinoma) are resistant to chemotherapy and radiotherapy. Interleukin-II and interferon-α may offer some benefit in metastatic disease.

48) e.

Excessive dialysis (whether haemodialysis or peritoneal dialysis) may produce hypophosphataemia. Prolonged hyperphosphataemia stimulates the parathyroid glands to produce metastatic calcification and results in pruritis as well. The use of oral phosphate binders may be sufficient treatment in this patient; otherwise, dialysis should be used.

49) d.
When there is strong family history of the adult polycystic kidney disease, other family members should be offered screening, usually in the form of abdominal ultrasound, starting at the age of 20 years. Younger patients may undergo genetic testing after careful genetic counselling. Affected individuals should have their blood pressure measured regularly. In at-risk individuals younger than 30 years of age, the presence of at least two cysts (in one or both kidneys) is sufficient to secure the diagnosis; in those aged 30–59 years, at least two cysts in each kidney; and in those older than 60 years, at least four cysts in each kidney.

50) b.
Defective platelet function and impaired coagulation are consequences of severe or prolonged hypophosphataemia. Diffuse muscle pain and weakness (including of the respiratory muscles, causing hypoventilation; even rhabomyolysis may result) and raised serum creatinine kinase, heart failure and arrhythmia, neurological dysfunction and encephalopathy (e.g. confusion, seizures), red cell haemolysis, hypercalciuria and hypermagnesuria are other consequences. Phosphate is essential for cell energy (ATP), the secondary messenger system (cAMP) and nucleic acid synthesis; therefore, phosphate deficiency can be expected to produce a variety of cellular dysfunction in many cell types.

51) d.
This patient's anion gap is 10, which is within the normal reference range (8–14); thus, this is a normal anion gap metabolic acidosis. Renal tubular acidosis, carbonic anhydrase inhibitors, ureterosigmoidostomy, diarrhoea or GIT fistulae, early uraemia and diabetic ketoacidosis (in the way of recovery) are the usual causes. Methanol or ethylene glycol poisoning results in a high anion gap metabolic acidosis with high osmolar gap.

52) b.
Type A lactic acidosis is associated with tissue hypoxia; any severe shock, respiratory failure, severe anaemia, and cyanide or CO poisoning are the usual causes. Type B is associated with impaired mitochondrial function; the usual causes are hepatic failure, ethanol or methanol poisoning, treatment with aspirin, metformin, sorbitol and isoniazid.

53) e.
Alport's syndrome is second only to adult polycystic kidney disease as an inherited cause of chronic renal failure (which results in hyperkalaemia). The other options are tubular syndromes of potassium loss. Liddle's syndrome involves an activated mutation in epithelial sodium channels which avidly absorb that cation; serum aldosterone is suppressed, hypokalaemia ensues and blood pressure rises, causing apparent aldosteronism.

54) a.
The overall picture is indicative of SIADH. In this condition, the urinary osmolality is usually in excess of 430 mosmol/kg, which is inappropriately concentrated for the profound systemic hypo-osmolality seen in this patient. The urinary osmolality should fall below 150 mosmol/kg when there is plasma hypo-osmolality.

55) c.
*Hyper*calcaemia, not hypocalcaemia, can result in nephrogenic diabetes insipidus. Note the failure of the urinary osmolality to rise following vasopressin injection in this patient with dilute urine and high plasma osmolality.

56) c.
As this is the first stone in this patient, only a limited number of investigations is required in the form of serum calcium and phosphate (and uric acid), serum urea and electrolytes, urine examination (for protein and blood) and chemical analysis of the stone; serum PTH is measured when there is hypercalcaemia. Recurrent stone formation requires further evaluation by measuring the 24-hour urine for calcium, oxalate, uric acid, sodium, urea and creatinine clearance, and the patient's urine should be tested for amino acids.

57) d.
This patient had a UTI which responded favourably to an oral antibiotic. Re-infection with the same organism or a new one is not uncommon, especially in young sexually active females. The initial response to ciprofloxacin in this UTI rules out a resistant organism and wrong initial diagnosis.

58) c.
Children with a nephrotic syndrome which has atypical features (impaired renal function, hypertension, haematuria or active urinary sediment) or those not responding to corticosteroids should undergo renal biopsy and histopathological examination.

59) c.
This woman has uncomplicated UTI in the form of cystitis; the uncomplicated nature of the disease does not justify the use of parenteral therapy. Oral co-amoxiclav, ciprofloxacin or trimethoprim are the empirical therapies of choice to start with. Oral vancomycin is not absorbed and is used in the treatment of pseudomembranous colitis.

60) c.
Urinary bladder squamous cell cancer occurs when the lining of the organ is chronically irritated and has undergone metaplasia due to a stone or schistosomiasis. Urinary bladder tumours are almost always of transitional cell type. As the bladder can store urine for a period of time, its lining is exposed to urinary carcinogens. Generally, patients with papillary tumours fare better than those with ulcerating ones.

4. Gastroenterology: Questions

1) A 43-year-old man accidentally ingested an alkaline fluid while at work. He was brought to A&E 1 hour later. Five months later, he reports some difficulty in swallowing, mainly of solid food. Which one of the following statements is true regarding this lye oesophageal stricture?

a. Mainly seen at the upper oesophagus
b. Predisposes patient to oesophageal squamous cell cancer
c. Alkalis do not produce oesophageal stricture when ingested accidentally
d. Total oesophagectomy is the treatment of choice
e. Oesophageal dilatation with bougienage is contraindicated

2) A 65-year-old woman presents with dysphagia to solids and progressive weight loss over 3 months. She reports coughing and regurgitation every now and then. Her GP has diagnosed achalasia of the cardia on the basis of her barium swallow appearance. What would you do?

a. Refer for Heller's myotomy
b. Arrange for endoscopic pneumatic dilatation
c. Do oesophago-gastroscopy
d. Give nitrates
e. Advise bougienage

3) A 54-year-old man presents with heartburn and regurgitation that he has had for many years. He is partially compliant with his lansoprazole. Otherwise, he is healthy and does not have hypertension or diabetes. Oesophagoscopy reveals a short-segment Barrett's oesophagus and biopsy examination shows mild mucosal dysplasia. What should you do for this complication of gastroesophageal reflux disease?

a. Frequent upper GIT endoscopy with biopsy taking
b. Refer for oesophagectomy
c. Endoscopic laser therapy
d. Oesophageal stent placement
e. CT scan of the chest with contrast

4) A 44-year-old woman presents with progressive dysphagia to solids. She smokes two cigarette packets per day and drinks alcohol occasionally. All of the following could be responsible for this difficulty in swallowing, except:

a. Oesophageal web
b. Achalasia of the cardia
c. Oesophageal ring
d. Oesophageal squamous cell cancer
e. Barrett's oesophagus

5) A 53-year-old patient presents with difficulty in swallowing and a weight loss of 10 kg over the past 4 months. He is pale and there is hard knobbly liver enlargement. Oesophagoscopy reveals a fungating mass in the lower oesophagus, biopsy of which reveals squamous cell cancer. Which one of the following is *not* implicated as a risk factor for this type of malignancy?

a. Coeliac disease
b. Tylosis
c. Lye stricture
d. Barrett's oesophagus
e. Cigarette smoking

6) A 45-year-old woman presents with epigastric pain and nausea. She was diagnosed with duodenal ulcer 2 weeks ago and has been given *H. pylori* eradication therapy in the form of omeprazole, metronidazole and clarithromycin. Urea breath test is still positive 2 weeks after starting the medications. She denies medication non-compliance. What is the reason for this medical treatment failure?

a. Non-compliance
b. Development of gastroesophageal reflux disease
c. Gastric cancer
d. Antibiotic resistance
e. *H. pylori* re-infection

7) A 51-year-old man with newly diagnosed duodenal ulcer presents with a 6-day history of diarrhoea after starting anti-*H. pylori* therapy. The stool is watery, without blood or pus. He reports abdominal cramps. What is the likely cause of this man's diarrhoea?

a. *Salmonella* food poisoning
b. Post-gastrectomy dumping syndrome
c. Anti-*H. pylori* medication
d. Gastrinoma
e. Bile reflux

8) A 47-year-old woman presents following an unintentional weight loss of 10 kg. She underwent gastric surgery for peptic ulcer disease 6 months ago, which was uncomplicated at that time. What is the reason for the current presentation?

a. Recurrent peptic ulcer disease
b. Small gastric remnant
c. Gastric cancer
d. Anorexia nervosa
e. Gastrinoma

9) A 51-year-old man with severe, recurrent, and extensive peptic ulceration is given a diagnosis of Zollinger–Ellison syndrome. Which of the following is true with respect to this syndrome?

a. Common cause of peptic ulcer disease
b. Never malignant
c. Should be treated by gastrectomy
d. Diarrhoea can be the presenting feature
e. Octreotide is contraindicated

10) A 34-year-old woman presents with upper abdominal pain and nausea that lessens with food ingestion. She underwent partial gastric removal surgery 6 months ago for peptic ulcer disease. You order serum gastrin level assessment which is found to be 1030 pg/L. Which one of the following is responsible for the hypergastrinaemia in this woman?

a. Retained gastric antrum
b. Chronic atrophic gastritis
c. Long-term lansoprazole therapy
d. Chronic renal failure
e. Gastrinoma

11) A 61-year-old man is referred to you because he is not responding to the medication prescribed by his GP for non-ulcer dyspepsia. The man admits to having weight loss and becoming pale lately. His original complaints were nausea, anorexia and epigastric pain. What is the best option to choose?

a. Give omeprazole
b. Arrange for barium swallow
c. Send for occult blood in stool
d. Do an upper GIT endoscopy
e. Check plasma CA-125 level

12) A 69-year-old man comes to see you because of early satiety and postprandial nausea. He reports upper abdominal discomfort and is losing weight. Urea breath test is positive. Gastroscopy reveals a small polypoidal mass in the gastric fundus and histopathological examination of a biopsy taken from it secures the diagnosis of MALToma. What is the best treatment?

a. CHOP regimen
b. ABVD regimen
c. Observation
d. Surgical resection
e. Anti-H. pylori therapy

13) A 33-year-old man complains of epigastric fullness and pain, nausea and vomiting, flushing, sweating and palpitations approximately half an hour after starting a meal. He was treated surgically for peptic ulcer disease 2 months ago. He has failed to respond to dietary manipulation to relieve these symptoms. How would you treat this patient?

  a. Refer for surgical opinion
  b. Metoclopramide
  c. Domperidone
  d. Octreotide
  e. Erythromycin

14) A 32-year-old man presents with daily watery diarrhoea. The stool is <1 litre/day and is devoid of pus or red blood cells. There is an osmolar gap of 180 mosmol/kg. The patient reports improvement with fasting. What is the likely diagnosis?

  a. Sorbitol food
  b. Travellers' diarrhoea
  c. Villous adenoma of rectum
  d. Somatostatinoma
  e. *Salmonella* food poisoning

15) A 31-year-old patient is referred to you for further evaluation of a gut disorder. He has bilateral pitting leg oedema. Precordial examination is unremarkable as is the JVP. Serum ALT is 12 U/L, total serum bilirubin is 0.8 mg/dl and urine is negative for protein, but serum albumin is 20 g/L. Which one of the following is *not* a potential cause of protein-losing enteropathy?

  a. Eosinophilic gastroenteritis
  b. Crohn's disease
  c. Whipple's disease
  d. Small bowel lymphoma
  e. *H. pylori*-associated peptic ulceration

16) One year after undergoing Billroth II gastrectomy, a 55-year old man presents with steatorrhoea. His serum vitamin B_{12} is low with increased plasma levels of folate. Which investigation would you choose to confirm your provisional diagnosis?

  a. Serum albumin
  b. ^{14}C-glycocholate breath test
  c. Jejunal biopsy
  d. Ascitic fluid aspirate
  e. Three-day stool fat content

17) A 23-year-old man with long-term coeliac disease presents with diffuse abdominal pain and vomiting. His abdominal wall is board-like rigid and he is in shock. He is poorly compliant with his gluten-free diet. What is the reason for this man's current presentation?

a. Small bowel perforation
b. Coeliac crisis
c. Refractory coeliac disease
d. Squamous cell oesophageal cancer
e. Selective IgA deficiency

18) Four months following the diagnosis of duodenal ulcer, a 28-year-old man presents to A&E with repeated vomiting of fresh blood. He is non-compliant with his antiulcer measures. Blood pressure is 80/40 mmHg, pulse rate is 130 beats/minutes and the haematocrit is 30%. What is the first step in your management plan?

a. Gastroscopy with thermotherapy
b. Surgical referral
c. Resuscitation
d. Send for blood urea and serum electrolytes
e. Terlipressin infusion

19) A 24-year-old patient is referred by his GP for further evaluation of diarrhoea. The patient has had loose stools six times a day for the past 2 months. What is the commonest cause of chronic diarrhoea?

a. *Salmonella* non-typhi
b. Amoebiasis
c. Irritable bowel syndrome
d. Ulcerative colitis
e. Coeliac disease

20) A 47-year-old woman has been receiving oral prednisolone for a relapsed ulcerative colitis for months. This is her third relapse within a 5-month period. Besides olsalazine, which one of the following would you prescribe?

a. Mesalazine
b. Methylprednisolone
c. Azathioprine
d. Infliximab
e. Folic acid

21) A 29-year-old man with ulcerative colitis attends for a scheduled follow-up. He has a rounded plethoric face, hypertension and skin striae. Because of back pain, an X-ray is ordered which reveals multiple wedged vertebral compression fractures. He denies loose stools or abdominal pain. What action would you take?

a. Continue his medical treatment
b. Do stool culture
c. Refer for surgical treatment
d. Advise an elimination diet
e. Add aledronate

22) A 29-year-old patient with inflammatory bowel disease is admitted with a severe and fulminant attack of colitis and fever. His plain abdominal X-ray shows a grossly dilated transverse colon of 8 cm in diameter. He is pale and has diffuse and severe abdominal pain. Which one of the following should be avoided?

a. Packed RBC transfusion
b. Intravenous fluids
c. Opiate analgesia
d. Intravenous antibiotics
e. Subcutaneous heparin

23) A 32-year-old woman has a 1-year history of pain-predominant irritable bowel syndrome that is not responding to spasmolytic medications. She had mild diarrhoea but this is now well-controlled. What would you prescribe?

a. High roughage diet
b. Loperamide
c. Amitriptyline
d. Lactulose
e. Mebeverine

24) A 65-year-old man develops extensive myocardial infarction and severe hypotension. A day later he develops diffuse abdominal pain, abdominal distension and bloody stool. Abdominal examination is unremarkable. He has hyperphosphataemia, leucocytosis, metabolic acidosis and elevated serum amylase. What is the diagnosis?

a. Ulcerative colitis relapse
b. Acute small bowel ischaemia
c. Warfarin-induced haemorrhage
d. DIC
e. Acute pancreatitis

25) A 33-year-old patient is referred from the haematology clinic. He has iron-deficiency anaemia associated with multiple oesophageal, gastric, small bowel and colonic polyps. Examination reveals alopecia, nail dystrophy and skin hyperpigmenation. What is the diagnosis?

a. Cronkhite–Canada syndrome
b. Familial adenomatous polyposis coli
c. Cowden's disease
d. Gardner's syndrome
e. Peutz–Jeghers syndrome

26) A 38-year-old man dies of cancer. He underwent prophylactic colectomy successfully at the age of 24 years because of positivity for familial adenomatous polyposis (FAP) genetic mutation. What type of cancer is he most likely to have had?

a. Oesophageal squamous cell cancer
b. Duodenal carcinoma
c. Colonic cancer
d. Thyroid cancer
e. Aggressive brain glioma

27) A 36-year-old woman presents with iron-deficiency anaemia. Because of a strong family history of colonic cancer (her older brother and father died of colonic cancer at the ages of 53 and 45, respectively), she undergoes colonoscopy which reveals a fungating mass in the caecum. Testing for FAP genetic mutation is negative. What is the cause of colonic cancer in this woman?

a. Familial adenomatous polyposis
b. Gardner's syndrome
c. Attenuated familial adenomatous polyposis
d. Hereditary non-polyposis colonic cancer
e. Sporadic colonic cancer

28) A 50-year-old man presents to A&E with severe upper abdominal pain radiating to the back, nausea and vomiting over 3 days. There is prominent epigastric tenderness but no guarding. His blood pressure is low and he is tachycardic. Plain abdominal X-ray is unremarkable. Serum amylase is marginally elevated but the urinary amylase:creatinine ratio is elevated. What is the diagnosis?

a. Perforated peptic ulcer
b. Acute pancreatitis
c. Bleeding duodenal ulcer
d. Acute intestinal ischaemia
e. Ruptured aortic aneurysm

29) A 71-year-old man still has upper abdominal pain six weeks after recovery from idiopathic acute pancreatitis. Examination reveals a rounded mass in the epigastrium. Serum amylase is persistently raised and has never fallen. What is the diagnosis?

a. Localized ascites
b. Pancreatic pseudocyst
c. Gastric cancer
d. Abdominal wall haematoma
e. Abdominal wall hernia

30) A 43-year-old patient with acute pancreatitis has developed a progressive abdominal distension. Abdominal bowel sounds are intact. You are considering a diagnosis of pancreatic ascites. Which one of the following would cast doubt upon this diagnosis?

a. Normal ascitic fluid amylase
b. Free collection of fluid
c. Ascitic fluid protein 50 g/L
d. Associated left-sided pleural effusion
e. Abdominal shifting dullness

31) A 69-year-old woman with gallbladder disease is referred to your hospital with acute pancreatitis. Your junior house officer asks what adverse prognostic factors this patient has. Which one of the following indicates a poor prognosis in acute pancreatitis?

a. Serum albumin 39 g/L
b. Random plasma glucose >5 mmol/L
c. PaO_2 <8 kPa
d. Age >35 years
e. Serum LDH <400 U/L

32) A 50-year-old man presents with a 1-year history of epigastric pain. The pain is continuous and relentless and is relieved by drinking alcohol. He admits to drinking heavily over the past 20 years. He is thin, has epigastric tenderness and there is erythema ab igne over the upper abdomen and back. Plain abdominal X-ray shows pancreatic calcification. All of the following are true regarding the management of chronic pancreatitis, except:

a. Avoid alcohol ingestion
b. Opiates carry the risk of addiction
c. Pancreatic enzyme supplements increase the pain severity
d. Coeliac plexus neurolysis can be used to alleviate pain
e. Median chain triglycerides are used in steatorrhoea

33) A 73-year-old man attends because of gnawing epigastric pain and pruritis. He has global wasting, epigastric mass, jaundice and a hard knobbly liver. Abdominal CT scan shows a pancreatic malignant-looking mass. All of the following are *untrue* regarding pancreatic cancer, except:

a. Associated with smoking
b. Majority of tumours are cystadenocarcinomas
c. Weight loss is unusual
d. Presentation as acute pancreatitis is common
e. 50% of tumours are amenable to surgery

34) A 33-year-old man is referred to you for further evaluation of unexplained jaundice and raised liver transaminases. Liver ultrasound examination is unremarkable. You are contemplating a liver biopsy. All of the following are contraindications to liver biopsy, except:

a. Severe COPD
b. Local skin infection
c. Marked ascites
d. Uncooperative patient
e. Platelets counts 150×10^9/L

35) A 44-year-old woman is found to have mild elevation of liver transaminases in a routine pre-employment screening. She denies any symptoms, or alcohol or illicit drug abuse. Her body mass index is 35 kg/m^2. Serum bilirubin and gamma-glutamyl transferase levels are within their normal reference range. Which one of the following is the most likely explanation for her abnormal liver function test?

a. Alcoholic liver disease
b. Acute hepatitis C infection
c. Fatty liver
d. Gilbert's syndrome
e. Haemolytic anaemia

36) A 16-year-old girl at secondary school comes with her parents to consult you. She reports jaundice every now and then but denies other symptoms like itching or abdominal pain. The indirect serum bilirubin is mildly elevated with normal ALT, AST and alkaline phosphatase. Blood film is unremarkable and there is a normal haemoglobin level. Coombs' test is negative. What is the treatment of choice?

a. Liver transplantation
b. Phenobarbital
c. Prednisolone
d. Azathioprine
e. No treatment is needed

37) A 45-year-old man presents with low-grade fever, arthralgia, hyper-pigmentation, steatorrhoea and weight loss. Examination reveals pallor, lymphadenopathy, ascites and pericardial friction rub. Jejunal biopsy reveals subtotal villous atrophy with dense infiltration of the lamina propria with PAS-positive macrophages. What is the likely diagnosis?

a. Intestinal lymphoma
b. Intestinal pseudo-obstruction
c. Whipple's disease
d. Coeliac disease
e. Tropical sprue

38) A 54-year-old man presents with confusional state. His last work-up revealed fulminant hepatic failure. His wife reports that he is other-wise healthy and has no chronic illnesses. Which one of the following would cast doubt on this man's diagnosis?

a. Absence of jaundice
b. Normal liver transaminases
c. Prominent splenomegaly
d. Myoclonus
e. Liver enlargement

39) A 41-year-old patient with liver cirrhosis presents requesting active treatment for his illness. He has surfed the internet and found that liver transplantation is a treatment option. You have reviewed him and found that he has a contraindication to this form of treatment. What is this contraindication?

a. Refractory itching
b. Fatigue interfering with many aspects of daily life
c. Recurrent variceal bleeding
d. Active alcohol misuse
e. Ascites not responding to drug therapy

40) A 52-year-old alcoholic man presents to the gastroenterology out-patient clinic with weight loss and fatigue. He has mild ascites, no encephalopathy, serum bilirubin 30 μmol/L, serum albumin 38 g/L and PT 15 seconds (control <13 seconds). This man's Child–Pugh grade is:

a. A
b. B
c. C
d. D
e. E

41) A 30-year-old woman with fulminant hepatic failure develops a number of complications while being managed in the intensive care unit. Which one of the following is *not* a recognized complication of this grave disease?

a. Blood sugar 300 mg/dl
b. Core body temperature 35°C
c. Raised serum amylase
d. Serum potassium 2.8 mEq/L
e. Serum potassium 6.0 mEq/L

42) A 47-year-old woman with alcoholic liver cirrhosis is brought to A&E in a shock state and with severe haematemesis. She underwent oesophagoscopy 4 weeks ago which revealed oesophageal varices. You resuscitate her. What is the next step?

a. Refer for shunt surgery
b. Discuss oesophageal transection
c. Use balloon tamponade
d. Do upper GIT endoscopy
e. Arrange for transjugular intrahepatic portosystemic stent shunt (TIPSS)

43) A 45-year-old man with hepatitis B-associated liver cirrhosis attends for a scheduled follow-up visit. He has received optimal medical treatment combined with a salt-free diet for his ascites. Abdominal examination reveals gross symmetrical abdominal distension with shifting dullness. What is the best way to treat him now?

a. Increase the dose of diuretics
b. Provide education in a low-salt diet
c. LeVeen shunt
d. Water restriction
e. Frequent abdominal paracentesis

44) A positive IgG anti-HBs antibody test is found during a routine pre-employment examination of a 32-year-old refugee from South East Asia. His English is not that good and you are unable to take a full history from him. What does this positive test imply?

a. Established acute hepatitis B infection
b. Co-infection with hepatitis D virus
c. Incubation period of hepatitis B infection
d. Past hepatitis B virus vaccination
e. Chronic infection

45) A difficult-to-manage 43-year-old male case is referred by his GP. The GP's report states that the patient has a positive test for HBs antigen and IgG anti-HBc, and his plasma viral DNA level is 10^9 copies/ml. How would you interpret his hepatitis B serological pattern?

a. Acute infection
b. Past vaccination
c. Chronic infection with a pre-core mutant strain
d. Chronic infection with high rate of replication
e. Prior infection with immunity

46) A 26-year-old homosexual man is referred from the STD clinic because of positive hepatic C virus (HCV) antibody testing using enzyme-linked immunoassay (EIA). After a thorough history taking and examination, you order anti-HCV antibodies testing using recombinant immunoblot assay (RIBA), which is found to be negative. How would you interpret this man's HCV serological testing?

a. Chronic HCV infection
b. Acute HCV infection
c. False-positive EIA
d. False-positive RIBA
e. Past vaccination

47) A 38-year-old woman with chronic hepatitis B infection is receiving interferon-α but has not responded to this therapy over the past 6 months. Which one of the following predicts a poor response to interferon-α treatment in this infection?

a. Female gender
b. Absence of frank cirrhosis on histology
c. Pre-core mutant form of the virus
d. Western origin
e. Low pre-treatment hepatitis viral DNA plasma level

48) A 44-year-old woman is being evaluated for an isolated elevation in serum ALT. The final diagnosis is obesity-associated fatty liver. Which one of the following is *not* a cause of hepatic macrovesicular steatosis?

a. Alcohol
b. Prolonged parenteral nutrition
c. Diabetes mellitus
d. Fatty liver of pregnancy
e. Rapid weight loss

49) A 30-year-old woman presents with fatigue, amenorrhea, cushingoid features and jaundice. Antinuclear antibodies are positive. Serum aminotransferases are elevated. Which one of the following would be inconsistent with type 1 autoimmune hepatitis?

a. Association with Graves' disease
b. Presence of HLA-DR3
c. Positive serum anti-LKM antibodies
d. Hypergammaglobulinaemia
e. Low serum albumin

50) A 55-year-old man is referred by his GP. You examine the patient and find that he has slate-grey skin hyperpigmentation and hepatomegaly. ECG reveals conduction disturbances and arrhythmia. Serum aminotransferases are elevated. Which one of the following is *not* seen in hereditary haemochromatosis?

a. Raised serum iron
b. Elevated serum ferritin
c. Transferrin saturation 90%
d. Chondrocalcinosis
e. Haemoglobin level 19 g/dl

51) A 50-year-old woman presents with a 3-year history of generalized itching. She has hepatomegaly, clubbing and hyperpigmentation. Serum anti-mitochondrial antibody testing is positive. What is the treatment?

a. Prednisolone
b. Ciclosporin
c. Azathioprine
d. Ursodeoxycholic acid
e. Plasma exchange

52) A 53-year-old man develops rapidly progressive right hypochondrial pain, tender hepatomegaly, and marked ascites. He states that he is otherwise healthy. He neither smokes nor drinks alcohol. Liver enzymes are elevated. Today you notice bilateral pitting leg oedema. What is the cause of leg oedema in this man's Budd–Chiari syndrome?

a. Treatment with vasodilators
b. Inferior vena cava thrombosis
c. Lymphoedema
d. Fluid overload
e. Bilateral calf deep venous thrombosis

53) A 48-year-old cirrhotic man has developed spontaneous bacterial peritonitis (SBP) and is about to be admitted to your medical ward to receive medical treatment. Which one of the following is true regarding this complication of cirrhosis?

a. Never presents as hepatic encephalopathy
b. Bowel sounds are hyperactive
c. Ascitic fluid neutrophil count is $>2.5 \times 10^9/L$
d. Usually polymicrobial
e. Prescribe daily norfloxacin on discharge

54) Three months following laparoscopic cholecystectomy, a 50-year-old woman presents with right upper abdominal quadrant pain, excessive flatulence and intolerance to fatty food. Abdominal ultrasound and ERCP fail to detect any residual stone or biliary stricture. What is the cause of this woman's presentation?

a. Small common bile duct stones
b. Cholangiocarcinoma
c. Peri-ampullary adenocarcinoma
d. Post-cholecystectomy syndrome
e. Choledochal cyst

55) A 45-year-old woman is found to have gallstones on abdominal ultrasonography that forms part of a pre-medical insurance examination. She is reasonably well and healthy and denies abdominal symptoms. She neither smokes nor drinks alcohol and there is no family history of note. Which of the following statements is true regarding this woman's gallbladder disease?

a. Emergency open cholecystectomy is required
b. Prophylactic laparoscopic gallbladder removal should be considered
c. Advise against cholecystectomy
d. Evaluate for surgery fitness
e. Refer to ERCP

Gastroenterology: Answers

1) b.
A lye stricture is seen mainly at the three physiological narrowing areas where the initial passage of the corrosive agent is delayed. Alkalis are *more* dangerous and more injurious to the oesophagus than acids; e.g. following gastrectomy, the refluxed alkaline duodenal fluid can induce severe oesophagitis. Induced vomiting is contraindicated in acute alkali ingestion but bougienage after 1 month may help prevent stricture formation. Alkali ingestion, whether accidental or intentional, can result in oesophageal stricture formation. Total removal of the oesophagus is rarely needed as the stricture usually has a short segment.

2) c.
This 65-year-old woman with an achalasia-like picture and 'regurgitation' has progressive weight loss and dysphagia within a relatively short period. All patients with radiographic suggestion of achalasia of the cardia should undergo upper GIT endoscopy; pseudoachalasia due to cancer at the oesophagogastric junction is at the top of the list of differential diagnoses. This woman is likely to have pseudoachalasia and proceeding with endoscopy would seem reasonable. Note that bougienage is contraindicated in achalasia, and that endoscopic pneumatic dilatation is as efficient as Heller's myotomy as a mode of treating achalasia. Botulinum toxin provides temporary relief in patients who are unfit for surgery.

3) a.
A common examination theme is the Barrett's oesophagus. It is clinically silent and is the endoscopic appearance of the metaplastic lower oesophageal mucosa. Its importance lies in its predisposition to oesophageal adenocarcinoma (the risk is increased 40–100 fold; 0.5% of patients per year will develop malignancy). The best management option in these patients is controversial, especially when high-grade dysplasia is present. If the biopsy shows mild dysplastic changes (which are common in severely inflamed mucosa), frequent enodoscopies and biopsies are indicated. If the biopsy reveals severe dysplasia, the risk of malignancy jumps to 25% and, unfortunately, there is no consensus regarding the management of this stage; referral for oesophagectomy versus endoscopic laser ablation versus aggressive PPIs therapy with frequent endoscopic surveillance are the treatment options.

4) e.
Barrett's oesophagus indicates many years of gastro-oesophageal reflux. The presence of metaplastic columnar lined epithelium that ascends from the gastro-oesophageal junction upward to a variable distance (short- and long-segment Barrett's oesophagus) is seen endoscopically. It is asymptomatic (per se), and its significance is that it is premalignant.

5) d.

Barrett's oesophagus predisposes to oesophageal adenocarcinoma. In the US, adenocarcinoma is responsible for 80% of all oesophageal cancers, with squamous carcinoma seen in the remaining 20%. Risk factors for the latter type of malignancy are cigarette smoking, alcohol ingestion, coeliac disease, tylosis, lye stricture, Plummer–Vinson syndrome and achalasia of the cardia.

6) d.

Antibiotic resistance ranks second to medication non-compliance on the list of causes of failure of medical therapy. Medication non-compliance can be excluded by the patient's history (although there is no evidence that the patient is fully compliant), and therefore bacterial resistance to antibiotics should be addressed now. This is becoming a major problem in the treatment of peptic ulcer disease; metronidazole has a resistance rate approaching 40% while that of clarithromycin is 10%. The patient should be retreated with another antibiotic(s) for a further 2-week period.

7) c.

Following initiation of anti-*H. pylori* therapy, 30–50% of patients will develop diarrhoea, which is usually mild; *Clostridium difficile* colitis is rarely responsible. Nausea, vomiting, diffuse cramping abdominal pains and headache are common side effects of the regimen.

8) b.

Following any gastric surgery, the majority of patients lose weight and up to 40% of them are unable to regain the lost weight. This is usually the aftermath of reduced intake because of the small gastric remnant, but diarrhoea and maldigestion also contribute.

9) d.

Zollinger–Ellison syndrome is a *rare* cause of peptic ulceration (0.1% of cases). It can be malignant and usually metastasizes to the liver. Some tumours are multifocal. The availability of high-dose PPIs has made gastrectomy unnecessary. In up to one-third of cases, the tumour is small and single and can be localized for successful resection. Diarrhoea is seen in 30% of cases and can be the presenting feature. Steatorrhoea may also occur. Octreotide and other long-acting somatostatin analogues reduce gastric secretion and be of benefit in some patients.

10) e.

Long-term PPI therapy and chronic atrophic gastritis are by far the commonest causes of raised serum gastrin. Persistently high serum gastrin following partial gastrectomy is usually due to retained gastric antrum or incomplete vagotomy; however, a very high serum gastrin level such as in this patient should always prompt a search for underlying gastrinoma. Mild hypergastrinaemia can be seen in uraemia, diabetes mellitus, rheumatoid arthritis, Sjögren's syndrome, ovarian cancer, massive small bowel resection, gastric cell hyperplasia, vitiligo and phaeochromocytoma.

11) d.
This man has many 'red flags' for non-ulcer dyspepsia. He is pale and is losing weight; besides, the occurrence of non-ulcer dyspepsia at this age is somewhat strange (it is usually seen in women before the age of 40 years). Gastric cancer can present simply with loss of appetite and nausea, and 50% of patients have an ulcer-like presentation. This man's presentation calls for upper GIT endoscopy; barium swallow is used in oesophageal diseases and barium meal lacks sensitivity and specificity for gastric cancers. Plasma CA-125 level is used in screening and follow-up of epithelial ovarian cancers.

12) e.
Gastric MALToma is a form of low-grade B-cell lymphoma that carries a good prognosis. Lymphoid tissue is absent in the gastric wall in normal situations; however, lymphoid aggregates develop in response to long-standing infection with *H. pylori*. This is the rationale for using *H. pylori* eradication therapy with close observation. High-grade tumours can be treated by surgical resection and chemotherapy. Primary gastric lymphoma accounts for about 5% of all gastric malignancies and 60% of all primary GIT lymphomas; the stomach is the commonest target for extranodal non-Hodgkin's lymphoma.

13) d.
This patient is manifesting early dumping syndrome following gastric surgery. Late dumping syndrome occurs after approximately 2 hours in the form of weakness, tremor and sweating. In both, the treatment involves dietary manipulation in the form of small frequent meals with low refined carbohydrate content, separating solid and liquid intake, and avoidance of hypertonic fluids. These measures usually suffice in the majority; however, if they fail, subcutaneous administration of octreotide 30 minutes before meals is usually helpful. Surgical treatment to slow this rapid gastric emptying has a limited role. Metoclopramide, domperidone and erythromycin are prokinetics and will aggravate the condition.

14) a.
This short scenario is typical of osmotic diarrhoea. An increased stool osmolar gap indicates the presence of osmotically active substance in stool; the normal stool osmolar gap is <50. Stool osmolar gap $= 290 - 2$ (stool Na + K). Travellers' diarrhoea, villous adenoma of the rectum and somatostatinoma can result in secretory diarrhoea. *Salmonella* is an invasive pathogen. Common causes of osmotic diarrhoea are antacids, sorbitol and lactase deficiency.

15) e.
Protein-losing enteropathy implies loss of plasma proteins into the gut lumen that is sufficient to cause hypoalbuminaemia (and its

consequences). It is seen in a multitude of gut disorders, notably those associated with mucosal ulceration. The presentation is usually with peripheral oedema in the context of normal liver function testing and in the absence of proteinuria, with or without features of the underlying disease. Other causes are radiation enteritis, ulcerative colitis, coeliac disease, bacterial overgrowth, tropical sprue, intestinal lymphangiectasia and chronic constrictive pericarditis. *H. pylori*-associated peptic ulceration is not a recognized cause of protein-losing enteropathy.

16) b.

The patient's operation puts him at risk of bacterial overgrowth. The serum vitamin B_{12} is low because it is consumed by the bacteria, while that of folate is raised because of increased production by the bacteria–this is the clue to the diagnosis in this scenario. Jejunal biopsy would reveal mucosal causes of malabsorption, and a 3-day faecal fat collection would confirm steatorrhoea, but neither would confirm the bacterial overgrowth per se. Jejunal aspirate with culture is the gold standard test for diagnosing bacterial overgrowth, but it is usually not done in clinical practice. The ^{14}C-glycocholate breath test is an easy non-invasive way of screening for the disease; the early rise in ^{14}C in breath suggests bacterial overgrowth and increased digestion of ^{14}C-glycocholate in the bowel lumen. Hypoalbuminaemia and ascites are consequences of malabsorption.

17) a.

This short scenario points towards peritonitis; coeliac patients may develop ulcerative jejunitis with small bowel strictures and/or perforations. Coeliac crisis and refractory coeliac disease implies severe disease with wasting, dehydration and electrolyte disturbances; these patients are usually managed in hospital and should be given glucocorticoids or another form of immune suppression to control the disease activity. Squamous cell oesophageal cancer is a complication of long-term celiac disease, but it would not result in this picture of peritonitis. Selective IgA deficiency occurs in 3% of coeliac patients, may result in recurrent sinopulmonary infections and predisposes to small bowel bacterial overgrowth and giardiasis.

18) c.

As is the case in status epilepticus, the first step is ABC resuscitation. All unstable patients should be immediately resuscitated on presentation in A&E and should be stabilized before any further intervention is carried out. This is a common theme in the MRCP examination. Terlipressin is used in oesophageal variceal bleeding.

19) c.

Infective bacterial diarrhoeas rarely last more than 10 days. Irritable bowel syndrome is by far the commonest cause of chronic/relapsing diarrhoea; the diarrhoea rarely occurs at night and often contains mucus, but is never bloody. Patients usually have increased frequency of defecation and the stool can be watery, loose or pelletty. Amoebiasis is a rare cause.

20) c.
Steroids are the drug of choice in acute relapses. Those who relapse frequently after stopping steroids, or need high doses for maintenance therapy, should be considered for receiving azathioprine. Mesalazine and olsalazine can be used to maintain remission in ulcerative colitis, but there is no rationale for combining them; sulfasalazine is rarely used nowadays because of its bad side effect profile. Infliximab is used in severe fistulating Crohn's disease.

21) c.
Surgical treatment for ulcerative colitis in the form of panproctocolectomy should always be considered in the following: (1) impairment of family life, schooling, occupation and education (the most important indication); (2) failure or complications of medical therapy (this patient has gross cushingoid features and osteoporotic fractures); (3) development of complications which are unresponsive to medical therapy, e.g. severe and extensive pyoderma gangrenosum; (4) severe mucosal dysplasia or development of carcinoma; and (5) fulminant colitis. Note that this form of treatment can be curative, unlike that for Crohn's disease.

22) c.
Opiates and antidiarrhoeal agents should be avoided in fulminant colitis. These would increase the colonic atony and augment the risk of colonic rupture. Intravenous methylprednisolone is used to control disease activity, but if the patient deteriorates rapidly, does not respond within a 1-week period, or the diameter of the transverse colon exceeds 6 cm, surgical treatment is indicated. Heparin is given because of the high risk of thrombotic complications.

23) c.
The patient is not responding to antispasmodics, and therefore, mebeverine can be ruled out. He has no constipation so there is no use for a high roughage diet or lactulose. The diarrhoea is well-controlled and there is no justification to prescribe loperamide. Pain-predominant irritable bowel syndrome that is not responding to antispasmodics can be treated with low-dose (10–25 mg/day) amitriptyline; if this fails, referral for relaxation therapy, biofeedback or hypnotherapy can be tried.

24) b.
Acute small bowel ischaemia is caused by cardiac emboli to the inferior mesenteric artery in 50% of cases; the remaining cases are due to severe hypotension (cardiogenic shock, acute blood loss, cardiac dysrhythmia) in the context of diffuse atherosclerotic disease (as in this patient). To start with, the patient's abdominal examination is relatively 'benign' in presence of severe abdominal pain; signs of peritonitis indicate advanced disease.

Note that many GIT diseases can result in elevation of serum amylase as well as diseases of the salivary gland.

25) a.

Gastrointestinal polyposis diseases and syndromes are commonly seen in the MRCP examination. Oesophageal polyps are seen in Cowden's disease (autosomal dominant) and Cronkhite–Canada syndrome (sporadic). The extraintestinal features in this patient are consistent with the latter diagnosis. Cowden's disease patients have oral and skin hamartomas and breast and thyroid tumours.

26) b.

Duodenal carcinoma is the commonest cause of death in colectomized FAP, especially peri-ampullary ones. Oesophageal squamous cell cancer is not a recognized cancer in FAP. Colonic cancer is ruled out because the patient does not have a colon! Thyroid cancer is seen in Cowden's disease and aggressive brain glioma in Turcot syndrome (gliomas and medulloblastomas + FAP).

27) d.

This woman fulfils the diagnostic criteria for hereditary non-polyposis colonic cancer: (1) three (or more) relatives with colonic cancer; at least one of whom a first-degree relative; (2) colonic cancer in two (or more) generations; (3) at least one member affected by the disease is under the age of 50 years; and (4) exclusion of familial adenomatous polyposis.

28) b.

The patient's scenario and the elevated urinary amylase:creatinine ratio are indicative of acute pancreatitis. Plasma amylase is easily excreted by the kidney, and its level can easily return to the normal reference range 1–2 days after the onset of acute attacks of pancreatitis; therefore, measuring the amylase:creatinine ratio in urine is a valuable tool to solidify the clinical diagnosis of acute pancreatitis by showing an elevated level. Serum amylase can be also be raised in acute parotitis, small bowel ischaemia and perforated peptic ulcer.

29) b.

The development of persistent epigastric pain and high serum amylase after acute pancreatitis should always prompt a search for pancreatic pseudocysts by ordering abdominal ultrasound or CT scan.

30) a.

The level of amylase enzyme is greatly elevated in pancreatic ascites; normal values suggest an alternative cause of the ascites. Abdominal shifting dullness is a sign of ascites regardless of its aetiology. Left-sided pleural effusion is commonly seen with pancreatic ascites. The collection of fluid is free which is exudative.

31) c.

Questions addressing poor prognostic factors are commonly seen in the MRCP examination, and acute pancreatitis is no exception. The Glasgow criteria, which predict severe disease and increased mortality, are a constellation of many laboratory test results with only one non-laboratory indicator (the patient's age). These are: patient's age >55 years, WBC count $>15 \times 10^9$/L, serum albumin <32g/L, plasma glucose >10mmol/L, ALT >200 U/L, corrected serum calcium <2mmol/L, PaO_2 <8kPa, blood urea >16mmol/L and serum LDH >600 U/L. Patients with more than three factors have severe disease.

32) c.

Pancreatic enzyme supplements reduce pancreatic secretions and their use with time may produce an analgesic effect. Avoidance of alcohol is a critical step that will dampen the progression of the disease and may reduce pain significantly. However, most patients fail to abstain from alcohol. Fifteen per cent of chronic pancreatitis patients become opiate-addicts because of the severity of the pain. NSAIDs can be used in early and mild cases. Coeliac plexus neurolysis is usually done in those who have abstained from alcohol and who have severe relentless pain. It can produce long-lasting pain relief; however, the majority of patients will eventually have a relapse of their severe pain. Median chain triglycerides are used together with dietary fat restriction and pancreatic enzyme supplements (with proton pump inhibitors).

33) a.

Pancreatic cancer is associated with chronic pancreatitis and smoking. Hereditary factors account for about 10% of cases (hereditary pancreatitis, hereditary non-polyposis colonic cancer and multiple endocrine neoplasias). Cystadenocarcinomas are rare tumors that are mainly seen in middle-aged women at the head of the pancreas. They are usually slowly growing. Profound weight loss and cachexia are seen. Most patients present with a variable combination of epigastric pain, weight loss and jaundice. Presentation with diabetes, steatorrhoea, acute pancreatitis and superficial thrombophlebitis is seen in a minority of patients. Around 15% of cases are amenable to surgery. The management is mainly palliative. Chemotherapy and radiotherapy offer little benefit.

34) e.

Liver biopsy is generally a safe procedure in experienced hands and complications are rare. It is a dangerous procedure in uncooperative patients (as the biopsy needle will move around and damage the surrounding structures) and the coagulation system should be dependable (platelets count $>100 \times 10^9$/L, PT prolongation <4 seconds of the control value); in addition, the following should be excluded: marked ascites, severe COPD, local skin infection, cystic liver lesions including hydatid cysts, ascending cholangitis, and severe anaemia).

35) c.

Haemolytic anaemia and Gilbert's syndrome are the commonest causes of isolated indirect hyperbilirubinaemia with otherwise normal liver function tests. Acute hepatitis C infection does not present with mild asymptomatic elevation in liver transaminases. The normal gamma glutamyl transferase argues against alcoholic liver disease. Obesity-related fatty liver changes are the commonest cause of isolated liver transaminase (particularly ALT) elevation.

36) e.

Differentiating Gilbert's syndrome from haemolytic anaemia is a common theme in the MRCP examination. The only abnormal investigation in this patient is mild elevation of the indirect serum bilirubin because of decreased hepatic conjugation. Gilbert's syndrome carries an excellent prognosis and no treatment is needed. It is the commonest cause of congenital non-haemolytic hyperbilirubinaemia; other congenital hyperbilirubinaemic syndromes and diseases are extremely rare. Phenobarbital can be used as a test to reduce indirect serum bilirubin, but it is not needed as a long-term therapy. Liver transplantation is an option for treating autosomal dominant (type II) Crigler–Najjar syndrome.

37) c.

Only Whipple's disease fits the scenario. The disease is rapidly fatal if not treated appropriately with penicillin or co-trimoxazole. Relapse is seen in 30% of cases and usually involves the CNS.

38) c.

Most patients with fulminant hepatic failure are jaundiced to some degree but the course can be rapidly progressive so as to cause death before the appearance of jaundice; this is seen especially in Reye's syndrome. Normal liver transaminases are an ominous sign which implies a very poor prognosis. Splenomegaly is rare in previously healthy individuals and is never prominent; prominent splenomegaly should cast doubt on the diagnosis. Focal and multifocal neurological signs are common and may be bilateral and/or alternating. Note that hepatic encephalopathy is the hallmark of fulminant liver failure. The liver is usually enlarged initially but it gradually shrinks and becomes impalpable. Note that papilloedema is a late sign, as well as ascites and leg oedema.

39) d.

The indications and contraindications to liver transplantation in liver cirrhosis need to be differentiated. Apart from active alcohol misuse, all the other options are indications for liver transplantation. Liver cirrhosis accounts for about 75% of cases referred for orthotopic liver transplantations. The usual contraindications are active substance or alcohol misuse, HIV infection, extrahepatic malignancy, sepsis and severe cardiorespiratory disease.

40) a.

Apart from mild ascites (which has a score of 2), other parameters in the Child–Pugh grading system each have a score of 1; the final score will be 6. This puts the patient in the grade A category which has 82% 1-year survival. There are no grades D or E!

41) a.

Acute liver failure can have a multitude of complications, which need to be anticipated and managed properly. Hypo-, *not* hyper-, glycaemia is seen because of impaired hepatic gluconeogenesis. Hyperglycaemia usually indicates pre-existent diabetes mellitus. Hypothermia can occur; however, infections are common and may result in fever. Acute pancreatitis is a well-recognized complication. A serum potassium of 2.8 mEq/L could result from repeated vomiting and poor oral intake, whereas a level of 6.0 mEq/L could be the result of acute renal failure. Note that both hyper- and hypo-kalaemia can occur. All patients need close monitoring of plasma electrolytes and acid/base status.

42) d.

All patients with upper GIT bleeding should undergo upper GIT endoscopy, even those who have pre-existent oesophageal varices. In the latter group, a non-variceal source is responsible for 20% of cases; usually from acute erosive gastritis, which needs a different management plan from the variceal one. When facing questions about upper GIT bleeding in the MRCP examination, three actions in succession should be kept in mind: resuscitation, then endoscopy and finally, specific treatment.

43) c.

Note that this man is already being optimally managed medically (with diuretics, salt and water restriction). The best treatment option would be liver transplantation (which is not an option in this question). However, LeVeen shunting can provide a favourable symptomatic response. This is the placement of a long tube with a one-way valve that allows peritoneal fluid to pass freely from the abdominal cavity to the internal jugular vein in the neck; the tube is placed subcutaneously. The benefit must be weighed carefully against the risk of shunt thrombosis, DIC, infection, superior vena cava thrombosis and pulmonary oedema. TIPSS can also be used in resistant ascites in selected patients. Frequent abdominal paracentesis would be highly inconvenient to the patient.

44) d.

Isolated anti-HBs antibodies positivity indicates past vaccination with development of immunity. Positive testing for HBs antigen (with IgG anti-HBc) is the hallmark of chronic hepatitis B infection. Positive anti-HBs with IgG anti-HBc reflects a prior exposure to the 'wild virus' and the presence of immunity.

45) c.

Positive HBe antigen testing is the hallmark of high infectivity with replication. Hepatitis B viral DNA levels $< 10^5$ copies/ml indicates chronic infection without replication. This patient's serological profile is typical of chronic infection with the pre-core mutant form of the virus (which lacks the HBe-antigen).

46) c.

There is no HCV vaccine! A negative RIBA with positive EIA reflects false-positive EIA and the patient has no true anti-HCV antibodies. Positive EIA with positive RIBA indicates the presence of true anti-HCV antibodies (but these antibodies do not necessarily indicate current infection). When the RIBA result is 'indeterminate' with a positive EIA, the patient is said to have 'uncertain antibody status'. Note that HCV RNA detection in plasma is the gold standard for diagnosing HCV infection; the RNA level in plasma does not reflect disease severity, but it is used to monitor disease response to medical treatment.

47) c.

The following predict poor response to interferon-α therapy for chronic hepatitis B infection: male sex, origin from the Far East, cirrhotic changes on histology, high pre-treatment HBV DNA plasma level and the presence of pre-core mutant form of the virus.

48) d.

Obesity and alcohol ingestion are the cause of the majority of cases of macrovesicular steatosis of the liver; other causes are starvation, intestinal bypass, malabsorption and minocyclin therapy. Microvesicular steatosis implies a more serious disease and is usually associated with mitochondrial dysfunction and impairment of β-oxidation of fatty acids; it is seen in Reye's syndrome, acute fatty liver of pregnancy, treatment with valproic acid and lysosomal acid esterase deficiency.

49) c.

Anti-smooth muscle antibodies as well as ANA are positive in type I autoimmune hepatitis, while anti-LKM antibodies are positive in type 2. Type I autoimmune hepatitis is associated with Graves' disease and other autoimmune diseases, like Coombs'-positive haemolytic anaemia, nephrotic syndrome and Hashimoto's thyroiditis. HLA-DR3 and HLA-DR4 are present. There is prominent elevation in IgG. Changes in serum albumin and PT reflect disease severity, while levels of serum aminotransferases indicate disease activity.

50) e.

A common mistake in the MRCP examination is to confuse hereditary haemochromatosis with polycythemia vera; in spite of oversaturation with iron, haemoglobin level is *not* raised in the former. A haemoglobin level of 19 g/dl is too high for hereditary haemochromatosis. Plasma iron, iron-binding capacity and transferrin saturation are all elevated in hereditary haemochromaotosis, as is the hepatic iron content. The disease is more common in men. Genetic testing and liver biopsy examination with quantification of hepatic iron content is the standard diagnostic approach. Liver iron concentration is usually in excess of 10 000 μg/g dry weight. Note that the disease has an autosomal recessive mode of inheritance and that only homozygous individuals will develop a clinical disease.

51) d.

This woman's primary biliary cirrhosis can be treated with ursodeoxycholic acid. This therapy has been shown to produce symptomatic and biochemical improvement and may slow the pace of progression of the histological changes; however, it does not improve the mortality rate or the need for liver transplantation. None of the other options has been shown to be of any benefit.

52) b.

No cause can be detected in up 50% of Budd–Chiari syndrome cases; the remaining cases are associated with hypercoagulable states, hepatic vein webs, inferior vena cava stenosis and involvement by a nearby malignancy. Sudden impediment to the hepatic venous outflow results in severe centrilobular venous congestion, followed gradually by necrosis and fibrosis. Cirrhosis develops over time in survivors. Tender hepatomegaly and marked ascites are the clinical hallmarks, and acute liver failure can ensue rapidly. Inferior vena cava thrombosis is reflected by the development of bilateral pitting leg oedema.

53) e.

Daily norfloxacin on discharge usually lessens recurrence (which is common) of SBP. One-third of patients with cirrhosis lack abdominal signs and symptoms and may present solely as hepatic encephalopathy in a previously well-compensated cirrhosis. This usually occurs in advanced cirrhosis with marked ascites and low ascitic fluid protein ($<15\,g/L$). Bowel sounds are *absent*. An ascitic fluid neutrophil count $>250/ml^3$ with positive ascitic fluid culture indicates SBP. The presence of positive ascitic fluid culture in the context of ascitic fluid neutrophils $<250/ml^3$ is called bacterascites; ascitic fluid neutrophil count and culture should be repeated at a later time using a new paracentesis. A negative ascitic bacterial culture with neutrophils $>250/ml^3$ is the so-called culture-negative neutrocytic ascites, which should be treated with antibiotics (like SBP). SBP is almost always *monomicrobial*; enteric organisms are the usual culprits and *E. coli* is the commonest one. Polymicrobial infection should always prompt a search for perforated viscus. Generally, it targets 10–20% of cirrhosis patients with ascites.

54) d.

This woman demonstrates the classical post-cholecystectomy syndrome, which affects one-third of cases following gallbladder removal. The disorder is usually seen in women, in those who have had chronic cholecystitis for >5 years and in those whose gallbladder was removed for acalculous disease. The negative imaging studies make small common bile duct stones highly unlikely. Note that residual common bile duct stones are the most important differential diagnosis for post-cholecystectomy syndrome.

55) c.

The patient looks healthy but has 'asymptomatic' gallstones. Prophylactic gallbladder removal has no place in the treatment of asymptomatic patients; exceptions are patients who are at risk of developing gallbladder cancer (e.g. choledochal cysts, porcelain gallbladder, Caroli disease) or who have increased risk of developing gallstone complications (e.g. hereditary spherocytosis, sickle cell disease, diabetes). Symptomatic gallstones are treated by surgical removal in surgically fit patients; otherwise medical treatment is instituted.

5. Endocrinology: Questions

1) A 76-year-old man presents with malaise, weight loss and anorexia. He has rapid atrial fibrillation and leg oedema. Which one of the following diagnoses is consistent with this picture?

   a. Hypothyroidism
   b. Cushing's syndrome
   c. Adrenal failure
   d. Hyperthyroidism
   e. Pituitary acidophil adenoma

2) A 43-year-old woman complains of feeling weak all the time, 9 months after finishing her pulmonary tuberculosis treatment. She is tanned and has postural hypotension. Which one of the following would cast doubt upon your provisional diagnosis?

   a. Amenorrhoea
   b. Hypokalaemia
   c. Weight loss
   d. Diarrhoea
   e. Loss of axillary hair

3) A 53-year-old man presents with headache and visual impairment. He has bitemporal hemianopia. His bloods reveal mildly elevated serum prolactin and low serum ACTH. Brain MRI shows a pituitary mass of 18 mm in maximum diameters. What is the likely diagnosis in this patient?

   a. Cushing's disease
   b. Phaeochromocytoma
   c. Non-functioning pituitary adenoma
   d. Secondary hyperthyroidism
   e. Acromegaly

4) A 54-year-old woman is started on medical treatment following a diagnosis of acromegaly. Which one of the following is indicative of active disease?

   a. Excessive sweating
   b. Polyuria
   c. Abdominal pain
   d. Arthropathy
   e. Goitre

5) A 27-year-old woman presents with anxiety and palpitations. Her serum TSH is suppressed with high free T$_4$ blood level. You start carbimazole. If she is compliant with her antithyroid medication, the serum TSH will normalize after how long?

a. 1 week
b. 4 weeks
c. 2 months
d. 6 months
e. 3 days

6) A 65-year-old woman is brought to A&E in a coma. She is obese with coarse facial features and a core body temperature of 29°C. Her past notes reveal delayed relaxation of ankle jerks, hypercholesterolaemia and macrocytosis. In addition to intravenous thyroid hormone replacement, which one of the following should be added?

a. Intravenous hydrocortisone
b. Oral thyroxin
c. Intravenous cefotaxime
d. Oral warfarin
e. Intravenous glucose water

7) A 71-year-old woman was diagnosed with primary atrophic hypothyroidism 2 years ago. She comes for a scheduled visit. She denies any symptoms, her serum TSH is 50 mU/L and her serum T$_4$ is 40 pmol/L. What is your interpretation of these laboratory results?

a. Treatment is satisfactory
b. She needs an increasing daily dose
c. She should lower her daily thyroxin
d. She erratically takes her thyroxin
e. She is hyperthyroid

8) A 34-year-old woman presents with sore throat and anal pain following a diagnosis of Graves' disease and initiation of its medical treatment. What investigation would you order?

a. Serum TSH
b. Complete blood count
c. Bone marrow examination
d. Carbimazole blood level
e. ASO titre

9) A 20-year-old woman presents with fatigue, constipation and amenorrhea. Examination reveals mucocutaneous hyperpigmentation and postural hypotension. Her serum ACTH is high. She has macrocytosis and hypercholesterolaemia. What additional test would you perform?

a. Serum potassium
b. Urinary catecholamines
c. Serum TSH
d. Serum calcium
e. Gastroscopy

10) A 45-year-old man is referred from the psychiatry clinic for further evaluation. His serum calcium is 2.8 mmol/L and serum phosphate is 0.7 mmol/L. What is the likely diagnosis?

a. Tertiary hyperparathyroidism
b. Chronic renal failure
c. Lithium-induced hyperparathyroidism
d. Iodine-induced hyperthyroidism
e. Malingering

11) A 17-year-old patient with chronic mucocutaneous candidiasis is suspected to have polyglandular failure type I. Which one of the following is consistent with this provisional diagnosis?

a. High serum TSH
b. Low serum parathyroid hormone
c. Low serum ACTH
d. High serum prolactin
e. Normal serum phosphate

12) A 54-year-old man with intermittent hypertension and headache has high 24-hour urinary metanephrins. He has a large right-sided suprarenal mass. Which one of the following indicates malignant phaeochromocytoma?

a. Size of the adrenal tumour
b. Blood supply of the adrenal mass
c. Presence of lung cannon ball masses
d. Histopathological examination of the adrenal tumour
e. Urination-induced hypertension

13) A 65-year-old heavy smoker presents with cough and pleural effusion which is found to be malignant due to small cell lung cancer. He is referred to you because of paraneoplastic Cushing's syndrome. Which one of the following would cast doubt upon the latter diagnosis?

a. Very high serum ACTH
b. Low serum potassium
c. Gross cushingoid features
d. High 24-hour urinary free cortisol
e. Normal brain MRI

14) A 29-year-old woman is having recurrent carpopedal spasms, which are found to be due to hypocalcaemia. Her serum phosphate is 1.8 mmol/L. Which one of the following could be responsible for this clinical picture?

a. Hypoalbuminaemia
b. Conn's syndrome
c. Acute pancreatitis
d. Vitamin D deficiency
e. Pseudohypoparathyroidism

15) A 49-year-old woman presents with polyuria and polydipsia. Her serum calcium is elevated with slightly suppressed serum PTH. All of the following might be responsible for these findings, except:

a. Metastatic breast cancer
b. Familial hypocalciuric hypercalcaemia
c. Thiazide abuse
d. Milk-alkali syndrome
e. Addison's disease

16) A 25-year-old woman presents with central obesity, rounded plethoric face, hypertension and abdominal striae. Her abdominal ultrasound examination reveals a mass in the left adrenal gland. You are considering Cushing's syndrome due to an adrenal tumour. Which one of the following would question your provisional diagnosis?

a. Raised 24-hour urinary free cortisol
b. High serum bicarbonate
c. Raised serum ACTH
d. Loss of circadian plasma cortisol
e. Normal pituitary gland on brain MRI

17) A 55-year-old woman presents with fatigue and amenorrhea. Her serum ACTH is very high. You ascribe her complaints to primary adrenal failure. Which one of the following is not a cause of primary adrenal failure?

   a. Metastatic lung cancer
   b. HIV infection
   c. Long-term metyrapone therapy
   d. Withdrawal of long-term prednisolone
   e. Haemochromatosis

18) A 31-year-old man is referred to the endocrinology clinic because of resistant hypertension. His blood pressure is 170/110 mmHg and is poorly responsive to multiple antihypertensive medications. His serum aldosterone is high with suppressed plasma renin activity. Imaging of the adrenals is normal. You suspect glucocorticoid-suppressible hyperaldosteronism after running a battery of investigations. What medication would you prescribe?

   a. Amiloride
   b. Spironolactone
   c. Dexamethasone
   d. Fludrocortisone
   e. Indometacin

19) A 26-year-old young woman presents with intermittent hypertension, headache, sweating and palpitations. Further work-up discloses the presence of bilateral adrenal phaeochromocytoma. Her older brother has asymptomatic hypercalcaemia. Which one of the following should be considered?

   a. Multiple endocrine neoplasia type I
   b. Polyglandular failure type II
   c. Albright syndrome
   d. Multiple endocrine neoplasia type IIa
   e. Neurofibromatosis type I

20) A 19-year-old woman is found to have 21-hydroxylase deficiency after being investigated for troublesome hirsutism. Which one of the following would suggest an alternative diagnosis to this autosomal recessive disease?

   a. Raised serum ACTH
   b. Blood pressure 160/100 mmHg
   c. Amenorrhoea
   d. Elevated serum 17OH-progesterone
   e. Positive family history

21) A 53-year-old man is started on a medication after securing a diagnosis of phaeochromocytoma. One day later, he develops severe hypertensive crisis. Which one of the following medications might this patient have been given?

a. Phenoxybenzamine
b. Propranolol
c. Labetalol
d. Phentolamine
e. Alpha-methyldopa

22) A 17-year-old obese girl is given a provisional diagnosis of polycystic ovarian syndrome because of oligomenorrhoea and cystic ovaries. Which one of the following would be suggestive of an alternative diagnosis?

a. Dyslipidaemia
b. Mild elevation of serum prolactin
c. Hyperglycaemia
d. Low serum LH
e. Infertility

23) A 21-year-old woman asks if there is any medication to tackle her troublesome facial hirsutism. She tires with physical measures. All of the following medications have an antiandrogen activity, except:

a. Flutamide
b. Oestrogen
c. Dexamethasone
d. Phenytoin
e. Cyproterone acetate

24) A 65-year-old woman was found to have a serum calcium of 2.8 mmol/L on a routine medical insurance assessment. She denies any symptoms, and she neither smokes nor drinks alcohol. There is no family history of a similar problem. Which of the following could be responsible for this abnormal biochemical finding?

a. Tertiary hyperparathyroidism
b. Furosemide abuse
c. Primary hyperparathyroidism
d. Sarcoidosis
e. Iodine excess

25) A 24-year-old woman presents with tremor, palpitations and hyperdefecation. Her serum TSH is suppressed. You are considering a diagnosis of factitious hyperthyroidism. Which one of the following would be *inconsistent* with your clinical suspicion?

a. No goitre
b. Normal serum thyroglobulin
c. Negligible radioiodine thyroid uptake
d. High T_4:T_3 ratio
e. No pretibial myxoedema

26) A 55-year-old man is given a diagnosis of acromegaly, following many years of excessive sweating, acral enlargement, hypertension, bilateral carpal tunnel syndrome and headache. Which one of the following is the first-line treatment?

a. Cabergoline
b. Pegvisomant
c. Surgery
d. External beam radiotherapy
e. Lanreotide

27) A 46-year-old patient is about to undergo assessment of his hypothalamic pituitary adrenal axis because of certain complaints. You are contemplating an insulin tolerance test. Which one of the following is true regarding this endocrinology test?

a. Used to detect Type I diabetes
b. Contraindicated in epilepsy
c. Useful in assessing severe hypopituitarism
d. Unhelpful in growth hormone deficiency
e. Insulin aspart is used in the test

28) A 67-year-old man presents because of enlarged breasts. He has multiple diseases for which he takes a variety of medications. Which one of the following does *not* result in gynaecomastia?

a. Digoxin
b. Spironolactone
c. Ranitidine
d. Diethylstilbestrol
e. Alpha methyldopa

29) A 54-year-old woman is found to have a suppressed serum TSH on pre-employment assessment and she is referred to the endocrinology clinic for further evaluation. She is reasonably well and healthy and denies any symptoms. Which one of the following is *not* a cause of this isolated suppression in serum TSH level?

a. Sub-clinical hyperthyroidism
b. Sick euthyroid syndrome
c. Dexamethasone therapy
d. Early in the course of treatment of hypothyroidism
e. First trimester of pregnancy

30) A 38-year-old woman attends your clinic because she feels tired and cold most of the day. She has primary atrophic hypothyroidism for which she takes daily thyroxin tablets. She is compliant with her medication. Which one of the following does *not* necessitate increasing the dose of daily thyroxin?

a. Sertraline therapy
b. Ferrous sulphate therapy
c. Aging
d. Coeliac disease
e. Pregnancy

31) A 43-year-old man has been recently diagnosed with severe hypertension. His plasma aldosterone is very high, and there is a left-sided adrenal mass. You are considering Conn's syndrome as his final diagnosis. Which one of the following would suggest an alternative diagnosis?

a. Serum bicarbonate 29 mEq/L
b. Raised plasma renin activity
c. Serum potassium 3.9 mEq/L
d. Normal renal artery Doppler study
e. No leg oedema

32) A 48-year-old man is about to undergo extensive evaluation because of a greatly raised serum growth hormone. Raised levels of growth hormone can be encountered in all of the following except:

a. Kallman's syndrome
b. McCune–Albright syndrome
c. Caney's complex
d. Multiple endocrine neoplasia type I
e. Laron's dwarfism

33) A 12-year-old girl has rounded face, short stature, short 4th and 5th metacarpals and low IQ. Her serum calcium is 2.3 mmol/L. What is the likely diagnosis?

   a. Idiopathic hypoparathyroidism
   b. Pseudohypoparathyroidism
   c. Multiple endocrine neoplasia type IIb
   d. Cushing's syndrome
   e. Pseudopseudohypoparathyroidism

34) A 51-year-old woman presents because of episodic cramping abdominal pain, diarrhoea, wheezes and facial flushing. What investigation would you choose to start with?

   a. Urinary catecholamines
   b. 24-hour urinary potassium
   c. Urinary hydroxyindoleacetic acid (HIAA)
   d. Abdominal ultrasound
   e. Chest CT scan

35) A 34-year-old man presents with ischaemic heart disease. His lower limb pulses are feeble with ulcers around the maleoli. There are many tubero-eruptive xanthomata and also palmer ones. What is the likely diagnosis?

   a. Apo CII deficiency
   b. Homozygous familial hypercholesterolaemia
   c. Remnant hyperlipidaemia
   d. Lipoprotein lipase deficiency
   e. Familial combined hyperlipidaemia

36) A 65-year-old man develops anterior wall myocardial infarction, for which he receives secondary prophylaxis, including fluvastatin. Which one of the following is true with respect to statins?

   a. Inactivate hepatic LDL receptors
   b. Decrease LDL catabolism
   c. Inhibit de novo cholesterol synthesis in the intestine
   d. Lower VLDL cholesterol
   e. They lower HDL cholesterol

37) A 22-year-old patient with severe hypertriglyceridaemia has failed dietary therapy, and you are considering adding a medication to lower serum triglyceride. Which one of the following is the most efficient in reducing this blood lipid?

a. Gemfibrozil
b. Niacin
c. Cholestyramine
d. Pravastatin
e. Metformin

38) A 3-year-old child has severe protein energy malnutrition (PEM). He is about to receive zinc supplements. Zinc replacement therapy in PEM has been found to produce all of the following effects, except:

a. Improves the overall sense of well-being
b. Hastens healing of skin lesions
c. Thymic atrophy
d. Better appetite
e. Reduces the overall disease morbidity

39) A 71-year-old vagrant man is brought to A&E with sudden painful right knee joint swelling. He has widespread perifollicular petechiae and spongy bleeding gums. What is the provisional diagnosis?

a. Acquired haemophilia A
b. Congenital haemophilia B
c. Scurvy
d. Idiopathic thrombocytopenic purpura
e. Elderly abuse

40) A 37-year-old obese woman is desperate for your help. She has surfed the internet and read about orlistat as a 'slimming' medication. She wants to take orlistat to induce weight loss. Which one of the following is true regarding the National Institute for Clinical Excellence (NICE) recommendations for the use of orlistat?

a. Patient should have lost 10 kg in the preceding 6 months
b. Patient's age is below 15 years
c. BMI should be between 25 and 30 kg/m^2
d. Dietary measures are not that important
e. Drug treatment should not exceed 24 months

41) A 22-year-old obese man has read in the newspaper that moderate weight loss may increase his life-expectancy. He asks about the benefits of losing 10 kg. Losing this magnitude of weight will result in all of the following, except:

a. Fall of 20 mmHg in the diastolic blood pressure
b. 50% fall in the fasting blood sugar
c. 1% fall in the total mortality
d. Fall of 10% in total cholesterol
e. Increase the HDL cholesterol by 8%

42) A 43-year-old woman has gained 40 kg in the preceding 6 months. She denies any excessive food intake or change in her daily food regimen. You are considering an obesity-promoting disease. All of the following can result in obesity, except:

a. Cushing's syndrome
b. Hypothyroidism
c. Insulinoma
d. Hypothalamic tumours
e. Adrenal failure

43) A 14-year-old girl takes large doses of daily vitamin A as she thinks this will make her healthier. This form of vitamin excess can lead to which one of the following?

a. Hepatic damage
b. Smooth wet skin
c. Watery eye
d. Macrosomic baby
e. Accelerated wound healing

44) A 34-year-old man presents with peripheral and autonomic neuropathy. He has heart block but his urine is negative for albumin. He has a strong family history for the same condition. Which one of the following types of amyloid protein is likely to be found in this patient?

a. AA amyloid
b. AL amyloid
c. Transthyretin
d. β-amyloid precursor
e. β_2-microglobulin

45) A 68-year-old man has recently been given a diagnosis of Type 2 diabetes and is about to receive treatment for it after failure of dietary measures. All of the following reduce the basal glycaemia, except:

a. Repaglinide
b. Miglitol
c. Tolbutamide
d. Metformin
e. Rosiglitazone

46) A 52-year-old administrator has had Type 2 diabetes for the last 2 years for which he takes metformin tablets, 850 mg thrice daily. His HbA 1c is 9.1%. His fundi are normal-looking and his supine blood pressure is 125/80 mmHg that becomes 115/80 mmHg upon standing. He is compliant with his daily anti-diabetic medication and denies exertional breathlessness. He smokes about a packet of cigarettes per day but does not drink alcohol. Which one of the following is *true* regarding this man's overall condition?

a. Autonomic function testing should be done
b. Give isosorbide dinitrate
c. Prescribe lisinopril
d. Add glibenclamide
e. Increase the dose of metformin

47) A 62-year-old Type 2 diabetic woman is receiving nateglinide and she asks for any useful advice regarding this form of therapy. What is your advice?

a. Omit a dose if you miss a major meal
b. Take immediately after each meal
c. Always combine it with insulin
d. Avoid in obese patients
e. Take a tablet when feeling hungry

48) A 23-year-old nurse has recurrent palpitations, sweating and headache. She denies illicit drug intake. Her serum insulin and C-peptide are elevated. Fasting blood glucose is 100 mg/dl. What investigation would you choose next?

a. Supervised prolonged fasting
b. Urinary toxicology for metformin
c. Plain abdominal X-ray
d. Repeat C-peptide level
e. Measure random plasma glucose

49) A 26-year-old man presents with recurrent headache, tremor, palpitations and sweating. His fasting plasma glucose tends to be low during these attacks. All of the following can result in reactive hypoglycaemia, except:

a. Idiopathic
b. Previous gastrectomy
c. Hyperthyroidism
d. Pancreatic β-cell adenoma
e. Soft tissue sarcoma

50) A 19-year-old man presents with recurrent abdominal pain, peripheral motor neuropathy and seizures. His serum sodium is low. Urinary porphobilinogen is raised and you are considering acute intermittent porphyria. Which one of the following would cast doubt upon this diagnosis?

a. Positive family history
b. Skin bullae
c. Psychosis
d. Autonomic neuropathy
e. Raised urinary γ-aminolevulinic acid

51) A 52-year-old alcoholic man presents with facial hypertrichosis, skin fragility, milia and hyperpigmentation. Which one of the following is *not* true regarding porphyria cutanea tarda?

a. May respond to regular phlebotomy
b. Chloroquine is contraindicated
c. Due to deficiency of the enzyme uroporphyrinogen decarboxylase
d. Hepatitis C virus may be implicated as a cause
e. Burning sensation in light-exposed areas

52) A 35-year-old female secretary presents with unintentional weight loss of 10 kg over the past 6 months in spite of having healthy meals. She has palpitations and she prefers cold weather. Her hands show fine and fast postural tremor. Which one of the following is *consistent* with your provisional diagnosis of hyperthyroidism?

a. Serum calcium 7.1 mg/dl
b. Serum creatine kinase 820 u/L
c. Random blood glucose 3.3 mmol/L
d. Total serum bilirubin 1.8 mg/dl
e. Serum ALT 930 u/L

53) A 62-year-old man is brought to A&E having severe global confusional state. His son says that his father has Type 2 diabetes and he takes a daily medication for it. He is not dehydrated but his breathing is rapid and deep. Random blood glucose is 210 mg/dl. His urine has mild ketonuria. Blood urea is 50 mg/dl and blood pH is 7.0 with an anion gap of 60. What is the likely diagnosis in this man?

a. Acute renal failure
b. Diabetic ketoacidosis
c. Non-ketotic hyper-osmolar diabetic coma
d. Distal renal tubular acidosis
e. Lactic acidosis

54) A 49-year-old man is referred to you for further evaluation of right iliac fossa mass. His abdominal ultrasound shows many small rounded liver masses in addition to the right iliac fossa mass. His 24-hour urinary 5-HIAA is prominently raised. Which one of the following could be part of this man's illness?

a. Unilateral rhonchus
b. Episodic facial pallor
c. Giant JVP v-wave
d. Fingers telangiectasia
e. Episodic constipation

55) A 22-year-old man develops a severe attack of acute intermittent por-phyria, two days after starting a medication prescribed by his GP. Which one of the following medications has *not* been prescribed by his GP?

a. Atenolol
b. Tolbutamide
c. Theophylline
d. Valproic acid
e. Dapsone

Endocrinology: Answers

1) d.
The presence of weight loss rules out hypothyroidism and Cushing's syndrome. Adrenal failure does not per se increases the risk of atrial fibrillation. Acromegaly has a different picture of acral enlargement, large tongue and nose, big doughy hands and prognathism. Apathetic hyperthyroidism is seen the elderly and presents with such a picture; cardiovascular decompensation is very common.

2) b.
Adrenal tuberculosis is a well-known cause of failure of that endocrine gland. *Hyper*kalaemia is expected, and normal serum potassium might be seen in early cases; however, a low serum potassium suggests another diagnosis or co-morbidity. Neutropenia, eosinophilia, raised blood urea, mild hypercalcaemia and hypoglycaemia can all be encountered as laboratory findings in Addison's disease.

3) c.
The low serum ACTH virtually excludes Cushing's disease. The relatively low serum prolactin is inappropriate for the large sellar mass; this rules out macroprolactinoma. As the question does not describe any particular endocrine hyperfunctioning, secondary hyperthyroidism and acromegaly can be ruled out. A non-functioning pituitary mass resulting in disconnection hyperprolactinaemia would be reasonable.

4) a.
Abdominal pain might indicate the development of colonic polyps or cancer, and arthropathy is a slowly progressive process; both of these are not indicative of disease activity, and nor is polyuria, which is usually the result of hyperglycaemia. Acromegaly results in large organs, e.g. large kidneys, large thyroid, large liver; the enlarged organ does not usually regress after cessation of disease activity, so it is not a useful marker for assessing activity. Excessive sweating, sebum production and to lesser extent, headache, are the usual pointers towards an active disease.

5) b.
Symptomatic improvement is noted 2 weeks after starting antithyroid medications; the biochemical normalization usually lags behind this for about a further 2 weeks. Serum thyroid hormones correct first, and serum TSH is the last to return to the normal range.

6) a.
Myxoedema coma has a mortality rate approaching 50%; a high index of suspicion in the appropriate clinical setting with early detection and treatment is the only method that has been shown to reduce this high

mortality rate. Contributory factors, like heart failure, chest infection and phenothiazines, should always be looked for and corrected if possible. In all cases, myxoedema coma should be assumed to be secondary to pituitary disease (unless a clear-cut marker for a primary disease exists, like thyroidectomy scar) and the patient should receive intravenous glucocorticoid replacement. High flow oxygen, broad-spectrum antibiotics, intravenous fluids and slow re-warming should also be used, but addition of intravenous hydrocortisone is the top priority here.

7) d.

Non-compliance with medications is a major problem when treating many diseases, and hypothyroidism is no exception. The serum free T_4 is elevated (normally 10–27 pmol/L), but, in addition, the serum TSH is greatly elevated. If the patient has been compliant with her medications for the past 2 years, the serum TSH should be within the normal range or only a little outside this range (depending on the daily dosing). Erratic thyroxin ingestion, or ingestion of larger doses of the hormone for a few days before a scheduled interview, will elevate the serum T_4 level, but the serum TSH needs a long time to fall. As some MRCP questions do not give the normal biochemical reference range, it is important to be familiar with the normal thyroid indices values. The objective of medical treatment of hyperthyroidism is to keep the serum free T_4 and TSH within their normal reference ranges. Note that the objective of treating primary hypothyroidism is to keep the serum TSH within its normal range, while that of free T4 should be kept in the upper part of the reference range (or even slightly above it).

8) b.

Carbimazole-associated agranulocytosis is unpredictable but reversible, and usually occurs within 1–4 weeks of starting the medication. All patients should be educated to stop their medication and contact their GP whenever fever or sore throat appears. Cross-sensitivity with other antithyroid medications is unusual; stopping the offending agent and using another antithyroid medication is all that is required. The objective of medical treatment is to keep the serum free T_4 and TSH within their normal range. There is no place for measuring serum levels of antithyroid medications in order to detect complications or compliance.

9) c.

This woman with Addison's disease has macrocytosis, which might point to coexistent pernicious anaemia or hypothyroidism; hypercholesterolaemia is consistent with the latter. Polyglandular failure can involve any organ to start with, and one or more organs can become involved later. Addison's disease occurs in type I and II syndromes; type II encompasses, in addition to Addison's disease, hypothyroidism, hypogonadism, Type 1 (not Type 2) diabetes mellitus, vitiligo and pernicious anaemia. The hallmark of type I syndrome is the mucocutaneous candidiasis. Patients with positive antimicrosomal and antithyroglobulin antibodies have a 2% annual incidence of overt hypothyroidism. The patient's scenario points towards hypothyroidism in addition to Addison's disease; serum TSH is the correct answer to detect hypothyroidism. Serum potassium can be raised in Addison's disease, but it does not pick up hypothyroidism.

10) c.

Lithium can result in a picture of hyperparathyroidism (and hypothyroidism) indistinguishable from the primary one (i.e. hypercalcaemia with normal or elevated serum PTH). This patient has hypercalcaemia with a serum phosphate that is in the lower normal range. Hyperphosphataemia is seen in tertiary hyperparathyroidism and chronic renal failure.

11) b.

The polyglandular syndrome type I encompasses primary hypoparathyroidism, Addison's disease and chronic mucocutaneous candidiasis. This patient should have a low serum level of PTH (with hypocalcaemia and hyperphosphataemia), while that of ACTH should be high (primary adrenal failure with loss of negative feedback control on ACTH secretion).

12) c.

As is the case for other endocrine tumours, histopathological examination of phaeochromocytoma fails to distinguish benign from malignant ones; the presence of metastasis strongly favours the latter (such as the presence of lung masses). Neither the tumour size nor the mass vascularity would be helpful with respect to this issue. Urination-induced hypertension is seen in urinary bladder tumours, whether benign or malignant.

13) c.

Paraneoplastic Cushing's syndrome of small cell lung cancer is usually a biochemical diagnosis with hypertension, hyperglycaemia and hypokalaemic alkalosis; gross cushingoid habitus is highly unusual. The patient is thin and pale, rather than obese, and plethoric. The serum ACTH tends to be very high, and because of the ectopic lung production of that hormone, the pituitary is normal-looking.

14) e.

This patient has hypocalcaemia and hyperphosphataemia (normal range 0.7–1.1 mmol/L). Three causes should be kept in mind: primary hypoparathyroidism, chronic renal failure and pseudohypoparathyroidism. A low serum albumin lowers the total, not the ionized, serum calcium, and the serum phosphate is normal. Acute pancreatitis may lower serum calcium (total and ionized) but with normal or low serum phosphate. Alkalosis (as in Conn's syndrome) lowers the ionized serum calcium (which may result in carpopedal spasm), but the total serum calcium and phosphate are normal. Vitamin D deficiency lowers serum calcium and phosphate. In all cases of low serum calcium, serum phosphate, albumin and PTH should be co-measured.

15) b.

Generally, there are four causes of hypercalcaemia with normal (which is inappropriate for the high serum calcium) or *elevated* serum PTH: primary hyperparathyroidism (with low serum phosphate), tertiary hyperparathyroidism (with hyperphosphataemia), lithium-induced hyperparathyroidism and familial hypocalciuric hypercalcaemia. The latter is an autosomal dominant disease with defective calcium receptors in the parathyroid glands, which is almost always asymptomatic. It is rare; some patients might have (wrongly) undergone surgical removal of the glands. The other options result in hypercalcaemia with suppressed serum PTH level.

16) c.

Adrenal causes (adenoma or carcinoma) of Cushing's syndrome are categorized as being ACTH-independent. The tumour secretes a large amount of glucocorticoid with a negative feedback on the pituitary; the serum ACTH is thus suppressed. Raised 24-hour urinary free cortisol and loss of circadian plasma cortisol are used in the screening of Cushing's syndrome, regardless of the aetiology.

17) d.

Secondary adrenal failure results from either hypothalamic-pituitary disease or withdrawal of long-term glucocorticoid therapy. The commonest causes of primary adrenal failure are autoimmune adrenalitis (sporadic or part of polyglandular syndromes), tuberculosis, metastatic cancer, HIV infection and surgical removal of both glands; other causes are rare in clinical practice, e.g. haemochromatosis, amyloidosis, lymphoma, congenital adrenal hyperplasias and drug-induced (ketoconazole, etomidate, aminoglutethimide and metyrapone).

18) c.

Glucocorticoid-suppressible hyperaldosteronism is a differential diagnosis of primary hyperaldosteronism of Conn's adenoma or idiopathic bilateral adrenal hyperplasia. It is a rare autosomal dominant disease with translocation between the ACTH-regulated promoter area of the 11β-hydroxylase gene and the coding area of aldosterone synthetase gene. The outcome is the synthesis and release of aldosterone in response to normal circulating levels of ACTH; plasma renin activity is secondarily suppressed. This process is extremely sensitive to ACTH release inhibition, such as with an exogenous steroid (like dexamethasone). Amiloride and spironolactone are effective in Conn's adenoma and bilateral idiopathic adrenal hyperplasia treatment. Fludrocortisone is used in adrenal failure or postural hypotension of autonomic failure to raise the blood pressure. Indometacin has a place in treating juxtaglomerular apparatus hyperplasia of Bartter's syndrome.

19) d.

Multiple endocrine neoplasia (MEN) type IIa encompasses primary hyperparathyroidism (seen in 50% of cases and is usually asymptomatic), medullary thyroid carcinoma and phaeochromocytoma. The disease is autosomal dominant with mutations in the *RET* proto-oncogene. Screening of first-degree relatives is by annual measurement of serum calcium, calcium-pentagastrin administration with calcitonin assessment and 24-hour urinary metanephrines. Genetic testing with pre-test counselling is available for type I and II. Type IIb has marfinoid habitus and mucosal neuromas. Type I and II syndromes should always be suspected in any patient with at least two hyperfunctioning endocrine systems, or one abnormal endocrine system plus a positive family history of another hyperfunctioning system.

20) b.

This late-onset or non-classical form of 21-hydroxylase deficiency results in hirsutism and may only be discovered after administration of exogenous ACTH to raise serum levels of 17OH-progesterone. Amenorrhea may occur. Deficiency of 11β-hydroxylase or 17-hydroxylase would result in hypertension. Idiopathic hirsutism and polycystic ovarian syndrome comprise at least 90% of cases of hirsutism.

21) b.

Initial treatment of high blood pressure in phaeochromocytomas should be with the long-acting α-blocker phenoxybenzamine. The aim of medical treatment is to prepare the patient for surgery. Unopposed β-adrenoceptor blocking action would result in severe hypertension; therefore, initiating treatment with beta-blockers is contraindicated. Because of its combined α- and β-adrenoceptor blocking action, labetalol might be used, but it should not be the first-line medication. Alpha methyldopa alone is not used in medical treatment of phaeochromocytoma.

22) d.

A multitude of endocrine and metabolic abnormalities are seen in polycystic ovarian syndrome. The serum LH is *raised*, while that of FSH is either normal or low; the net result is a LH:FSH ratio of 2.5:1. Serum prolactin is usually mildly elevated. Elevated androgen levels might result in hirsutism. There may be hypertension, hyperglycaemia and dyslipidaemia. Patients usually have oligomenorrhoea or secondary amenorrhea rather than primary amenorrhea. In spite of amenorrhea, these patients are not at risk of osteoporosis and do not need hormonal replacement therapy, as the endogenous levels of oestrogens and progestins are high.

23) d.

Phenytoin has no antiandrogen activity; besides, it produces facial hypertrichosis. Cyproterone acetate, flutamide and spironolactone act on androgen receptors. Cyproterone acetate and flutamide may cause hepatic dysfunction. The former also has progesterone agonistic activity and may result in dysfunctional uterine bleeding. 5α-reductase inhibitors, like finasteride, are not recommended for hirsutism and have no proven efficacy. Oestrogen might be used alone (usually with cyproterone) or as part of conventional oral contraceptives. Dexamethasone suppresses ACTH and is useful in the hirsutism of congenital adrenal hyperplasias.

24) c.

Primary parathyroidism is responsible for up to 90% of cases of outpatient hypercalcaemia. This woman is otherwise healthy and sarcoidosis would have produced symptoms before presenting as hypercalcaemia (rarely the presenting feature on its own). Thiazides decrease the urinary excretion of calcium and may result in hypercalcaemia; furosemide has the opposite effect. Tertiary hyperparathyroidism has a long history of secondary hyperparathyroidism (with hypocalcaemia) before entering the tertiary phase. Iodine excess can result in hyperthyroidism in susceptible individuals.

25) b.

Exogenous thyroid hormone suppresses the endogenous TSH, resulting in suppression of thyroid hormone synthesis and release; there is no goitre and serum thyroglobulin is low. Almost all of the peripheral T_3 comes from the peripheral conversion of T_4, creating a $T_4:T_3$ ratio of 70:1. Radioiodine uptake is suppressed because of the low TSH and suppressed follicular activity. The combination of low serum thyroglobulin, low radioiodine thyroid uptake and very high $T_4:T_3$ ratio would be highly consistent with factitious hyperthyroidism.

26) c.

Surgical resection is the first-line treatment of acromegaly regardless of the size of the tumour, but the tumour size governs the approach; transfrontal versus trans-sphenoidal. Persistent disease activity after surgery calls for radiotherapy to shrink the tumour remnant; however, many patients go on to develop hypopituitarism and this form of therapy only slowly reduces serum growth hormone. Medical treatment is a second-line policy if surgery fails to reduce the serum growth hormone to <5 mU/L. Long-acting somatostatin analogues, like octreotide or lanreotide, can be given every few weeks in the form of intramuscular injections. Growth hormone receptor blockers, like pegvisomant, are showing good results in treatment. Dopamine agonists are especially helpful if there is co-secretion of prolactin, as they are weakly effective in acromegaly. Medical treatments do not shrink the tumour size (unlike in macroprolactinomas).

27) b.

The insulin tolerance test is used in the assessment of hypothalamic pituitary adrenal axis and growth hormone deficiency whenever conventional tests prove inconclusive. The test uses soluble insulin intravenously and the objective is to produce symptoms of hypoglycaemia and blood glucose of <2.2mmol/L; intravenous glucose must be available. The test is contraindicated in epilepsy, ischaemic heart disease and severe hypopituitarism. The test is not involved in the diagnosis of Type 1 diabetes or Type 2 diabetes.

28) c.

Cimetidine, not ranitidine, may result in gynaecomastia. The commonest causes of gynaecomastia are idiopathic and physiological (neonatal, pubertal and in the elderly). Drug-induced cases rank the third. Oestrogen- and hCG-secreting tumours are rare causes.

29) d.

A primary hypothyroid patient with suppressed TSH indicates over-treatment; the serum thyroid hormones must be elevated. During recovery from hyperthyroidism (from any cause) or early in the course of treating *hyper*thyroidism, the serum TSH usually lags behind T_4 and T_3 normalization. Sick euthyroid syndrome (or non-thyroidal illness) produces a variety of abnormal T_4, T_3 and TSH combinations. During an illness, the serum TSH may be low, while during recovery it may be elevated, wrongly pointing towards subclinical hypothyroidism. In this syndrome, the synthesis and affinity of thyroid hormone-binding proteins are altered, and there is reduction in the peripheral conversion of T_4 to T_3; besides, many medications may affect the thyroid axis, like glucocorticoids or dopamine. Causes of isolated elevation in serum TSH are subclinical hypothyroidism, sick euthyroid syndrome and during recovery from hypothyroidism. The patient's age excludes pregnancy.

30) c.

Patients receiving thyroxin may require dose reduction or dose escalation at some point in their life-long therapy. Dose *escalation* is required whenever there is (1) increased thyroid hormone clearance (e.g. when taking medications like phenytoin, carbamazepine, rifampicin, sertraline and chloroquine); (2) interference with intestinal absorption of the orally ingested hormone (as in malabsorption, or when taking certain medications, like colestyramine, ferrous sulphate, calcium carbonate and aluminium hydroxide); (3) an increase in the thyroid hormones binding globulins (as in pregnancy or the use of oestrogen); or (4) gradual reduction in functioning thyroid tissue over time (as in post-ablative cases). Dose *reduction* is required with aging (as there is reduced thyroxin clearance) and when the thyroid antibodies switch from blocking to stimulating (converting hypothyroidism to Graves' disease).

31) b.

The increased aldosterone secretion by the adenoma is independent of the plasma renin activity; renin is thus secondarily suppressed. Raised plasma renin activity should cast strong doubt upon the diagnosis of Conn's syndrome. Hypokalaemia is seen in 70% of cases; normokalaemia is seen in the rest and small doses of diuretics can easily induce hypokalaemia in these cases; a normal serum potassium therefore is not inconsistent with the diagnosis. In spite of hypertension and hypernatraemia, pitting leg oedema is highly unusual and would suggest secondary aldosteronism. The renal artery is not affected. Conn's syndrome is one of the differential diagnoses of hypertension with hypokalaemic alkalosis.

32) a.
Kallman's syndrome is idiopathic hypogonadotrophic hypogonadism; growth hormone is not affected. Laron's dwarfism is a syndrome of growth hormone resistance; serum growth home levels are expected to be high. McCune–Albright's syndrome is due to an activating mutation in the G protein, resulting in endocrine hyperfunctioning, like Cushing's syndrome and precocious puberty, with polyostotic fibrous dysplasia and skin café-au-lait spots. Carney's complex is an autosomal dominant disease with cardiac myxoma and skin hyperpigmentation.

33) e.
The phenotype is suggestive of pseudohypoparathyroidism but the serum calcium is normal; this is pseudopseudohypoparathyroidism. Hypocalcaemia would be seen with idiopathic hypoparathyroidism and pseudohypoparathyroidism. Patients with multiple endocrine neoplasia type IIb have a marfinoid habitus (i.e. tall and thin). Patients with Cushing's syndrome do not have short metacarpals.

34) c.
This woman's overall clinical picture is suggestive of carcinoid syndrome. Starting with a 5-HIAA assessment in urine would be reasonable for a biochemical diagnosis; localization with adominal ultrasound or chest CT scan is the next step.

35) c.
Apo CII deficiency and lipoprotein lipase deficiency result in hypertriglyceridaemia early in childhood. The constellation of premature coronary artery disease, peripheral vascular disease and palmer xanthomata is highly suggestive of remnant hyperlipidaemia (or dysbetalipoproteinaemia). The disease results from accumulation of intermediate density lipoproteins and chylomicrons. Patients are homozygous for $apoE_2$ alleles; this leads to less avid binding to LDL receptors, lessening the clearance of chylomicrons and affecting the catabolism of IDL to LDL. The diagnosis relies upon the demonstration of $apoE_2$ homozygosity or unusual cholesterol enrichment in VLDL particles. The disease is extremely sensitive to weight reduction, use of a low-cholesterol diet and lipid lowering therapy (especially gemfibrozil). The xanthomata of this disease differ from those of familial hypercholesterolaemia by being soft and triglyceride-rich and they tend to irritate the skin.

36) d.
HMG-CoA reductase inhibitors inhibit the rate-limiting enzyme of cholesterol biosynthesis. This inhibits the de novo synthesis of

cholesterol in the liver, lowers the intracellular cholesterol level and activates cell-surface LDL receptors. The outcome is increased LDL catabolism, and decreased LDL, VLDL and total cholesterol. Serum triglyceride is also reduced. Serum HDL cholesterol is increased to some extent (5–10%).

37) a.
Gemfibrozil lowers serum triglyceride by 30–50%, and niacin ranks second in efficiency (20–30%). Statins are less efficient; they lower blood lipid by 10–20%. Statins should not be used primarily to treat hypertriglyceridaemia. Patients with combined hyperlipidaemia should have their total and LDL cholesterol reduced first; serum triglyceride comes next.

38) c.
Zinc is an important part of many body enzymes, like alkaline phosphatase and alcohol dehydrogenase. Zinc deficiency can produce apathy, dermatitis-like lesions (especially around body orifices) and diffuse scalp thinning. Chronic zinc deficiency, which can occur in alcoholism and malabsorption states, impairs wound healing and atrophies the thymus gland.

39) c.
Scurvy is the clinical phenotype of vitamin C deficiency. Vitamin C deficiency impairs wound healing and platelet adhesion, produces haemorrhagic manifestations (e.g. perifollicular haemorrhage, bruises, haemarthrosis, GIT bleeding), and may result in anaemia (which may respond to oral iron and/or folate). The gum is spongy and bleeds easily.

40) e.
Orlistat inhibits gastric and pancreatic lipases and reduces the absorption of dietary triglycerides. The medication itself is not absorbed, and its side effect profile mainly results from fat non-absorption, resulting in excessive flatulence, anal soiling, faecal urgency and fat-soluble vitamin malabsorption. The NICE recommendations for the use of orlistat are: (1) BMI should be >30 (or >28 if there is any co-morbidity); (2) age should be between 18 and 75 years; (3) patient should have lost at least 2.5 kg in the preceding month; (4) the medication should be used *with* other weight management plans; (5) treatment should be stopped if the patient fails to lose at least 5% of their body weight after 3 months; (6) treatment should be stopped if the patient fails to lose at least 10% of their body weight after 6 months, and (7) the medication should never be used for >2 years.

41) c.
Sustained loss of at least 10 kg results in >20% fall in total mortality, >30% fall in diabetes-related deaths and >40% fall in obesity-related cancer deaths. It also has a favourable effect on lipid profile: reducing the total cholesterol by 10%, LDL-cholesterol by 15% and triglyceride by

30%, and increasing the HDL-cholesterol by around 8%. The systolic blood pressure falls by at least 10% and diastolic pressure by 20%.

42) e.
Adrenal hypofunctioning results in weight loss and anorexia, with diarrhoea and/or constipation. As well as the other options, an increase in bodyweight is seen with valproic acid, sulphonylureas, tricyclics and some oral contraceptives.

43) a.
Vitamin A abuse damages the bone and liver, dries the skin and mucosal surfaces, and is teratogenic (an important consideration when treating acne in females using vitamin A products). Maternal hyperglycaemia can cause fetal macrosomia.

44) c.
Familial amyloidoses result from mutations in the transthyretin gene. The disease has many variants, with different ages of complaint onset. Unlike primary AL and secondary AA amyloidoses, renal involvement is rare but with prominent peripheral and autonomic neuropathies. Hepatic transplantation is the cornerstone in the treatment. β_2-microglobulin accumulates in patients with long-term haemodialysis, mainly in bones and around joints (carpal tunnel syndrome is the classical presentation). Alzheimer's disease accumulates β-amyloid precursor in the brain.

45) a.
Antidiabetic medications, apart from meglitinides and amino acid derivatives, reduce the basal glycaemia. Alpha glucosidase inhibitors have a slight effect on basal glycaemia. Post-prandial glycaemia can be reduced by all antidiabetic medications. Risk of hypoglycaemia is encountered with insulin, sulphonylureas and meglitinides. Insulin has the most favourable lipid profile; metformin and alpha glucosidase inhibitors impose a slight favourable effect, while sulphonylureas have no effect and actually promote weight gain. TZDs have a variable impact.

46) d.
He is taking the maximum daily doses of metformin, yet his blood glucose is poorly controlled as evidenced by the elevated HbA1c of 9.1% (the target should be < 7.0). Simply, to control this hyperglycaemia, add another anti-diabetic medication (option d). The postural drop in the systolic blood pressure does not exceed 20 mmHg; therefore, testing for dysautonomia is not warranted. Note that autonomic dysfunction in diabetics is mainly related to the duration of diabetes and that proper control of hyperglycaemia rarely improves symptoms of autonomic neuropathy. Diabetic autonomic neuropathy does not necessarily need to be associated with somatic peripheral neuropathy. He is not hypertensive and we don't know his urinary protein status (like microalbuminuria); therefore, no need to give an ACE inhibitor. Nothing in the question

points towards ischemic heart disease; hence, there is no place to prescribe isosorbide dinitrate.

47) a.

Repaglinide and nateglinide are non-sulphonylurea secretagogues belonging to a class of oral antidiabetic mediations called meglitinides. These medications directly enhance endogenous insulin secretion and therefore, they should be taken immediately before meals. They are metabolized in the liver and can be given to patients with renal impairment. They are a good option to choose in patients with modest post-prandial hyperglycaemia and those who have erratic meals (with frequent meal 'skipping', e.g. long-distance drivers, businessmen). They lower the HBA_{1c} by about 0.5–2%. Compared with sulphonylureas, they have a lower incidence of hypoglycaemia and weight gain.

48) a.

The differential diagnosis of this recurrent hypoglycaemia and raised plasma levels of endogenous insulin and C-peptide is between insulinoma and surreptitious sulphonylureas ingestion. Toxicology screen in blood and urine would help detect the latter, but it is not mentioned in the question (metformin carries no risk of hypoglycaemia). The secretion of insulin by an insulinoma may be erratic, and a random or fasting blood glucose sample may well fall within the normal reference range. Prolonged supervised fasting would help detect hypoglycaemia symptoms. Another method is to measure the plasma pro-insulin level. Normally it is 10–20% of the total insulin; in insulinoma, this fraction rises to 80%, while that of factitious sulphonylurea ingestion is within its normal value. Up to 80% of cases of insulinoma syndromes have single islet beta-cell adenoma, and 10% have multiple adenomas. Around 5% are due to islet beta-cell carcinoma, and an additional 5% have diffuse beta-cell hyperplasia. About 5–10% of insulinomas are part of MEN type I.

49) e.

Sarcomas may be associated with *fasting* hypoglycaemia, but not a reactive one. Reactive hypoglycaemia is mainly due to a 'reaction' towards refined carbohydrates (like glucose and sucrose); rarely, the reaction occurs to other substances (like galactose, fructose and leucine). Note that insulinomas may result in fasting and/or reactive hypoglycaemia.

50) b.

Acute intermittent porphyria (AIP) is a relatively rare autosomal dominant disease, with deficiency of the enzyme porphobilinogen deaminase. This syndrome only develops with at least 50% reduction in enzyme activity; accordingly, many deficient individuals never develop AIP attacks. AIP has no skin manifestations (unlike variegate porphyria, which has acute attacks and skin manifestations).

51) b.

Porphyria cutanea tarda is usually an acquired disease seen in alcoholic liver disease and chronic hepatitis C infection, and has prominent cutaneous manifestations. Skin fragility and photosensitivity are the hallmarks of the disease. Regular phlebotomy is an effective mode of treatment, and severe cases may require the addition of chloroquine.

52) d.

Hyperthyroidism can produce many "non-specific" lab abnormalities. These abnormalities are usually mild and are not helpful at distinguishing various causes of this thyroid dysfunction. They usually resolve when hyperthyroidism is well-controlled; therefore, their persistence after controlling hyperthyroidism justifies further testing. Hyperthyroidism can produce all of the following: mild hypercalcaemia, mild elevation in liver functions (ALT, gamma glutamyl tranferase, serum bilirubin, and even alkaline phosphatase), hyperglycaemia (from secondary diabetes), and lag-storage glucose tolerance testing. *Hypothyroidism* can elevate muscle serum markers (creatine kinase, AST, and LDH). Option e reflects severe hepatocellular injury that is not seen in hyperthyroidism. Neither hypoglycaemia (option c) nor hypocalcaemia (option a) are seen in hyperthyroidism. Serum bilirubin of 1.8 mg/dl can be encountered in hyperthyroidism of any aetiology.

53) e.

Diabetic ketoacidosis does not occur in those with Type 2 diabetes. Renal tubular acidosis (whether proximal or distal) produces a normal anion gap (8–14). The mildly elevated blood urea (normal 15–40 mg/ld) argues against acute renal failure that produces such a degree of brain dysfunction. The absence of profound dehydration points away from option c. Lactic acidosis is a rare metabolic complication that is seen in Type 2 diabetic patients taking metformin. Those patients look very ill with rapid sighing breathing and clouded consciousness. Their urine has mild or no ketones and their breath has no odour of acetone. Their blood shows profound acidaemia (blood pH is usually < 7.2) with high anion gap. Confirmation of lactic acidosis is by measuring serum lactic acid which usually returns very high (in excess of 50 mmol/L). The objective of treatment is raised blood pH above 7.2 by giving intravenous sodium bicarbonate. Sometime, intravenous sodium dichloroacetate is given to lower the blood levels of lactate. Insulin and glucose are also part of the treatment plan. Unfortunately, the mortality rate is high (>50%).

54) c.

This brief scenario is pointing towards carcinoid syndrome resulting from hepatic metastases belonging to a gastrointestinal (most likely a terminal ileal one) carcinoid tumour. Episodic facial flushing with bilateral wheezes and cramping abdominal pain and diarrhoea are the cardinal features of carcinoid syndrome. Right-sided cardiac involvement can produce tricuspid regurgitation (with giant JVP *v*-wave) and/or pulmonary valvular stenosis. Unilateral chest wheeze reflects partial bronchial obstruction by a tumour or an inhaled foreign body (which could be seen in bronchial (not GIT) carcinoid tumours. Facial (not fingers) telangiectasia develops in long-standing cases. The small bowel tumour may produce intestinal obstruction that is likely to have progressive constipation (not episodic).

55) a.

Beta-blockers, gabapentin, phenothiazines and opioids are safe in acute intermittent porphyrias. Beta-blockers are useful in controlling the hyperadrenergic features (tachycardia and hypertension). Opioids are effective in pain control, which might be severe. Phenothiazines are helpful in controlling agitation and psychotic symptoms. Seizures are common and can be controlled by gabapentin (phenytoin, carbamazepine and alproic acid are unsafe).

6. Clinical haematology and oncology: Questions

1) A 16-year-old girl consults you because of progressive pallor and poor exercise tolerance. She has had dysfunctional uterine bleeding for several months. Her haemoglobin is 6.5 g/dl. Which one of the following would be inconsistent with iron-deficiency anaemia in this girl?

   a. Thrombocytosis
   b. Low serum iron
   c. Low serum ferritin
   d. Reticulocyte percentage 10%
   e. Transferrin saturation 9%

2) A 21-year-old patient is referred for further evaluation. He has pallor and recurrent infections. His referral states aplastic anaemia with pancytopenia. Which one of the following would cast doubt upon the diagnosis of aplastic anaemia?

   a. Progressive pallor
   b. Dry tapping of the bone marrow aspirate
   c. Haemorrhagic bullae on gums
   d. Hypercellular marrow
   e. No splenomegaly

3) A 65-year-old man has recently been diagnosed with pernicious anaemia because of pallor, jaundice and lassitude. He has blue eyes and grey hair. Which one of the following would be consistent with this diagnosis?

   a. Direct serum bilirubin 4 mg/dl
   b. Mean corpuscular volume 65 fl
   c. Elevated serum LDH
   d. Reticulocyte count 9%
   e. Decreased bone marrow stores of iron

4) A 13-year-old boy with sickle cell disease presents with severe pallor and malaise. His haemoglobin is 5 g/dl with a reticulocyte count of 0.1%. What has developed in this boy?

   a. Sequestration crisis
   b. Haemolytic crisis
   c. Aplastic crisis
   d. *Salmonella* septicaemia
   e. Acute chest syndrome

5) A 5-year-old child with progressive pallor from the age of 6 months has since been diagnosed with beta-thalassaemia major. His transfusion requirements are gradually increasing to four packed RBC transfusions/month. What is the best step to take?

a. Continue the transfusions
b. Add iron chelation therapy
c. Polyvalent pneumococcal vaccination
d. Give hydroxycarbamide
e. Refer for splenectomy

6) A 16-year-old boy presents with rapidly progressive pallor and dark urine. He has low haemoglobin, raised serum LDH, elevated indirect serum bilirubin, and bite and blister cells on peripheral blood film. What is the diagnosis?

a. Clostridial septicaemia
b. Falciparum malaria
c. G6PD deficiency
d. Megaloblastic anaemia
e. Paroxysmal nocturnal haemoglobinuria

7) A 34-year-old woman presents with recurrent attacks of severe right upper abdominal colicky pains. Examination reveals a tinge of jaundice, pallor and palpable spleen. Spherocytes are seen on blood film. Coombs' test is negative, with raised serum LDH and indirect serum bilirubin. Her older brother has the same disease. What is the best treatment you can offer this woman?

a. Regular blood transfusion
b. Splenectomy
c. Cholecystectomy
d. Daily folic acid
e. Prednisolone

8) A 34-year-old woman has declined splenectomy as a mode of treatment for her acquired immune haemolytic anaemia. She has had three relapses of the disease following steroid tapering. What would you do next?

a. Increase the dose of prednisolone
b. Continue to advise removal of the spleen
c. Prescribe azathioprine
d. Give daily folic acid
e. Arrange for regular packed RBC transfusions

9) A 29-year-old immigrant from South East Asia presents with mild pallor and hypochromia. He has failed to respond to oral iron therapy. His stool examination is unremarkable as is his upper GIT endoscopy. His haemoglobin is 9.5 g/dl and MCV is 60 fl. Haemoglobin A_2 is 1.2%. What is the likely diagnosis in this man?

a. Hook worm infestation
b. Malabsorption
c. Beta thalassaemia minor
d. Hereditary spherocytosis
e. Alpha thalassaemia minor

10) A 71-year-old man presents and states that his fingers and toes become bluish in colour and are painful upon cold exposure. He has been diagnosed with stage A low-grade lymphoma for which he receives no medication. His blood count shows macrocytosis. What is the reason for this man's presentation?

a. Vitamin B_{12} deficiency
b. Chronic cold agglutinin disease
c. Idiopathic Raynaud's disease
d. Paroxysmal nocturnal haemoglobinuria
e. Paroxysmal cold haemoglobinuria

11) A 52-year-old man is given a diagnosis of idiopathic aplastic anaemia after developing progressive pallor, mucocutaneous bleeding and recurrent fever with hypocellular marrow. Which of the following indicates 'severe' aplastic anaemia?

a. Recurrent gum bleeds
b. Severe chest infection
c. Neutrophil count 0.3×10^9/L
d. Anaemia with corrected reticulocyte count <4%
e. Bone marrow cellularity >40%

12) A 54-year-old woman with recently diagnosed aplastic anaemia is referred from the gastroenterology department after receiving treatment for portal vein thrombosis. She reports dark urine in the morning every few days. Which one of the following is a possible diagnosis in this patient?

a. Myelodysplastic syndrome
b. Cold agglutinin disease
c. Paroxysmal nocturnal haemoglobinuria
d. Idiopathic aplastic anaemia
e. Chronic myeloid leukaemia

13) A 64-year-old man presents with left hypochondrial heaviness, fever, night sweats and fatigue. The liver is impalpable and there is no lymphadenopathy. Leucocyte count is 70×10^9/L with full spectrum of leucocyte cell series. Which one of the following is incompatible with the diagnosis of chronic myeloid leukaemia?

a. Eosinophilia
b. High serum LDH
c. Hyperuricaemia
d. High leucocyte alkaline phosphatase score
e. Hypercellular bone marrow

14) A 69-year-old man attends for a check-up. The patient denies any symptoms. His blood counts reveal a white cell count of 50×10^9/L with the majority of cells being mature-looking lymphocytes. His haemoglobin is 14 g/dl and there is a normal count of platelets. Which one of the following is true with respect to the management of this man's chronic lymphocytic leukaemia (CLL)?

a. Start CHOP chemotherapeutic regimen
b. Bone marrow transplantation
c. Observation
d. Whole body irradiation
e. Low dose chlorambucil

15) A 17-year-old girl presents with persistent right upper neck swelling that is finally proved to be due to Hodgkin's disease involving the upper cervical lymph node chain. What is the best treatment option?

a. Local radiotherapy
b. ABVD chemotherapy
c. Observe
d. Stem cell transplantation
e. Surgical debulking

16) A 61-year-old man presents with increasing fatigue, bone pains and weight loss. He has multiple myeloma for which he receives melphalan and prednisolone. His blood counts show leucocytosis with 90% plasma cells. His urinary Bence–Jones protein is positive and his plasma paraprotein level is high. There is mild renal impairment and hypercalcaemia. Plasma alkaline phosphate level is normal. What is the cause of this man's current presentation?

a. Flare-up of multiple myeloma
b. Plasma cell leukaemia
c. Amyloid renal disease
d. Pathological bone fractures
e. Monoclonal gammopathy of undetermined significance

17) A 70-year-old man has diffuse bone pain and pathological fracture of his right humerus. There are multiple lytic bony lesions, raised total serum protein and prominent M-band on serum protein electrophoresis. Urine is positive for Bence–Jones's protein. Bone marrow aspirate reveals hypercellularity with 38% plasma cells, and the ESR is 110 mm/hour. Which one of the following does *not* portend a bad prognosis in this multiple myeloma?

a. Thrombocytosis
b. Haemoglobin <7 g/dl
c. High serum β_2-microglobulin
d. Severe hypoalbuminaemia
e. Intractable renal failure

18) A 53-year-old man presents with ill health for a few weeks. He has a prominently enlarged spleen but no palpable lymph nodes. He has neutropenia and monocytopenia with a very high leucocyte alkaline phosphatase score. The leucocyte acid phosphatase staining is resistant to the action of tartrate. What is the best treatment?

a. Imatinib mesylate
b. Regular venesection
c. Cladribine
d. Prednisolone
e. Hydroxycarbamide

19) A 67-year-old man with stage B chronic lymphocytic leukaemia presents with a rapidly downhill course of ill health and weight loss. There is rapid enlargement of his upper mediastinum and progressive increment in serum LDH level. Which one of the following can explain this man's recent complaints?

a. Acute leukaemia
b. Richter's lymphoma
c. Hodgkin's lymphoma
d. Prolymphocytic leukaemia
e. Myelodysplastic syndrome

20) A 54-year-old man is found to have M-band on serum protein electrophoresis done as part of his health insurance examination. Which one of the following is not consistent with the diagnosis of monoclonal gammopathy of undetermined significance (MGUS)?

a. No bone lesions
b. Serum calcium 9 mg/dl
c. Serum paraprotein 1 g/dl
d. Hypogammaglobulinaemia
e. Blood urea 30 mg/dl

21) A 70-year-old man presents with progressive exercise intolerance and fatigue. He reports early satiety and upper left abdominal fullness. Examination reveals gross hepatosplenomegaly but no lymphadenopathy. His bloods reveal anaemia and a leucoerythroblastic blood picture with abundance of tear-drop anisopoikilocytosis. Which one of the following is true with respect to this man's illness?

a. The prognosis is excellent
b. Philadelphia chromosome is present in the majority
c. Fever and weight loss are the earliest symptoms
d. Hydroxycarbamide is contraindicated
e. Intracranial haemorrhage is one of the causes of death

22) A 43-year-old man with newly diagnosed acute myeloid leukaemia presents with rapidly progressive shortness of breath, profound hypoxemia, and bilateral pulmonary interstitial and alveolar infiltrates. His AML is of M_2 subtype, with 120×10^9 blasts/L, mild anaemia, and platelets count of 80×10^9/L. What is the reason for this man's grave presentation?

a. Intrapulmonary haemorrhage
b. Leucostasis syndrome
c. *Pneumocystis carinii* pneumonia
d. Transfusion-related acute lung injury
e. Pulmonary embolism

23) A 47-year-old man has been diagnosed with AML M_3 subtype after presenting with progressive pallor and fatigue. His blood results are haemoglobin 8 g/dl, WBCs 120×10^9/L and platelets 67×10^9/L. After starting treatment, he develops cardiopulmonary collapse with diffuse pulmonary infiltrates. What is the likely explanation for this man's deterioration?

a. Bone marrow failure
b. Bilateral pneumothoraces
c. Retinoic acid syndrome
d. Irradiation pneumonitis
e. Anthracylin-induced heart failure

24) A 10-year-old boy has been started on a chemotherapeutic regimen for his newly diagnosed acute lymphoblastic leukaemia L_2 subtype. His white cells count is 90×10^9/L with 95% blasts. From day 2 of treatment, he develops progressive renal impairment. Why?

a. Protracted chemotherapy-induced vomiting
b. Gram-negative septicaemia
c. Drug anaphylaxis
d. Tumour lysis syndrome
e. Disseminated intravascular coagulation

25) A 63-year-old man presents with pruritis after having a bath. He reports headache, mental cloudiness and features suggestive of TIAs. His haemoglobin is 19 g/dl, while his previous notes reveal 'normal' haemoglobin. After a few months of follow-ups, his haemoglobin returns to 14 g/dl. His red cell mass is increased, with splenomegaly, ESR 2 mm/hour, MCV 65 fl and raised serum level of vitamin B_{12} level. What is the reason for this haemoglobin normalization?

a. Stopping smoking
b. Iron-deficiency anaemia
c. Progression to acute leukaemia
d. Laboratory error
e. Over treatment with phlebotomy

26) A 67-year-old man comes with progressive pallor and fatigue for his fifth scheduled packed RBC transfusion. His haemoglobin is in the range 6–8 g/dl, with short-lived improvement following blood transfusions. His bloods reveal leucopenia with hypogranular hypolobulated neutrophils, and there is macrocytosis with thrombocytopenia and zero blasts. Bone marrow study shows hypercellular marrow with dysplastic changes in all three cell lines with 16% blasts. What is the diagnosis?

a. Vitamin B_{12} deficiency
b. Chronic myeloid leukaemia
c. Myelodysplastic syndrome subtype refractory anaemia
d. Acute myelomonocytic leukaemia
e. Myelodysplastic syndrome subtype refractory anaemia with excess blasts

27) A 27-year-old man with severe aplastic anaemia asks about the possible treatment options. He has declined a bone marrow transplantation because of its risks. What is the best treatment option?

a. Refer for counselling
b. Continue to advise a bone marrow transplantation
c. High-dose cyclophosphamide
d. Growth factor injections
e. Ciclosporin and antithymocyte globulin

28) A 65-year-old man with newly diagnosed multiple myeloma is referred to you for further management. He reports diffuse bone pain. Bone scanning is unremarkable with no focal areas of increased uptake. What is your next step?

a. Repeat bone scanning
b. Add pamidronate
c. Do urinary Bence–Jones protein test
d. Measure serum alkaline phosphatase
e. Give calcium and vitamin D

29) A 61-year-old man presents with confusion, epistaxis and visual disturbances. Examination reveals bruises, retinal haemorrhages and splenomegaly. The bone marrow is infiltrated with lymphoid cells and prominent mast cells. Which one of the following would suggest a diagnosis other than Waldenström's macroglobulinaemia?

a. Hypercalcaemia
b. Peripheral neuropathy
c. Hyperviscosity
d. Acrocyanosis
e. Cryoglobulinaemia

30) A 54-year-old woman with rheumatoid arthritis presents with fatigue and pallor. She takes daily sulfasalazine and diclofenac. She has hypochromic microcytic anaemia that is attributed to 'chronic diseases' by a haematologist. Which one of the following would suggest iron-deficiency anaemia rather than anaemia of chronic diseases in this woman?

a. Normal serum ferritin
b. Elevated serum soluble transferrin receptor level
c. Low serum iron
d. Low MCV
e. Low total iron binding capacity

31) A patient has been referred to you for further evaluation of a long history of recurrent mucocutaneous bleeding. His referring paediatrician is considering an inherited disorder. Which one of the following is *not* responsible for this patient's presentation?

a. May–Hegglin anomaly
b. Thrombocytopenia-absent radii syndrome
c. Haemophilia A
d. Alport's syndrome
e. Wiskott–Aldrich syndrome

32) A 32-year-old man with acute lymphoblastic leukaemia in the remission consolidation phase has severe epistaxis. Six units of platelet transfusions fail to produce a clinical response. Previous episodes of mucocutaneous bleedings have responded well to platelets. After 1 hour of this transfusion, his platelets count is $8 \times 10^9/L$. What is the reason for this treatment failure?

a. Disseminated intravascular coagulation
b. Sepsis
c. Fever
d. Alloimmunization
e. Amphotericin B

33) A 12-year-old child presents with epistaxis, gum bleeding and skin bruising 2 weeks after an apparently benign common cold. He has haemorrhagic bullae in his mouth, but fundoscopy is normal. His platelets count is 15×10^9/L. Which one of the following is consistent with a diagnosis of acute immune thrombocytopenic purpura in this boy?

a. Pancytopenia
b. Splenomegaly
c. Increased peripheral reticulated platelets
d. Cervical lymphadenopathy
e. Leucoerythroblastic blood picture

34) A 29-year-old woman with chronic fluctuating immune thrombocy-topenic purpura is not demonstrating any improvement following the administration of *Rho*GAM infusions. She underwent splenect-omy 1 year ago. What are you going to do?

a. Increase the frequency of *Rho*GAM infusions
b. Search for an accessory spleen
c. Stop *Rho*GAM
d. Start prednisolone
e. Arrange for bone marrow transplantation

35) A 43-year-old woman presents with widespread skin petechiae one week after undergoing splenectomy for a traumatic splenic rupture. She is otherwise reasonably well and lives peacefully with her healthy 10-year-old boy. Her platelets count is 10×10^9/L. What has developed in this woman?

a. Acute lymphoblastic leukaemia
b. Warfarin-induced skin bleeding
c. Post-transfusion purpura
d. Idiopathic thrombocytopenic purpura (ITP)
e. Domestic violence

36) A 56-year-old man develops acute left lower limb ischaemia 6 days following treatment of right calf deep venous thrombosis provoked by a recent knee surgery. His ECG shows sinus rhythm. His past records reveal a healthy man with right knee osteoarthritis and unre-markable medical, surgical and family history. His platelets count is 65×10^9/L. What is the best option for short-term anticoagulation?

a. Continue heparin
b. Use warfarin
c. Lepirudin
d. Inferior vena cava filter
e. Enoxaparin

37) A 31-year-old man with confusion, fever and skin rash is referred from another hospital with a provisional diagnosis of thrombotic thrombocytopenic purpura (TTP). He has not yet undergone any blood test. Which one of the following would point to an alternative diagnosis?

a. Prolonged PT and aPTT
b. Mild renal impairment
c. Platelets count 30 x 10^9/L
d. Raised serum LDH
e. Reticulocytosis

38) A 62-year-old man presents with a platelets count of 40×10^9/L 1 day after undergoing coronary arteries bypass grafting. He is doing well and is having no active bleeding. How would you explain this result?

a. DIC
b. Dilutional thrombocytopenia
c. Post-transfusion purpura
d. HELLP syndrome
e. Thrombotic thrombocytopenic purpura

39) A 7-year-old girl presents with recurrent epistaxis and ecchymosis. She has mild thrombocytopenia with large platelets and prolonged bleeding time. There is decreased cell surface expression of the platelet GPIb/IX. What is the diagnosis?

a. Glanzmann's thrombosthenia
b. Aspirin abuse
c. Bernard–Soulier syndrome
d. Uraemic platelets dysfunction
e. Michael–Albert syndrome

40) A 10-year-old boy presents with recurrent severe mucocutaneous bleeds. He has oculocutaneous albinism. There is mild thrombocytopenia with severe reduction in the number of dense platelets granules. His history does not include recurrent pyogenic infections. What is the likely explanation for these bleeds?

a. Chédiak–Higashi syndrome
b. Hermansky–Pudlak syndrome
c. Gray platelets syndrome
d. Von Willebrand's disease
e. Haemophilia B

41) A 21-year-old man has recurrent nose bleeds. He reports excessive bleeding following dental extraction. His mother has the same illness. Today, he presents with gum bleeding and his blood counts reveal mild thrombocytopenia. The house officer is considering the administration of DDAVP but the consultant has declined this therapy because it is contraindicated in this man. Which one of the following types of von Willebrand's disease does this man have?

a. Type 1
b. Type 2A
c. Type 2M
d. Type 2B
e. Type 5

42) A 16-year-old patient is referred from a rural hospital because of excessive gum bleeding and severe right knee haemarthrosis. His notes mention that he has haemophilia A. Ristocetin cofactor activity and vWF antigen are normal. The patient shows no response following high-dose infusions of high-purity factor VIII concentrate, but does demonstrate a favourable response following vWF concentrate infusion. Which one of the following types of von Willebrand's disease does this patient have?

a. Type 3
b. Type 2N
c. Type 1
d. Type 4
e. Type 2M

43) A 65-year-old man with multiple myeloma presents with mucocutaneous bleeding. His platelet counts are normal but the bleeding time is prolonged. The aPTT is marginally prolonged and vWF antigen is reduced. There is absence of larger vWF multimers in the plasma. The patient shows a favourable response following intravenous immunoglobulin infusion. What is the reason for his bleeding tendency?

a. Acquired von Willebrand's disease
b. Haemophilia B
c. Excessive anticoagulation
d. Acquired haemophilia A
e. Type 3 von Willebrand's disease

44) A 19-year-old man has been referred to the haematology outpatient clinic because of prolonged PT. The referring physician does not mention the aPTT value. Deficiency of which one of the following coagulation factors is responsible for this man's presentation?

a. XIII
b. High molecular weight kininogen
c. IX
d. VII
e. Prekallikrein

45) A 16-year-old boy presents with recurrent haemarthrosis and muscle haematomas. His aPTT is prolonged. Which one of the following coagulation factor deficiencies is *not* responsible for this boy's bleeding?

a. Factor X
b. Factor V
c. Factor XII
d. Factor XI
e. Factor IX

46) A 23-year-old man with haemophilia A presents with acute left-sided knee joint swelling. The joint is extremely painful and warm. Factor VIII concentrate infusions do not produce any response. You are considering factor VIII inhibitors and their assessment reveals an activity of 11 BU. Which one of the following is *not* used to tackle these inhibitors?

a. Recombinant factor VIIa
b. Intravenous immunoglobulin
c. Immune suppressants
d. FEIBA
e. Recombinant factor XIII concentrate

47) A 19-year-old patient presents with excessive bleeding following skin cuts and tooth extraction. His PT, aPTT and platelet counts are normal. Apart from this bleeding, he is healthy, reasonably well and enjoys an independent life. He denies any spontaneous nose or gum bleed or skin bruising. What is the likely cause of this bleeding?

a. Mild von Willebrand's disease
b. Haemophilia B
c. Idiopathic thrombocytopenic purpura
d. Systemic vasculitis
e. Occult dexamethasone ingestion

48) A 6-year-old boy is brought by his mother to consult you. He bled excessively following an apparently uncomplicated tonsillectomy 1 week ago and his mother was advised by his surgeon to see you. She says that there was a late umbilical stump bleeding during his early neonatal period. Platelets count, bleeding time, PT and aPTT are normal. Which of the following tests should be ordered?

a. Repeat his aPTT
b. Bone marrow examination
c. Serum immune electrophoresis
d. Urea clot solubility test
e. Factor VIII inhibitors assay

49) A 23-year-old woman presents with a second episode of left leg swelling up to the upper thigh that pits on pressure. The right leg appears to be normal. Extensive evaluation uncovers an activated protein C mutation cleavage site at Arg 306. What is the cause of this deep venous thrombosis?

a. Factor V Leiden
b. Deficient protein C
c. Factor V Cambridge
d. Prothrombin gene mutation
e. Dysfibrinogenaemia

50) A 17-year-old boy is referred to the haematology clinic for further evaluation. He has been given a diagnosis of antithrombin III deficiency. Which one of the following would make you question his diagnosis?

a. Intracranial cerebral venous sinus thrombosis
b. Bilateral lower limb DVT
c. Femoral artery thrombosis
d. Family history of thrombophilia
e. His age of presentation

51) A 65-year-old man with rheumatoid arthritis presents with right lower limb deep venous thrombosis. Acute anticoagulation with heparin has been instituted. The aPTT fails to be prolonged despite using 50 000 units/day. What is the reason for this anticoagulation failure?

a. Expired heparin
b. Wrong method of administration
c. Heparin resistance
d. Antiphospholipid antibodies
e. Protein S deficiency

52) A 45-year-old man is receiving warfarin because of unprovoked deep venous thrombosis with resultant pulmonary infarction 3 weeks ago. His surgeon insists on carrying out elective cholecystectomy 6 days from now. The surgeon consults you and the patient does not know what to do. What is your response?

a. Continue warfarin
b. Stop warfarin 1 day before the elective surgery
c. Add heparin to warfarin
d. Stop warfarin today and place an inferior vena cava filter
e. Stop warfarin and start nadroparin

53) A 35-year-old multiparous woman presents with a 1-day history of low-grade fever, jaundice and pallor. Serum LDH and indirect bilirubin are raised and there is reticulocytosis. She underwent peptic ulcer surgery 1 week ago which was complicated by massive bleeding. What is the reason for the current presentation?

a. Subphrenic abscess
b. Major ABO incompatibility transfusion reaction
c. Transfusion-related CMV infection
d. Delayed haemolytic transfusion reaction
e. Transfusion-related hepatitis C infection

54) A 23-year-old woman has postpartum haemorrhage following vaginal delivery of a macrosomic baby. Three hours after starting blood transfusion, she develops fever, breathlessness and diffuse pulmonary infiltrates. Pulmonary capillary wedge pressure is 8 mmHg. You start high-flow oxygen. What has developed in this woman?

a. Over-transfusion
b. Major ABO incompatibility
c. Pulmonary aspiration
d. Re-expansion pulmonary oedema
e. Transfusion-related acute lung injury

55) A 48-year-old man with acute leukaemia develops fever, chills, headache, flushing, tachycardia and chest tightness one hour after starting blood transfusion because of anaemia. He reports 'similar things' whenever he receives blood transfusion. What is the best action now?

a. Continue the transfusion
b. Call the resuscitation team
c. Stop the transfusion
d. Give paracetamol
e. Epinephrine (adrenaline) injection

Clinical haematology and oncology: Answers

1) d.
The reticulocyte count in iron-deficiency anaemia is inappropriately low for the degree of haemoglobin, indicating poor bone marrow response to anaemia (but a reticulocyte 10 represents gross reticulocytosis). Transferrin saturation <15% is highly suggestive of iron-deficiency anaemia. Other features are hypochromia, microcytosis, low serum iron and increased total iron-binding capacity. Thrombocytosis is common.

2) d.
Pancytopenia with hypercellular marrow indicates myelodysplastic syndromes, peripheral immune cytopenias (as in SLE), megaloblastic anaemia or bone marrow infiltration (by tumour, granuloma). Aplastic anaemia has *hypo*cellular marrow. Haemorrhagic bullae on gums indicates severe thrombocytopenia.

3) c.
Elevated serum LDH is a marker of red cell destruction. In pernicious anaemia the *indirect* serum bilirubin is raised because of red cell haemolysis. There is macrocytosis (MCV >98 fl, usually >120). Bone marrow stores of iron are increased because of ineffective erythropoiesis. Megaloblastic anaemia is one of the causes of hypoproliferative anaemia, i.e. low haemoglobin with low reticulocyte count.

4) c.
The poor bone marrow response in this scenario fits with an aplastic crisis (note the reticulocyte count). Nothing in this brief scenario points towards a sequestration crisis (recent rapid hepatomegaly), *Salmonella* septicaemia (fever, rigor, osteomyelitis, low blood pressure) or acute chest syndrome (dyspnoea, hypoxemia, pulmonary infiltrates). Haemolytic crisis would have rapidly rising reticulocytosis and deepening jaundice.

5) e.
The high transfusion requirement calls for splenectomy to remove the site of red cell destruction; this is an effective means of reducing the monthly transfusions. All patients should receive daily folic acid and considered for iron chelation therapy. Although the latter is an adjunctive step to prevent or treat transfusion-induced haemosiderosis, it is not the best step at this time. With an already high number of monthly transfusions, it would never be acceptable simply to continue the transfusions. Hydroxycarbamide raises the haemoglobin F and is used as an adjunctive. Polyvalent pneumococcal vaccination is used in sickle cell anaemia.

6) c.

Patient scenarios are very common in the MRCP examination; however brief, there is always a single clue. Bite and blister cells are highly suggestive of G6PD deficiency. The overall picture is of severe intravascular haemolysis; note the dark urine.

7) b.

This woman has Coombs'-negative haemolytic anaemia with symptomatic gallstones; the latter calls for splenectomy in this hereditary spherocytosis. The anaemia itself appears mild. Other indications for splenectomy in hereditary spherocytosis are recurrent severe crisis, growth retardation in children, family history of death because of the disease and symptomatic cholecystitis. Symptomatic gallstones are best treated by surgery, but this is not the correct option for the long-term control of the disease.

8) c.

Patients who fail steroid therapy or are steroid-dependent should be considered for splenectomy. This will remove the site of red cell destruction and antibody production, and produces a favourable clinical response in up to 70% of cases. Patients who are unfit for or decline surgery should be offered an alternative mode of immune suppression; azathioprine is an excellent choice and a response is seen within 3 months (much slower than with steroids).

9) e.

Hook worm infestation and malabsorption might well be responsible for failure of oral iron therapy, but these are ruled out by the unremarkable stool examination and normal upper GIT endoscopy. The discrepancy between the mildly reduced haemoglobin and the profoundly decreased MCV are suggestive of alpha- or beta-thalassaemia minor; the normal haemoglobin A_2 rules out the latter leaving alpha-thalassaemia minor as the most probable diagnosis in this man. Note that the iron-deficiency in beta-thalassaemia minor 'normalizes' the level of haemoglobin A_2! Hereditary spherocytosis does not reduce the MCV value.

10) b.

Chronic cold agglutinin disease is usually seen in elderly people with low-grade B-cell lymphomas. Patients develop agglutination of red blood cells upon cold exposure; this is mainly seen in the fingers, toes, nose and ear lobules, producing acrocyanosis. The monoclonal IgM antibodies are directed against the red blood cell 'I' antigen. The RBC agglutination produces spurious elevation in the MCV with automatic analysers. Treatment should be directed against the underlying lymphoma and the troublesome acrocyanosis may respond to prednisolone.

11) c.

Severe aplastic anaemia is defined as: (1) peripheral blood count reveals at least two of the following: anaemia with corrected reticulocyte count

<1%, neutrophil count <0.5 x 10^9/L and platelet count <20 x 10^9/L; and (2) bone marrow cellularity <25% (usually 5–10%). Clinical features do not form part of the definition.

12) c.
The occurrence of thrombotic phenomenon (especially at abnormal sites) in the context of aplastic anaemia and 'early morning dark urine' should always prompt a search for paroxysmal nocturnal haemoglobinuria. The treatment is largely supportive; however, young patients should strongly be considered for allogenic stem cell transplantation.

13) d.
The chronic phase of myeloid leukaemia has mildly reduced haemoglobin, thrombocytosis, leucocytosis (with a full spectrum of leucocyte series with prominence of neutrophils and myelocytes), hyperuricaemia (increased cell turnover), *low* leucocyte alkaline phosphatase score and high serum LDH (elevated levels indicate poor prognosis in haematological malignancies). Eosinophilia is common and basophilia usually marks the start of the accelerated phase.

14) c.
The scenario fits stage 'A' CLL; there is no anaemia or thrombocytopenia and there are fewer than three areas of lymph node enlargement. Observation is the best approach and most patients have normal life-expectancy. All patients should be reassured.

15) a.
The scenario does not mention any symptoms (fever, weight loss, night sweats) nor organomegaly or sites of lymph node enlargement other than the neck. This patient has stage IA Hodgkin's disease; the best approach is local radiotherapy. Note that the presence of symptoms calls for chemotherapy regardless of the disease stage.

16) b.
Plasma alkaline phosphatase is normal in multiple myeloma unless there is a coexistent bone fracture. The patient has multiple myeloma and now presents with plasma cell leukaemia, which portends a very poor prognosis; note the very high blood plasma cell level. Monoclonal gammopathy of undetermined significance is ruled out the patient's diagnosis of multiple myeloma.

17) a.
Thrombocytopenia is a sign of poor prognosis, as is the presence of plasma cell leukaemia, haemoglobin level <7g/dl at the time of the diagnosis, intractable renal failure, high serum β_2-microglobulin and severe hypoalbuminaemia.

18) c.
Cladribine (as well as deoxycoformycin) usually produces long-lasting remission in hairy cell leukaemia, which is a chronic lymphoproliferative B-cell disorder, although the cells express CD25 and CD103.

19) b.
CLL rarely transforms to aggressive diffuse large B-cell lymphoma, called Richter's lymphoma (or transformation), which has a very poor prognosis. Note that transformation to acute leukaemia is extremely suspicious as is the presence of hyperuricaemia (cell turnover is slow).

20) d.
The presence of immune paresis, renal impairment, hypercalcaemia, lytic bony lesions, high level of plasma paraprotein and progressive increment in the latter are suggestive of multiple myeloma. Approximately 20% of MGUS patients develop multiple myeloma and 10% will develop solid tumours and therefore, all MGUS patients need close and regular follow-ups.

21) e.
Poor prognostic signs in agnogenic myeloid metaplasia are age >60 years, anaemia, thrombocytopenia, leucocytosis, increased number of circulating blasts, bone marrow cytogenic abnormalities, presence of systemic symptoms and hepatomegaly. Generally, the prognosis is poor. Philadelphia chromosome should be *absent* in agnogenic myeloid metaplasia. Constitutional symptoms indicate an advanced disease. Hydroxycarbamide is useful to control leucocytosis and thrombocytosis. Leukaemic transformation is seen in up to 10% of cases. Other causes of death are heart failure, infections and pulmonary embolism.

22) b.
Intrapulmonary haemorrhage is definitely a differential diagnosis, but it usually occurs with much lower platelets counts. Leucostasis occurs with very high circulating blast numbers (usually $>100 \times 10^9$/L) that result in injury to the vasculature of the lung, causing diffuse bilateral infiltrates and acute respiratory distress syndrome. Packed RBCs transfusion is contraindicated in patients with high circulating blast numbers because of high risk of precipitating leucostasis. *Pneumocystis carinii* pneumonia is a risk in lymphoblastic leukaemias. Acute respiratory distress syndrome can occur after blood transfusion but the question does not mention any blood or blood component transfusion. The patient is at risk of haemorrhagic complications!

23) c.
Acute promyelocytic leukaemia differs from other AML subtypes by having a special cytogenic abnormality–translocation t(15,17), which arrests maturation of the leucocytes at the level of promyelocytes. ATRA has been shown to overcome this arrest and to enhance the differentiation of immature leucocytes into mature neutrophils. Acute

cardiopulmonary collapse with severe hypoxaemia and pulmonary infiltrates, the retinoic acid syndrome, is seen when starting ATRA in those with high pre-treatment leucocyte count. Mediastinal radiotherapy is not a mode of treatment in acute myeloid leukaemias. Anthracyclins have a dose-dependent cardiac toxicity; first time exposure is unlikely to produce heart failure.

24) d.

All patients with high pre-treatment blast count should receive prophylactic regimen in the form of a few days' proper hydration and alkalization of urine to prevent the development of tumour lysis syndrome. Rapid destruction of large number of blast cells release their intracellular contents resulting in hyperuricaemia (and renal damage because of renal tubular precipitation), hyperkalaemia and hyperphosphataemia.

25) b.

The overall picture in this man is that of polycythemia vera. The 'normalization' of haemoglobin with prominent reduction in the MCV should always prompt a search for coexistent iron-deficiency anaemia, which is very common in these patients and usually results from occult upper GIT peptic ulcer bleeding and iron overconsumption in the bone marrow (which is used to synthesize the expanded RBC population). Other causes of haemoglobin reduction are the development of acute leukaemia (which has a short history and grave prognosis) and progression to secondary myelofibrosis. Although the question states 'a few months of follow-up' it does not mention any form of treatment, i.e. the patient has not been given any active treatment, which eliminates over treatment with phlebotomy. Such scenarios are common in the MRCP examination, so take care when reading the question.

26) e.

Megaloblastic anaemia is one of the most important differential diagnoses of myelodysplastic syndromes, as both may present with pancytopenia, dysplastic changes and hypercellular marrow. The patient has refractory anaemia with 5–20% marrow blasts; this would put him in the category of MDS subtype refractory anaemia with excess blasts. Marrow blasts of 20–30% would suggest refractory anaemia with excess blasts in transformation, while exceeding the 30% blasts cut-off in the bone marrow is frank leukaemic process. Hypogranulated hypolobulated neutrophil with bilobed nuclei is the pseudo-*Pegler-Huët* anomaly; this cell type should always be suspected to be present when automated analysers report an abnormally increased number of band form cells.

27) e.

All young patients with an HLA-matched sibling should be strongly considered for allogenic bone marrow transplantation. For older patients or those who have no HLA-matched donor, the objective of treatment is to control the immune response causing the bone marrow damage. This patient declines stem cell transplantation and thus going for ciclosporin and antithymocyte globulin is the most appropriate next step. G-CSF and erythropoietin injections are generally useless, but might be effective in severe cases to maintain peripheral cell count; however, this should not be the sole treatment in this young man. Some patients who recover from aplastic anaemia may go on to develop leukaemia, myelodysplasia or paroxysmal nocturnal haemoglobinuria; all of which are marrow clonal stem cell disorders.

28) b.

The increased osteoclastic activity in multiple myeloma is not coupled with an increased osteoblastic activity; therefore, serum alkaline phosphatase and isotope bone scanning are normal, unless there is a fracture. The patient has undergone bone scanning which is normal; serum alkaline phosphatase would add nothing, as it is also most likely to be normal. Bisphosphonates have been shown to reduce bone pain and skeletal events in multiple myeloma and may induce apoptosis of the malignant cells.

29) a.

Hypercalcaemia and lytic bony lesions are extremely rare and suggest an alternative diagnosis. Peripheral neuropathy is a demyelinating type, and may antedate the appearance of the malignant disease. The paraprotein is of IgM type which is an intravascular and increases the plasma viscosity. A percentage of patients with Waldenström's macroglobulinaemia have cold agglutinin syndrome with acrocyanosis. Ten per cent of the IgM paraprotein has properties of cryoglobulins.

30) b.

Differentiation between iron-deficiency anaemia and anaemia of chronic diseases is crucial because their treatment and prognosis are totally different. Serum iron is reduced in both because of deficiency in the former and impairment of iron kinetics in the latter. Serum ferritin is usually raised in anaemia of chronic diseases; however, levels down to $100\,\mu g/L$ may well indicate associated iron-deficiency anaemia, although it is not 100% accurate. The best approach is testing serum soluble transferrin level as this is elevated in the plasma in iron-deficiency anaemia. Around 25% of anaemia of chronic diseases is hypochromic microcytic.

31) c.

The scenario points towards a 'platelet type' of bleeding in this child. Giant platelets and Döhle bodies (basophilic inclusion bodies in platelets and WBCs) are seen in May–Hegglin anomaly. Thrombocytopenia-absent radii syndrome is a congenital defective production of megakaryocytes in the bone marrow. Alport's syndrome is a renal disorder that is accompanied by congenital hypoproductive thrombocytopenia. Wiskott–Aldrich syndrome is characterized by immune deficiency, eczema and neurological disorder, accompanied by thrombocytopenia with small platelets. Haemophilia A is a disorder of secondary haemostasis with deep tissue haematomas and haemarthroses.

32) d.

The six platelet units would be expected to increase the platelets count by 30–60 x 10^9/L. Failure of the count to increase can be attributed to fever, sepsis, DIC, graft-versus-host disease, treatment with amphotericin B and alloimmunization. Obtaining a 1-hour post-transfusion platelets count will help differentiate between the first five causes and the last one. With the exception of alloimmunization, the 1-hour post-transfusion platelet count would be expected to rise normally and then to fall steeply over the next few hours. Alloimmunized patients will have a minimal rise or even no rise because of rapid platelet destruction. This patient needs type-specific platelets (by donor screening with platelet cross-matching or HLA-matching) to minimize any clearance caused by the ABO determinants carried on the platelet surface.

33) c.

An increase in the percentage of the so-called reticulated platelets in the circulation is highly suggestive of destructive (especially immune-mediated) thrombocytopenia. The young platelets have a relatively high granule content to provide better haemostatic function. The presence of fever, hepatomegaly, splenomegaly, lymph node enlargement, pancytopenia or abnormal peripheral cells should suggest an alternative diagnosis (e.g. leukaemia and bone marrow infiltration by a tumour or granuloma), or a primary bone marrow disorder.

34) c.

*Rho*GAM is an antibody directed against the *Rh* D antigen. This antibody usually induces a mild degree of haemolysis and presumably causes FC receptor blockade of the reticuloendothelial system and thereby decreases platelets uptake by the liver and spleen; therefore, it is generally of no value in splenectomized patients. It should be given only to *Rh*-positive individuals. Some of these patients may respond to anti-CD20 monoclonal antibody. An accessory spleen is a very rare cause of treatment failure after splenectomy. This patient has definitely not responded to steroids in the past; note the splenectomy! Adding an immune suppressant agent, like cyclophosphamide, would be reasonable. The fault in immune thrombocytopenic purpura does not lie in the bone marrow; there is increased peripheral destruction of the platelets rendering their lifespan short.

35) c.

Post-transfusion purpura is a form of alloimmune thrombocytopenia following exposure to a platelet alloantigen, usually the Pl(A1), which is absent on the patient's native platelets. Most cases are females who are sensitized to this platelets antigen through pregnancy (or rarely previous blood transfusion) and homozygous for Pl(A2) antigen. This woman has had a major operation for a ruptured vascular organ; she must have been given blood transfusion. Upon re-exposure, the recipient's alloantibodies will destroy the donor's residual platelets and surprisingly, the recipient's own native platelets which do not carry the Pl(A1) alloantigen. Treatment is with intravenous immunoglobulins and future transfusions (or further transfusions if needed) should be derived from Pl(A2) homozygous donors. ITP is unlikely here and the other options do not fit the scenario.

36) c.

The overall picture is suggestive of heparin-induced thrombocytopenia. Heparin must be *stopped* immediately and an alternative form of short-term anticoagulation should be instituted. Warfarin should not be used in the short-term setting; after using the appropriate medication for acute short-term anticoagulation, warfarin can be used for long-term anticoagulation. The indications for the inferior vena cava filter are failure of anticoagulation, difficult anticoagulation or contraindications to the use of anticoagulation. Heparin-PF4 antibodies do not cross-react with the direct thrombin inhibitors lepirudin and argatroban. They do cross-react with low molecular weight heparins in 80% of cases, while 15% of antibodies will cross-react with heparinoids. This patient should be started on a direct thrombin inhibitor.

37) a.

The classical pentad of fever, skin rash, neurological dysfunction, renal impairment and microangiopathic haemolytic anaemia is seen in only 25% of cases of TTP. Defective vWF-cleaving protease function (whether inherited or acquired) leads to decreased clearance and increased blood levels of the larger high molecular weight vWF multimers. The latter will increase platelet adhesion and clearance without activating the coagulation cascade; the PT and aPTT will be within their normal reference range. They are prolonged in DIC (the top-ranking differential diagnosis). Thrombocytopenia is often severe. A raised serum indirect bilirubin and LDH and reticulocytosis provide evidence of haemolysis. The degree of the acute renal impairment in TTP is usually mild; severe renal impairment is more suggestive of haemolytic uraemic syndrome (HUS).

38) b.

Dilutional thrombocytopenia is seen whenever there is prominent haemodilution. Clinically, this is usually seen with massive blood transfusion (especially in trauma patients) or when using cardiopulmonary bypass (as in this patient). Bleeding is uncommon and is usually mild. A rebound increase in the platelet count is seen within 48–72 hours. Patients with clinically significant bleeding should receive platelet transfusion.

39) c.

In Glanzmann's thrombosthenia there is decreased expression (or rarely defective function) of the platelets GPIIb/IIIa (the receptor for both fibrinogen and vWF). Aspirin abuse is highly unlikely in this girl as the surface GPIb would then be normal in number. The GPIb is a receptor for vWF only; therefore, there is no platelet aggregation response to ristocetin despite the normal levels of vWF. No clue is given in the synopsis to renal failure. There is no such syndrome as Michael–Albert syndrome–this is a distraction! Most cases of Bernard–Soulier syndrome are characterized by decreased expression or defective function of the platelet cell surface receptor GPIb/IX; rarely, defective GPV is the cause of this platelet dysfunction syndrome.

40) b.

The differential diagnosis of this inherited platelet storage pool disease with defective dense granules and oculocutaneous albinism is between Chédiak–Higashi syndrome and Hermansky–Pudlak; the absence of recurrent pyogenic infections points to the diagnosis of Hermansky–Pudlak.

41) d.

There is no type 5–a distraction! Type 2B has abnormal vWF molecules that have a high affinity for platelets; the net result is the loss of high molecular weight multimers from the plasma, and thrombocytopenia. DDAVP has been shown to increase the release of this abnormal vWF in this type and is therefore contraindicated here because it aggravates thrombocytopenia; instead, vWF concentrate should be used.

42) b.

There is no type 4–a distraction! Type 2N has abnormal vWF molecules that have a low binding affinity for factor VIII, resulting in a shortening of factor VIII survival; the presentation is haemophilia A-like. Ristocetin cofactor activity and vWF antigen are normal because the mutation in the factor VIII binding site does not affect vWF function or survival.

43) a.

Type 3 vWD has a complete deficiency of vWF due to the inheritance of two abnormal vWF alleles. The bleeding time and PTT are markedly prolonged and there is severe reduction in factor VIII activity. Acquired vWD results from abnormal and rapid clearance of larger multimers of vWF from the plasma. This is usually seen in monoclonal gammopathies (like multiple myeloma), lymphoproliferative disorders, or malignant diseases and myeloproliferative disorders characterized by thrombocytosis. This patient has a vWF type 2A-like presentation. Apart from treating the underlying disorder, IVIG can successfully stop the bleeding tendency.

44) d.

Questions addressing prolonged PT and/or PTT are commonly encountered in the MRCP examination. In factor VIII deficiency PT, PTT and TT are characteristically normal. In deficiency of high molecular weight kininogen PT and TT are normal, and the aPTT is prolonged; similar results are seen for prekallikrein deficiency. Similar to factor XI deficiency, factor IX deficiency has normal PT and TT but prolonged aPTT. In factor VII deficiency PT is prolonged; the aPTT and TT are normal. Note that factor XII, high molecular weight kininogen and prekallikrein deficiencies do not present with bleeding tendency.

45) c.

Factor XII, high molecular weight kininogen and prekallikrein deficiencies do not present with bleeding tendency. The other options present with haemophilia-type bleeding, i.e. recurrent joint bleeding and deep tissue hematomas.

46) e.

Factor inhibitors develop in about 25% of haemophilia A patients and 5% of haemophilia B patients. An inhibitor is an antibody that has an activity that is measured in Bethesda units (BU). Each BU means that the inhibitor is able to neutralize around 50% of the coagulation factor in vivo. A level of > 10 BU renders coagulation factor infusion virtually useless. This blocking step can be bypassed during clinical bleeding settings by using factor VIII inhibitor bypass activity (FEIBA) infusion or infusing recombinant factor VIIa. Long-term measures to decrease the plasma levels of the factor inhibitors are regular IVIG infusion and/or the use of immune suppressants. There is no recombinant factor XIII concentrate for use in clinical practice.

47) a.

Some patients present with generalized bleeding tendency with normal screening tests (platelets count, PT, and aPTT). Apart from vascular purpura, mild von Willebrand's disease is the commonest cause in clinical practice in young otherwise healthy individuals; the bleeding time, however, is usually marginally prolonged. Mild coagulation factor deficiencies may present with normal PT and aPTT; specific factor assay usually demonstrates levels below the normal reference range. Factor XIII deficiency has normal PT, aPTT, and TT. In haemophilia B the patient's aPTT is normal but patients demonstrate joint and deep tissue bleedings. The normal platelet count rules out ITP and systemic vasculitis does not fit the picture. No clue is given in the scenario to point to occult dexamethasone ingestion; besides such patients bruise easily but do not have platelet-type of bleeding.

48) d.

Factor XIII deficiency does not prolong PT, aPTT or TT, but results in clot instability. The patient's clot dissolves easily in 8mol/L urea; if the test is positive, ELISA assay for factor XIII must be done next. Treatment is with fresh frozen plasma. The other options are of no value as the history is suggestive of an inherited tendency to bleed.

49) c.

Factor V Leiden is a common theme in the MRCP examination as it affects 5% of the general population. The mutation targets the cleavage site (at Arg 506) of activated protein C (APC) resulting in an ability to inactivate factor Va, which makes the prothrombinase complex relatively active; the net result is increased thrombin generation and thrombophilia. A similar mutation at Arg 306 produces factor V Cambridge. The third cause of APC resistance is lupus anticoagulant. Dysfibrinogenaemia results in bleeding tendency!

50) c.
By the age of 25 years, around 50% of heterozygous individuals deficient in antithrombin III (ATIII) will have had at least one episode of thrombosis that occurs exclusively in the venous circulation; there are few reports of arterial thromboses associated with mutations at the heparin binding site of ATIII (this should not stop you from giving this as the answer). Acquired cases have been associated with nephrotic syndrome (loss in urine as part of gross proteinuria) and severe hepatic veno-occlusive disease following stem cell transplantation (ATIII is consumed in the damaged liver microvasculature).

51) c.
Heparin resistance is defined as the daily administration of >40 000 units with the inability to achieve a therapeutic aPTT level. This is commonly seen in inflammatory diseases when heparin-binding proteins and factor VIII levels are elevated in plasma (as part of increased positive phase reactants). ATIII deficiency is a rare cause of heparin resistance.

52) d.
A common clinical dilemma is how to prepare hypercoagulable patients who are taking anticoagulants to surgery; the objective is to weigh the need for secured haemostasis during and immediately after surgery against the danger of anticoagulation after surgery. In patients with recent thromboembolic phenomenon and anticoagulation of <4 weeks, elective surgical procedures should be postponed if at all possible; if not, stopping the anticoagulant and placement of an inferior vena cava filter is the best option in clinical practice. Continuing with warfarin is totally unreasonable. It should be stopped 4 days before an elective operation to allow the INR to fall below 1.5; a level that is safe for surgery. Adding heparin to warfarin will definitely increase the risk of bleeding. Stopping warfarin and starting nadroparin will change nothing.

53) d.
The woman has had previous pregnancies and this might well be responsible for her RBC antigen sensitization and formation of antibodies against the Rh or Kidd RBC antigens. These antibodies are usually undetectable because of their low titre, but upon re-exposure, the titre rises rapidly, usually within 5–10 days, resulting in delayed haemolytic transfusion reaction. One-third of patients are clinically asymptomatic (with laboratory evidence of haemolysis) while the remaining patients present with fever, rigor, jaundice and progressive pallor. The incidence is 1/4000 blood transfusions. This woman has had a bleeding event while

undergoing surgery and she must have been given blood transfusion. Subphrenic abscess is a possibility in this scenario but it does not explain the laboratory evidence of haemolysis. Major ABO incompatibility transfusion reaction occurs acutely, not after a week. Delayed haemolytic transfusion reaction takes longer to manifest. Transfusion-related hepatitis C infection, which has an incidence of 1/800 000–2 000 000 transfusions, has a longer incubation and haemolysis is not a feature.

54) e.
Transfusion-related acute lung injury (TRALI) is usually under-diagnosed and ranks third in list of causes of transfusion-related deaths. The presentation is similar to adult respiratory distress syndrome and usually occurs 1–6 hours following the initiation of transfusion. It can be due to leucoagglutinins or HLA-specific lymphotoxic antibodies in the donor plasma that activate neutrophils and complements, ending with diffuse pulmonary microvascular damage. All patients should receive oxygen therapy and severe cases should receive a PEEP-assisted type of mechanical ventilation. The prognosis is generally good and a clinical improvement is usually seen within 24–48 hours. The mortality rate is 5–7%. Over-transfusion is the most important differential diagnosis of TRALI. It results in hypervolaemia and elevated PCWP. Major ABO incompatibility has a different presentation (fever, rigor, flank pain, dark urine with haemoglobinuria; severe breathlessness with diffuse pulmonary opacities would be a highly unusual feature). The patient has no risk factor for aspiration, e.g. caesarean section and aspiration during induction of anaesthesia. There is no mention of treatment for pneumothorax or pleural effusion (which would point to re-expansion pulmonary oedema).

55) c.
Transfusion reactions are very common in the MRCP examination. Although the history is suggestive of febrile non-haemolytic transfusion reaction (note the past reactions) in this patient, the current reaction could still be a major ABO incompatibility one; the best approach would be to stop the transfusion immediately and evaluate further. Prevention is by using blood filters.

7. Neurology, psychiatry and ophthalmology: Questions

1) A 46-year-old woman with mitral stenosis presents with dense right-sided hemiplegia and global aphasia. Her radial pulse is rapid and irregular. Brain CT scan shows cerebral infarction and she is admitted to the neurology ward to receive treatment for embolic stroke. Which one of the following arteries is likely to be occluded?

   a. Main stem of the left middle cerebral artery
   b. Lower posterior branch of the right middle cerebral artery
   c. Left anterior cerebral artery
   d. Top of the basilar artery
   e. Left vertebral artery

2) A 14-year-old boy presents with three generalized tonic-clonic seizures over the past 4 weeks. These fits start suddenly with tonic posturing and are followed by generalized body twitching. He regains consciousness after 10 minutes with headache and some confusion. His older brother has the same illness. He denies illicit drug abuse and past head trauma. Brain imaging is normal. What is the boy's likely diagnosis?

   a. Petit mal attacks
   b. Temporal lobe epilepsy
   c. Benign Rolandic epilepsy
   d. Idiopathic grand mal epilepsy
   e. Malingering

3) A 32-year-old woman consults the neurologist because of recurrent attacks of left arm numbness. She states that each attack lasts for about 1 week and improves spontaneously over the next week, and that attacks are separated by an average of 2 months. Examination reveals loss of joint position and vibration senses in the left arm, bilateral up-plantars and pale discs with central scotoma. She is anxious and desperate for your help. What does this woman have?

   a. Primary progressive multiple sclerosis
   b. Right parietal meningioma
   c. Relapsing–remitting multiple sclerosis
   d. Pseudotumour cerebri
   e. HIV encephalopathy

4) A 17-year-old boy is brought to you by his parents with progressive stance and gait ataxia. The mother states that the boy's cousin has similar features. After a thorough history and examination, your provisional diagnosis is Friedreich's ataxia. The presence of which one of the following features would cast doubt upon your provisional diagnosis?

a. Bilateral extensor plantars
b. Double vision
c. Mini-mental status examination score of 29
d. Impaired glucose tolerance test
e. Absent ankle jerks

5) A 39-year-old man has distal weakness and wasting of both hands with positive percussion thenar myotonia. His deceased mother had a disease affecting her muscles. Which one of the following is consistent with the diagnosis of myotonia dystrophica?

a. Thigh muscle fasciculation
b. Extensor plantars
c. Raised serum LH and FSH
d. Hypertrophy of both sternomastoids
e. Hypergammaglobulinaemia

6) A 65-year-old man presents with fluctuating cognitive function, formed visual hallucinations and parkinsonian features. He scores 24 during a mini-mental status examination. Brain MRI shows prominence of cortical sulci and compensatory hydrocephalus. What does this man have?

a. Alzheimer disease
b. Normal pressure hydrocephalus
c. Lewy body dementia
d. Depressive pseudodementia
e. Paraneoplastic limbic encephalitis

7) A 56-year-old woman has progressive spastic paraparesis. Her dorsal spine MRI is unremarkable. Serum vitamin B_{12} is within its normal reference range. There is no family history of note and she is HIV-negative. What would you do next?

a. Repeat the dorsal MRI with contrast
b. Plain X-ray of the cervical spine
c. Brain CT scan with contrast
d. Thigh muscle biopsy
e. Nerve conduction studies of both lower limbs

8) A 32-year-old woman has double vision while reading. Her visual acuity is normal. You are considering a diagnosis of myasthenia gravis. Which one of the following would point to another diagnosis?

a. Left-sided partial ptosis
b. Intact joint position in both lower limbs
c. Fixed-dilated pupil
d. Normal deep tendon reflexes
e. Dysphagia

9) A 62-year-old man with recurrent TIA presents with sudden mild left-sided weakness. He is admitted in the neurology ward and is given treatment for stroke. His carotid Duplex study reveals 80% stenosis involving the proximal right internal carotid artery. At discharge, what would you *not* do?

a. Give aspirin
b. Start simvastatin
c. Refer for carotid artery surgery
d. Do an ECG
e. Do a lumbar puncture

10) A 54-year-old woman is admitted to the neurology ward following a subarachnoid haemorrhage. At day 9, she develops right-sided hemi-paresis and up-going plantar. Her brain CT scan, done after 1 hour, reveals a trace of blood at the basal cisterns. What is the cause of this new feature?

a. Cardioembolic stroke
b. Carotid artery plaque rupture
c. Vasospasm
d. Acute hydrocephalus
e. Syndrome of inappropriate secretion of ADH

11) A 65-year-old man presents with a 9-month history of hand clumsi-ness and calf stiffness. After examining him in your clinic, you refer him for EMG testing for a suspected motor neurone disease. Which one of the following would lead you to revise your provisional diagnosis?

a. Exaggerated deep tendon reflexes
b. Hypoactive ankle jerks
c. Positive Hofmann's sign in the hands
d. Diminished pinprick sensation in the feet
e. Thigh wasting

12) A 65-year-old man is diagnosed as having lateral medullary ischae-mic stroke syndrome after being evaluated in A&E and undergoing brain CT scan. Which one of the following is inconsistent with this diagnosis?

a. Arm ataxia
b. Vomiting
c. Extensor plantar
d. Dysphagia
e. Vertigo

13) A 29-year-old woman with relapsing–remitting multiple sclerosis presents with an attack of transverse myelitis at C5–6 segments of the cord. Examination reveals an additional Horner's syndrome. Which one of the following would be an unexpected finding in Horner's syndrome in this woman?

a. Partial ptosis
b. Slight elevation of the lower lid
c. Pupillary narrowing
d. Loss of spinociliary reflex
e. Heterochromia iridis

14) A 65-year-old woman with a past history of head trauma presents with progressive cognitive decline. Her examination and brain imaging is suggestive of normal pressure hydrocephalus. Which one of the following would suggest an alternative diagnosis?

a. Dilated cerebral aqueduct
b. Urinary incontinence
c. Elevated CSF opening pressure
d. Subcortical type of dementia
e. Transient improvement after removing 50 ml of the CSF

15) A 61-year-old woman presents with rapidly progressive memory loss, behavioural abnormalities, gait ataxia, extensor plantars and startle myoclonus. Her brain CT scan is relatively normal. What is the likely diagnosis?

a. Cerebral glioblastoma multiforme
b. Creutzfeldt–Jacob disease
c. Pick's dementia
d. Multiple sclerosis
e. AIDS–dementia complex

16) A 51-year-old man complains of excessive right eye tearing while eating. Detailed history taking is likely to reveal which one of the following past histories?

a. Left-sided frontal lobe stroke
b. Right-sided disc swelling
c. Right-sided facial palsy
d. Left-sided Horner's syndrome
e. Bilateral ptoses

17) A 43-year-old man presents with bilateral foot drop. Sensory examination is unremarkable. All of the following can result in predominantly motor neuropathy, except:

a. Porphyria cutanea tarda
b. Lead poisoning
c. Dapsone ingestion
d. Guillain–Barré syndrome
e. Imipramine therapy

18) A 43-year-old man presents with severe lower limb weakness and thigh pain but intact sensory examination, 2 weeks after apparently benign diarrhoea. Which one of the following is inconsistent with the diagnosis of Guillain–Barré syndrome?

a. 5 neutrophils in the CSF
b. CSF protein of 60 mg/dl in the first week of the illness
c. Normal nerve conduction study in the first week of the illness
d. Symmetrical lower limb weakness
e. Bilateral facial weakness

19) A 38-year-old woman presents with a 3-year history of double vision when reading. Examination reveals bilateral asymmetrical fatigable ptosis with normal limb examination. Which one of the following statements is true?

a. Pupillary reactions should be impaired
b. Respiratory compromise is common
c. Thymectomy is contraindicated
d. Antiacetylcholine receptor antibodies should be negative
e. Brain MRI is usually abnormal

20) A doctor reviews a 25-year-old female patient diagnosed with idiopathic pseudotumour cerebri visits and no longer considers this diagnosis appropriate. Which one of the following might have been observed on review?

a. Bilateral disc swelling
b. Right-sided extensor plantar
c. Enlargement of the physiological blind spot
d. Left-sided abducens palsy
e. Intact facial sensation

21) A 21-year-old man has a long history of distal weakness and pes cavus. Family history reveals the same disease in many family members. You are considering a diagnosis of Charcot–Marie–Tooth disease. Which one of the following would suggest an alternative diagnosis?

a. Bilateral hand wasting
b. Contracture of Achilles tendon
c. Exaggerated ankle jerks
d. High stepping gait
e. Stork-like legs

22) A woman is referred to the neurology clinic for further evaluation of her hand wasting. All of the following might be responsible for this woman's presentation, except:

a. Motor neurone disease
b. Bilateral cervical ribs
c. Syringomyelia
d. Facioscapulohumeral dystrophy
e. Cervical spondylosis

23) A 63-year-old man with small cell lung cancer has weakness. His overall clinical picture points towards Lambert–Eaton myasthenic syndrome (LEMS). Which one of the following indicates an alternative diagnosis?

a. Positive serum antivoltage gated calcium channel antibodies
b. Dry mouth
c. Impotence
d. Exaggerated reflexes
e. Incremental response on repetitive EMG testing

24) A 29-year-old patient has asymmetrical upper limb wasting and fasciculation. Biceps reflexes are lost and there is dissociated sensory loss in both hands. Syringomyelia may be associated with all of the following, except:

a. Arnold–Chiari malformation
b. Spina bifida
c. 'Inverted champagne bottle' legs
d. Scoliosis
e. Hydrocephalus

25) A 27-year-old female patient with multiple sclerosis patient has right-sided internuclear ophthalmoplegia (INO) detected during her routine check-up. Which one of the following would be seen on ocular examination?

a. Left-sided partial ptosis
b. Impaired left medial rectus action
c. Ataxic nystagmus in the left eye
d. Small pupils
e. Impaired right-sided eye depression

26) A 43-year-old man presents with impaired hearing, and diminished right corneal reflex and pinprick sensation over the right side of the face. Brain CT scan shows a mass in the right cerebellopontine angle. What is the commonest cause of this triangular area mass lesion?

a. Secondary tumour
b. Acoustic neuroma
c. Cholesteotoma
d. Basilar artery aneurysm
e. Meningioma

27) A 41-year-old patient with brainstem pathology is referred to the neurologist for further evaluation. He has bulbar palsy. Which one of the following might be demonstrated on physical examination?

a. Conical tongue
b. Donald duck speech
c. Exaggerated jaw jerk
d. Tongue fasciculation
e. Emotional lability

28) A 45-year-old man has central disc prolapse in the lower spine. Examination is consistent with cauda equina syndrome. Which one of the following features points to an associated conus medullaris lesion?

a. Loss of right ankle jerk
b. Hypoactive left knee
c. Saddle anaesthesia
d. Bilateral extensor plantars
e. Overflow incontinence

29) A 19-year-old patient with myoclonic epilepsy has been started on a new antiepileptic medication by his GP. His myoclonic jerks seem to be increased in frequency and severity. Which one of the following medications has been added by the GP?

a. Carbamazepine
b. Valproic acid
c. Gabapentin
d. Phenobarbital
e. Clonazepam

30) A 17-year-old female patient with a known conversion disorder presents with repetitive wild thrashing movements but no loss of consciousness or incontinence. Her EEG during these attacks shows no organized epileptiform activity. You suspect pseudo-seizures. Which one of the following is the most important differential diagnosis?

a. Petit mal seizures
b. Complex partial status epilepticus
c. Frontal lobe seizures
d. Salaam attacks
e. Tardive dyskinesia

31) You suspect subarachnoid haemorrhage in a 53-year-old man because of sudden severe thunder-clap headache a few hours ago, and are contemplating lumbar puncture. CSF xanthochromia starts to appear after:

a. 8–12 hours
b. 1–day
c. 2–3 week
d. $\frac{1}{2}$ hour
e. 7 days

32) A 64-year-old woman presents with repetitive lancinating facial pains on the right side that are brought about by toothbrushing and chewing. Examination is unremarkable. What would you prescribe?

a. Carbamazepine
b. Aspirin
c. Donepezil
d. Nimodipine
e. Riluzole

33) A 45-year-old man presents with weakness that involves both upper and lower limbs, proximally and distally. He reports pain and paraesthesia in his limbs. He has had these symptoms for the past 8 months. Neurophysiological studies reveal widespread demyelination and secondary axonal degeneration. CSF protein is greatly elevated. What is this man's diagnosis?

a. Guillain–Barré syndrome
b. Diphtheritic neuropathy
c. Chronic inflammatory demyelinating polyradiculopathy
d. Acute intermittent porphyria
e. Charcot–Marie–Tooth disease

34) A 23-year-old woman has impaired vision and headache. Her GP has diagnosed conversion disorder with psychogenic blindness. However, her optokinetic response is impaired on the right side. You are considering an intracranial mass lesion. Where is the lesion?

a. Bifrontal
b. Right parietal
c. Right temporal
d. Left occipital
e. High midbrain

35) A 56-year-old man is referred for further evaluation because of up-gaze palsy associated with other neurological deficits. He is about to undergo MRI examination of the brain with contrast administration. Where do you think the lesion lies?

a. Lower medulla
b. Midbrain
c. Midpontine
d. Right pontomedullary junction
e. At the level of foramen magnum

36) A 54-year-old man is referred from the ophthalmology clinic because of bilateral optic nerve head swelling. Which one of the following is *not* a potential cause of this ocular finding?

a. Hypercapnia
b. Parietal glioblastoma multiforme
c. Normal pressure hydrocephalus
d. Methanol intoxication
e. Malignant hypertension

37) A 42-year-old alcoholic man is referred from a rural hospital for further management. His referral report suggests Wernicke's encephalopathy. You examine him thoroughly. Which one of the following would reject the diagnosis of Wernicke's encephalopathy?

a. Nystagmus
b. Global confusion
c. Combined horizontal and vertical gaze palsies
d. Right-sided facial palsy
e. Left-sided abducens palsy

38) A 67-year-old woman is brought by her son to consult you. He states that his mother is becoming forgetful and does not participate in family activities. She admits to having difficulty concentrating. Which one of the following would point to pseudodementia rather than Alzheimer's disease?

a. Progressive cognitive decline
b. Insidious onset
c. No past history of depression
d. Prominent vegetative symptoms
e. Abnormal neurological examination

39) A 61-year-old man is brought by the police to A&E in a state of agitation that he has had for a few hours. You meet the man who is perplexed and keeps asking, 'Where am I?' He knows his identity and this was useful to allow review his past records which reveal a prior ischaemic stroke. What is your provisional diagnosis?

a. Korsakoff's amnesic psychosis
b. A new stroke
c. Dissociative amnesia
d. Occult head trauma
e. Transient global amnesia

40) A 23-year-old woman presents at A&E with severe right-sided head-ache. This is her fifth visit this month. She says that she has had migraine with aura since adolescence. She is given appropriate treatment and recovers before discharge. What is your advice with respect to her illness?

a. Avoid excessive red meat
b. Increase milk ingestion
c. Use sunscreens
d. Take daily amitriptyline
e. Take the rest of the week off

41) A 55-year-old woman presents with apathy, headache and impaired vision. Her right optic disc is atrophied while the left one is swollen. Brain CT scan with contrast administration reveals a semi-rounded mass in the right frontal lobe, 4×5 cm in dimensions and without surrounding brain oedema, which takes the contrast homogenously. What is your provisional diagnosis?

a. Craniopharyngioma
b. Anaplastic astrocytoma
c. Osteoma
d. Meningioma
e. Pituitary adenoma with suprasellar extension

42) A 67-year-old man comes for his annual check-up. Apart from right knee osteoarthrosis, he denies any symptoms. He does the shopping and cleans the house every week without feeling short of breath. You detect a left carotid bruit. Duplex study of the carotids reveals 43% stenosis in the proximal left internal carotid artery. What would you do next?

a. Refer for cerebral angiography
b. Start warfarin
c. Give aspirin
d. Refer for carotid endarterectomy
e. Do a brain CT scan

43) A 16-year-old boy with recently diagnosed Wilson's disease comes with his parents to see you. He has been given penicillamine tablets. He says that his complaints have worsened, especially his dystonias. What is the likely reason for this?

a. Wrong diagnosis
b. Penicillamine therapy
c. Surreptitious administration of an illicit drug
d. End of dose phenomenon
e. Coexistent hepatic encephalopathy

44) A 61-year-old diabetic man presents to A&E with a 3-hour history of mild left-sided weakness. His GP attributes this to hypoglycaemia but his random blood glucose was 180 mg/dl at that time. You order a brain CT scan which reveals no haemorrhage. His blood pressure is 160/95 mmHg. What would you do regarding his stroke?

a. Aspirin
b. Thrombolytic therapy
c. Enalapril
d. Atrovastatin
e. Wait and see

45) A 64-year-old man is referred by his GP for review of a diagnosis of Parkinson's disease. The GP states that his patient has not improved with escalating doses of Sinemet®. Which one of the following would cast strong doubt on the diagnosis of idiopathic Parkinson's disease?

a. Asymmetric hand tremor
b. Jaw tremor
c. Blepharospasm
d. Depression
e. Ankle clonus

46) A 19-year-old nurse presents with recurrent breast abscesses which respond well to surgical evacuation and antibiotics. Pus culture always uncovers Gram-negative enteric organisms. She is sexually inactive, single and has no children, and her history and bloods are not suggestive of any of the immune compromised states. What is the likely explanation for her presentation?

a. Chronic myeloid leukaemia
b. Somatization disorder
c. Factitious disorder
d. Conversion disorder
e. Iatrogenic faults

47) A 16-year-old secondary school girl has been assessed thoroughly by a psychologist who notices that she is indecisive, has difficulty with daily responsibilities, demands constant support from others and has many unstable relationships. Which one of the following types of personalities would fit her?

a. Narcissistic
b. Histrionic
c. Dependent
d. Obsessional
e. Schizoid

48) An 18-year-old man presents with extreme emaciation. He admits to having lost interest in sex but denies being thin. He has hypotension, bradycardia and blue peripheries. During weight checking on the scale, he was caught hiding heavy objects in his clothing. What does this man have?

a. Graves' disease
b. Kallman's syndrome
c. Anorexia nervosa
d. Coeliac disease
e. Heart failure

49) A 21-year-old woman presents with recurrent bouts of binge-eating and self-induced vomiting. Which one of the following is not usually seen in bulimic patients?

a. Normal weight
b. Regular menses
c. Serum bicarbonate 12 mEq/L
d. Serum potassium 2.9 mEq/L
e. Erosion of dental enamel

50) A 17-year-old girl is brought to A&E by her single mother. All of a sudden the girl remembers nothing, including her name and address, and even her mother. Her mother states that her daughter is healthy, has no chronic illnesses and she does not take drugs as far as she knows. What does this girl have?

a. Surreptitious amfetamine ingestion
b. Accidental morphine ingestion
c. Hysterical amnesia
d. Subdural haematoma
e. Early-onset Alzheimer's disease

51) A 31-year-old man has fear of open spaces, especially when crowded. When confronted with such a situation he becomes anxious, tachycardic and sweaty. What type of phobia does he have?

a. Panic attacks
b. Social phobia
c. Agoraphobia
d. Obsession
e. Conversional

52) A 32-year-old woman presents with a 4-week history of low mood most of the day, weight loss, early morning insomnia, loss of interest in everyday activities and feelings of excessive guilt. Which one of the following would *not* call for electroconvulsive therapy in this woman?

a. Long duration of the illness
b. Depressive stupor
c. Failure of medical therapy
d. Severe malnutrition
e. Attempted suicide

53) A 29-year-old man has been recently diagnosed as having schizophrenia and is receiving an antipsychotic medication. You notice that he is much better now and his family confirms your impression. Which one of the following would portend a bad prognosis?

a. Acute onset of the symptoms
b. Normal premorbid personality
c. Catatonic features
d. Prominent affective symptoms
e. No precipitating factor

54) A 31-year-old schizophrenic patient still has many negative features of the disease after receiving many medications for 7 months. Which one of the following is *not* a negative symptom in schizophrenia?

a. Apathy
b. Poverty of speech
c. Auditory hallucinations
d. Flat affect
e. Social withdrawal

55) A 54-year-old individual was unsuccessful at terminating his life by hanging himself. After his failed attempt, his wife found a letter with a will stating that it is better for him to be dead as his life is hopeless and helpless. All of the following are risk factors for committing suicide after a suicidal attempt, except:

a. Living alone
b. Unemployed
c. Married
d. Male sex
e. Alcohol abuse

56) A 21-year-old woman gave birth to a full-term baby 3 days ago. Her husband says that his wife is anxious and has mood lability, irritability, poor concentration and tearfulness. Her symptoms peak on the fifth postpartum day. She improves gradually with reassurance and psychological support during the next 10 days. What is the likely diagnosis in this woman?

a. Postpartum depression
b. Schizophrenia
c. Surreptitious drug abuse
d. Postnatal blues
e. Conversion reaction

57) A 19-year-old man asks the surgeon to prescribe him oestrogen pills. The man is convinced that he is actually female and he wishes to live the rest of his life as a woman. What does this man have?

a. Delusional disorder
b. Trans-sexualism
c. Exhibitionism
d. Transvestism
e. Paedophilia

58) A 31-year-old woman repeatedly visits her dermatologist stating that he is not helping her get rid of a parasitic disease that has infested her body. The dermatologist refers her to you for further evaluation and his referral states that her skin is totally normal. Blood tests are normal and she denies illicit drug or alcohol abuse. What is the likely explanation for this woman's attitude?

a. Munchausen syndrome
b. Psychogenic pruritis
c. Hypochondriasis
d. Schizoid personality
e. Somatization disorder

59) A 21-year-old woman visits you for the first time. She has abdominal pain, backache, and headache for the past 3 years. Her weight is constant and her stool and appetite are unchanged. She says that GPs have failed to uncover the reason for these complaints and she is desperate for your help. After thorough history taking, examination and investigations, no apparent pathology is found. What is the likely cause of her recurrent complaints?

a. Somatization disorder
b. Conversion disorder
c. Fibromyalgia
d. Chronic fatigue syndrome
e. Munchausen syndrome

60) A 63-year-old man is brought by his son to consult you. The son states that his father is not behaving himself lately and he forgets many things. Examination reveals a well-kempt man, who is apathetic and has significant impairment of short-term memory. Long-term memory is impaired to a lesser extent. He has nystagmus and mild gait ataxia. His past history is notable for malnutrition following successful cure of stage 1B Hodgkin's disease. The man tries to reassure you that he is OK. What is the explanation for this man's presentation?

a. Early Alzheimer's disease
b. Paraneoplastic limbic encephalitis
c. Korsakoff's syndrome
d. Relapse of Hodgkin's disease
e. Major depression

61) A 33-year-old woman presents with rapidly progressive lower limbs weakness. All of the following might be implicated as a cause, except:

a. Botulism
b. Shellfish poisoning
c. Myasthenia gravis
d. Becker's muscular dystrophy
e. Periodic paralysis

62) A 40-year-old man consults you because of involuntary hand shaking movements. These movements have been present from the age of 14 years and are somewhat socially embarrassing. You find postural tremor in his hands with head and voice tremor. What is the likely cause of this man's presentation?

a. Early onset Parkinson's disease
b. Motor neurone disease
c. Juvenile Huntington's disease
d. Essential tremor
e. Wilson's disease

63) A 25-year-old woman is referred to you by her GP because of recurrent unconsciousness. The GP states that this woman loses consciousness all of a sudden without any prodrome, but has never injured herself or had incontinence. The period of unresponsiveness is long, during which the patient is not pale or blue-looking, and is followed by immediate full recovery with headache or confusion. What do you think this young woman has?

a. Recurrent tachyarrhythmia
b. Complex partial seizures
c. Psychogenic syncope
d. Mitral valve prolapse
e. Grand mal epilepsy

64) A 48-year-old woman is referred by the optometrist because of visual field defect. Neurological examination is unremarkable. Which one of the following is *not* implicated as a cause of the faulty field detection by the optometrist?

a. Partial ptosis
b. Uncorrected refractive error
c. Lens opacity
d. Papilloedema
e. Miosis

65) A young man's father's eyesight is impaired because of retinal disease. This 23-year-old college student consults you to ask about the nature of the disease, possible prognosis and treatment options of age-related macular degeneration. He is afraid that his eyes might also be affected. Which one of the following is the earliest fundoscopic finding in this disease?

a. Temporal optic nerve head pallor
b. Retinal drusen
c. Lens opacities
d. Choriodal neovascular tuft
e. Macular oedema

66) A 19-year-old man presents with defective dark adaptation and night blindness. Fundoscopy reveals perivascular pigmentary changes in a bone–spicule configuration. Which one of the following is *not* a recognized cause of this disease?

a. Usher's syndrome
b. Refsum's disease
c. Hunter's mucopolysaccharidosis
d. Kearns–Sayre syndrome
e. Diabetes mellitus

67) A 61-year-old man presents with constant boring pain in his left eye. He had ischaemic central retinal vein occlusion (CRVO) 3 months ago which resulted in severe loss of vision to hand movements. What is the cause of this eye pain?

a. Recurrent minor attacks of CRVO
b. Neovascular glaucoma
c. Optic nerve head swelling
d. Giant cell arteritis
e. Uveitis

68) A 24-year-old man has multiple skin neurofibromas, axillary freckling and 10 café-au-lait macules. He is hypertensive and his seizures are well-controlled with carbamazepine. You examine his eyes and find many iris hamartomas. Which one of the following is true regarding these Lisch nodules?

a. They are premalignant
b. Do not affect vision
c. Present in 90% of young children with this disease
d. Predict the development of optic nerve glioma
e. Cannot be seen with the indirect ophthalmoscope

69) A 15-year-old boy has long extremities, with arm span greater than height, flat sternum and dorsal spine, aortic reflux and hypermobile joints. He is about to undergo eye examination. He says that he has lens dislocation in an upward direction. Which one of the following would be an unexpected ocular finding in this boy?

a. Myopia
b. Iridodenesis
c. Blue sclera
d. Hypoplasia of dilator pupillae
e. Snow-flake cataract

70) A 59-year-old man with long-standing Type 2 diabetes presents for his annual check-up. Fundoscopy reveals scattered dot haemorrhages and a few hard exudates in the macular area. He states that his vision is not that good but he is coping with it and that his eye glasses are not helpful. Which one of the following is true?

a. He has proliferative retinopathy
b. He has pre-proliferative retinopathy
c. He should be referred to the ophthalmologist
d. He should be referred for pars plana vitrectomy
e. Reassure and ask him to return next year

Neurology, psychiatry and ophthalmology: Answers

1) a.

Cardiogenic emboli are usually large enough to lodge in and occlude the main stem of one of the middle cerebral arteries (MCA), resulting in a devastating stroke. The global aphasia indicates involvement of the dominant hemisphere. Occlusion of the upper anterior branch of the MCA would result in Broca's aphasia and hemiplegia, while occlusion of the lower posterior division would result in Wernicke's type of aphasia and upper quadrantic homonymous field defect. Occlusion of the top of the basilar artery is usually embolic but would result in quadriplegia, decerebrate (or decorticate) posturing and profound impairment of consciousness (a differential diagnosis of transtentorial herniation). Vertebral artery occlusion usually results in lateral medullary syndrome of Wallenburg.

2) d.

The scenario is typical of idiopathic grand mal epilepsy. Absence attacks present with sudden staring and no such profound motor movements. Temporal lobe epilepsy has repetitive stereotypical aura, followed by impaired consciousness and automatism; there is no profound body twitching unless there is secondary generalization. Nothing in the clinical picture points to the boy malingering.

3) c.

This woman fits the diagnostic criteria of relapsing–remitting multiple sclerosis: two or more attacks of white matter dysfunction, each lasting for at least 24 hours, with an interval of at least 4 weeks; and the examination shows two or more white matter signs at different sites (i.e. dissemination in time and place). As she has no progressive deterioration in the absence of relapses, primary progressive multiple sclerosis can be ruled out. The other options have a totally different clinical picture.

4) b.

The presence of ocular weakness, seizures and extrapyramidal signs is highly suggestive of an alternative diagnosis. Ophthalmoplegia and diplopia are seen in spinocerebellar ataxia (SCA) type-3 (Machado–Joseph). The other options are consistent with a diagnosis of Friedreich's ataxia. Bilateral extensor plantars result from degeneration of the spinal cord's pyramidal tracts (one of the causes of up-plantars and lost ankles). As well as absent ankle jerks, there is loss of kinesthesia from large fibre peripheral neuropathy. Patients have no cognitive decline (dementia features are seen in SCA type-2 and 3). Overt diabetes mellitus occurs in 10–20% of cases (be aware of diabetic retinopathy in Friedreich's ataxia patients in the MRCP examination). Note cardiomyopathy, diabetes and skeletal manifestations are consistent with Friedreich's ataxia rather than other types of SCA.

5) c.
The raised LH and FSH in males with myotonia dystrophica indicates testicular atrophy and hypergonadotrophic hypogonadism. There is also *atrophy* of facial, sternomastoid, and distal limb muscles. Hypertrophy of certain muscle groups is seen in myotonia congenita. Thigh muscle fasciculation is seen in motor neurone disease from chronic denervation and reinnervation. Extensor plantars will not be seen as the pyramidal system is intact. Peripheral nerves should be intact in myotonia dystrophica; however, features of symmetrical peripheral neuropathy may occur from long-standing Type 2 diabetes (seen in 20% of cases). *Hypo*gammaglobulinaemia may be seen and predisposes the patient to recurrent chest infections.

6) c.
Lewy body dementia fits the scenario as, unlike in Alzheimer's disease, there is no prominent early memory impairment. (These patients are extremely sensitive to neuroleptics, which may be prescribed for the visual hallucinations, but should be avoided.) The first signs of Alzheimer's disease are prominent forgetfulness and impairment of short-term memory. In normal pressure hydrocephalus the patient would show gait deficit, incontinence and dementia. The dilated ventricles would efface the cortical sulci. Prominent vegetative symptoms would be seen with depressive pseudodementia; there are no parkinsonian features. Paraneoplastic limbic encephalitis is an inflammatory degenerative disease of the grey matter of the brain that typically precedes the diagnosis of small cell lung cancer. Patients typically demonstrate profound impairment of recent memory (corresponding to the inability to store new information), and have some impairment in long-term memory as well. Some patients may confabulate. Complex partial seizures may occur. The disease gradually progresses to global dementia.

7) c.
Spastic paraparesis results from diseases of the dorsal spine or pathologies that affect the paramedian area of both leg cortices (e.g. tumours and sagittal sinus thrombosis). As this patient has a normal dorsal spine MRI, proceeding to brain imaging would be reasonable. Spastic paraparesis does not result from primary muscle disease and thigh biopsy would be of no value. Nerve conduction studies for peripheral nerves would be expected to be normal (as peripheral nerves are unaffected); however, EMG studies may reveal a poor recruitment pattern of motor neurones (which is seen in any pyramidal weakness and would not diagnose the cause).

8) c.
In myasthenia gravis pupillary size, reactivity and shape should be *normal* (pupillary abnormalities are seen in Lambert–Eaton myasthenic

syndrome). Ptosis is usually partial, uni- or bi-lateral, and is mainly asymmetrical. It is a disease of the motor endplate; peripheral nerves and neurones are unaffected. Deep tendon reflexes are normal (or sometimes exaggerated). Hypoactive reflexes are seen in severe advanced cases. Dysphagia, nasal speech and dysarthria are seen.

9) e.
A lumbar puncture has no place in this patient. It may have a place in infectious and inflammatory causes of stroke, especially in young patients. Aspirin should be given to this patient to prevent further attacks. Simvastatin is used as a secondary prophylaxis in atherosclerosis vascular disease. This patient should be referred for surgery as he has significant symptomatic stenosis. An ECG is useful to look for cardiac arrhythmia (which might be responsible for this stroke) or to detect ischaemic changes (myocardial infarction is the usual killer in these patients).

10) c.
Any deterioration in patients with subarachnoid haemorrhage should prompt a search for re-bleeding, vasospasm and acute/subacute hydrocephalus. The focal nature of the deficit in this patient with unremarkable brain CT scan points towards vasospasm.

11) d.
Motor neurone disease can have a combination of upper and lower motor neurone signs, as well as bulbar or pseudobulbar palsy. The presence of sensory signs, cerebellar deficits, extrapyramidal features or cognitive decline call for a review the diagnosis.

12) c.
The pyramidal tracts lie anteriorly and near to the midline in the medulla oblongata. They are not affected in lateral medullary syndrome. Their involvement indicates either a wrong diagnosis, or combined medial and lateral medullary syndromes. In addition to arm ataxia, vomiting, dysphagia and vertigo, other features that could be expected in this patient are ipsilateral facial sensory deficit, contralateral spinothalamic deficit, ipsilateral Horner's syndrome and hiccough.

13) e.
Heterochroma iridis is the hallmark of congenital cases. In Horner's syndrome, partial ptosis reflects paralysis of levator palpebrae superioris; slight elevation of the lower lid reflects paralysis of the lower tarsal muscle of Muller; and pupillary narrowing reflects sympathetic denervation to the sphincter pupillae. Loss of the spinociliary reflex will mean that pinching of the lower neck will fail to produce dilatation of the ipsilateral pupil.

14) c.
In normal pressure hydrocephalus the CSF opening pressure is *normal or low*, and there is no papilloedema. The ventricular system is dilated in a

'communicating' pattern. Gait disorder is usually the initial manifestation. The dementia is typically mild and is usually preceded by the gait disorder. It begins with apathy and mental slowness and is followed gradually by more global dementia. The cortex is not degenerated and focal cortical signs (aphasia, agnosia) are very rare; however, bilateral spasticity and extensor plantaris may be seen in some patients. Urinary incontinence is usually a late sign and most patients are unaware of it. Faecal incontinence is extremely rare. With CSF removal, transient improvement can be seen in the cognitive function, incontinence or gait; this is the best predicator of a favourable response to shunting surgery.

15) b.

Creutzfelt–Jacob disease fits the clinical scenario. Memory loss is invariably present at the time of diagnosis. The EEG shows triphasic complexes with sharpened outlines that occur once per second and is seen in 65–95% of cases. Cerebral glioblatoma is ruled out by the normal brain CT scan. In Pick's dementia prominent behavioural and personality changes with minimal memory impairment would be seen. There is atrophy of the frontal and temporal lobes. A subcortical type of dementia can be seen in advanced cases of multiple sclerosis but the history would be totally different from that given for this patient. The scenario could fit presentation with an AIDS-defining illness but the question does not mention any risk factors for HIV infection.

16) c.

Crocodile tears, or facial synkinesis, is a syndrome of 7th cranial nerve misrouting upon recovery from a facial nerve palsy. The net result is ipsilateral lacrimation in response to normal facial movement stimuli (like eating).

17) a.

Porphyria cutanea tarda is not associated with neurological dysfunction. Acute intermittent porphyria is associated with motor and autonomic neuropathy during attacks.

18) a.

The presence of even a single neutrophil in the CSF is inconsistent with a diagnosis of Guillain–Barré syndrome. In this syndrome, the CSF white cell count is minimally elevated (or normal) and is lymphocytic. The CSF protein may be markedly elevated, but it can also be normal or minimally raised in the first week. The demyelinating process may not produce any detectable abnormalities during neurophysiological studies in the first week. After the end of that week, however, signs of demyelination appear (e.g. conduction slowing and block, dispersion of compound muscle action potential and prolonged distal latencies). The disease is symmetrical. Slight asymmetry may be encountered in 9% of cases; strict unilateral signs are totally incompatible with the diagnosis. Bilateral facial weakness is seen in around 50% of cases.

19) c.

The clinical scenario fits pure ocular myasthenia (the disease should be limited to the eye muscles for at least 2 years, with no involvement of facial, bulbar and limb muscles). Pure ocular myasthenia is one of the contraindications of thymectomy. Pupillary reactivity is *intact* in myasthenia gravis. There is no involvement of trunk muscles or the diaphragm. Antiacetylcholine receptor antibodies are positive in around 50% of pure ocular myasthenia (while they are positive in 80–85% of generalized myasthenia). Brain MRI is always *normal*.

20) b.

Apart from uni- or bi-lateral abducens palsy, the presence of any focal or lateralizing sign should question the diagnosis. Florid papilloedema is seen in about 95% of cases of idiopathic pseudotumour cerebri at the time of diagnosis, with enlargement of the physiological blind spot and later development of peripheral visual field constriction. Bilateral central scotomas with bilateral disc swelling would point to papillitis. Left-sided abducens palsy is a false localizing sign; it results in double vision. The trigeminal nerve and central midbrain sensory pathways should be intact.

21) c.

In Charcot–Marie–Tooth disease (CMT) ankle jerks are lost; exaggerated ankles rule out this diagnosis. CMT is one of the differential diagnoses of bilateral hand wasting. Achilles tendon contracture responds well to tenotomy. A high stepping gate is seen because of bilateral foot drop. 'Inverted champagne bottle' legs (also called stork legs) are seen in advanced cases; the wasting stops suddenly at the mid-thighs.

22) d.

In fascioscapulohumeral dystrophy hand muscles are preserved. In motor neurone disease there is a mixture of upper and lower motor neurone signs and intact sensation. With bilateral cervical ribs there may be vascular manifestations (e.g. Raynaud's phenomenon and embolic features) as well as hand wasting. Advanced cases of syringomyelia with bilateral Horner's syndrome may also show a cape-like distribution of dissociated sensory loss. In cervical spondylosis there is also neck or occipital pain radiating to the shoulders and down the arms.

23) d.

The deep tendon reflexes are *hypoactive* in LEMS, but with repetitive tapping, improvement occurs (the EMG is similar to botulism; a decremental EMG response is seen in myasthenia gravis). The exaggerated reflexes indicate a different diagnosis. The P/Q type of serum antivoltage gated calcium channel antibody is highly sensitive and specific for LEMS of any aetiology. In LEMS, dry mouth and impotence result from autonomic dysfunction.

24) c.

'Inverted champagne bottle' legs are seen in advanced Charcot–Marie–Tooth disease. Skeletal manifestations are common in syringobulbia. The dissociated sensory loss in syringobulbia involves the face in an onion-skin pattern with vertigo and wasting of the tongue.

25) c.

In right-sided INO, the right globe adduction (i.e. medial rectus action) is impaired when the patient is asked to look to the left. The left eye is 'disconnected' from the right during this horizontal gaze and will have 'ataxic' nystagmus. The reverse is seen in left INO. Bilateral INO is highly suggestive of multiple sclerosis. INO in the elderly is seen with brainstem strokes and tumours.

26) b.

Acoustic neuroma accounts for 80–85% of cases of cerebellopontine angle masses. The tumour arises from the neurilemmal sheath of the vestibular portion of the 8th cranial nerve in the internal auditory canal. It is usually a sporadic tumour and occurs as an isolated lesion in those between 30 and 50 years of age; bilateral tumours are the hallmark of neurofibromatosis type II.

27) d.

An atrophied fasciculated tongue is seen in bulbar palsy together with nasal speech and loss of gag reflex. A conical tongue indicates spastic tongue that is not atrophied; a sign of pseudobulbar palsy. Donald duck speech is thick, laboured, indistinct speech, as if the patient is trying to speak from the back of the mouth; a sign of pseudobulbar palsy. Exaggerated jaw jerk results from degeneration of the corticonuclear fibres; a sign of pseudobulbar palsy. Emotional lability is the classical pseudobulbar affect.

28) d.

Cauda equina syndrome involves damage to a variable combination of the lumbosacral nerve roots. The clinical findings are bizarre, bilateral and asymmetric, and involve lower motor neurone signs, sensory deficits and sphincteric changes. Upper motor neurone signs would suggest involvement of the lower spinal cord segments (conus medullaris).

29) a.

Carbamazepine and phenytoin appear to exacerbate myoclonic jerks and petit mal seizures. Valproic acid is a broad-spectrum antiepileptic and is useful in the treatment of patients with more than one type of seizure (as in juvenile myoclonic epilepsy, where patients may have additional generalized seizures).

30) c.

Frontal lobe seizures usually have midline movements (e.g. bicycling or pelvic thrusting), a very short postictal phase and very minor EEG changes that might well escape detection; this type of seizure is the most important differential diagnosis of pseudoseizures. Petit mal seizures and complex partial status epilepticus have no gross involuntary movements. The scenario is inconsistent with Salaam attacks (sudden flexion or extension of the trunk that is usually seen in infants) and tardive dyskinesia (continuous involuntary purposeless movements that usually target the face and tongue in those receiving dopamine depleting agents).

31) a.

The differential diagnosis of a grossly bloody CSF is between traumatic tap and subarachnoid bleed. Detection of xanthochromia is one of the differentiating methods; the enzymatic degradation of the CSF RBCs will convert haemoglobin to bilirubin in situ and the supernatant fluid will be yellow–white; it is clear following traumatic CSF tapping. Xanthochromia takes 8–12 hours to appear after the ictus, peaks within 2–4 days and disappears after 2–3 weeks.

32) a.

Carbamazepine is the first-line agent in idiopathic trigeminal neuralgia. Brief lancinating neuropathic pains respond well to it. Aspirin is used in ischaemic strokes; donepezil in mild Alzheimer disease; nimodepine to prevent cerebral vasospasm following subarachnoid haemorrhage; and riluzole confers a modest survival benefit in motor neurone disease.

33) c.

The temporal profile, the patterned weakness and the neurophysiological studies are consistent with chronic inflammatory demyelinating polyradiculopathy. The following are well-documented features but are clinically uncommon: dysarthria (9%), dysphagia (9%), impotence (4%) and incontinence (2%). Most of these patients respond to glucocorticoids, plasmapharesis or intravenous immunoglobulins. In Guillain–Barré disease there is acute/subacute motor weakness, which does not exceed 6 months, and no sensory signs. Diphtheritic neuropathy is a pure peripheral demyelinating motor neuropathy. Acute intermittent porphyria is an acute peripheral motor neuropathy with autonomic dysfunction, seizures, psychosis and abdominal pain. Features of Charcot–Marie–Tooth disease are many years of foot weakness and wasting, foot drop, pes cavus and stork-like (inverted champagne bottle) legs.

34) b.

The optokinetic response reflects the ability to perceive movements and/or contour, and therefore is useful to detect visual perception in newborns and in psychogenic blindness. This woman had unilateral impairment of this reflex and this indicates a pathology affecting the parietal lobe. She needs brain imaging.

35) b.

The centre controlling vertical gaze lies in the midbrain, while that governing horizontal eye movements and gaze lies in the pons. Down-beating nystagmus is seen with lesions at the level of the foramen magnum.

36) c.

In normal pressure hydrocephalus there is normal intracranial pressure and no papilloedema. It is thought to result from intermittent impairment of the CSF absorption at the level of arachnoid granulations. Hypercapnia results in intracranial vasodilatation with increased blood flow and pressure. Parietal glioblastoma multiforme is an aggressive malignancy that acts as a space-occupying lesion, raising the intracranial pressure. Methanol intoxication causes bilateral optic neuritis with gradual atrophy. Malignant hypertension causes grade IV hypertensive retinal changes.

37) d.

Right-sided facial palsy should cast doubt on the diagnosis. Some patients with Wernicke's encephalopathy may have hypothermia, hypotension and lost ankle jerks (from associated peripheral neuropathy). Nystagmus is very common, and some degree of nystagmus may persist after recovery. Mild anisocoria and subtle pupillary abnormalities are occasionally seen. Global confusion is seen with prominent disorder of immediate recall and recent memory. Progression to frank coma is uncommon. Combined horizontal and vertical gaze palsies or isolated horizontal gaze palsy are seen. There is left-sided or bilateral abducens palsy. Note that ataxia is primarily of gait but limb ataxia is uncommon, as is dysarthria.

38) d.

A classical MRCP question concerns the differentiation of early Alzheimer's disease and depressive pseudodementia; however, they may coexist! The presence of prominent vegetative symptoms (e.g. abnormalities in weight, appetite, sleep, sexual drive) is strongly associated with depressive pseudodementia. There is a more or less *abrupt* onset in depressive pseudodementia, with a *plateauing* of dysfunction. A personal and/or family history of depression may be seen in depressive pseudodementia, and neurological examination should be *normal*. The demented patient is typically unaware of the deficit and does not complain of memory loss; actually he denies such a thing and is cooperative when examined. The depressive patient is aware of the deficit, and may even exaggerate his complaints, and admits to having poor concentration and memory; he is usually uncooperative with the examiner, has many somatic complaints and hypochondriasis is common.

39) e.

Transient global amnesia is a primary disorder of short-term memory that lasts for minutes to days (usually a few hours), and is typically seen in middle-aged or elderly people with diffuse atherosclerosis and a past history of ischaemic stroke (usually in the posterior circulation). The patient cannot form new memories (which accounts for this patient's repetitive questions); however, personal indentity, remote memory and registration are well preserved. Patients with Korsakoff's amnesic psychosis have difficulty in forming and storing new memories, but long-term ones are intact. They may confabulate, but they do not forget their 'house' or the street where they live. Amnesic types of strokes are usually devastating and involve both inferiomedial parts of the temporal lobes with occlusion of both posterior cerebral arteries. Dissociative amnesia has a characteristic isolated or disproportionate amnesia of traumatic or stressful personal events. Despite a patient's apparent distress and disorientation to person, orientation to place and time is usually well preserved. Post-traumatic amnesia may have some degree of retrograde amnesia and is one of the differential diagnoses of transient global amnesia. The question, however, does not describe or hint at any risk factor for head trauma.

40) d.
Prophylaxis for migraine attacks should be strongly considered if there are three or more attacks per month, highly disabling attacks (regardless of the frequency) and interference with various life aspects (schooling, marriage, job). Tricyclics, valproic acid, beta-blockers and calcium channel blockers are the useful agents.

41) d.
The patient has Foster–Kennedy syndrome with a frontal lobe meningioma (an anterior fossa mass lesion with ipsilateral optic atrophy and contralateral optic nerve head swelling). The imaging study describes a benign meningioma (note the scarce brain oedema and the diffuse homogeneous contrast intake).

42) c.
This man has asymptomatic carotid artery stenosis and bruit. Carotid bruit is present in 7% of normal healthy individuals over the age of 65 years, while carotid duplex/Doppler study detects carotid stenosis in up to 30% of those older than 70 years. Asymptomatic carotid artery stenosis has a 2.5% annual risk of ipsilateral stroke, and a lower risk of contralateral stroke, but a higher risk of myocardial infarction. The best approach for asymptomatic carotid artery stenosis is aspirin.

43) b.
Up to 50% of patients with Wilson's disease will have some degree of worsening following initiation of penicillamine therapy. This should always be kept in mind, especially when treating severe cases. This is usually followed by gradual improvement over the next few months.

44) a.
The scenario most likely describes an early and mild ischaemic stroke (rather than a TIA). It does not mention any speech or sensory deficits, and a pure motor lacunar stroke syndrome would fit the picture. The

mild deficit is an exclusion criterion for the use of thrombolytic therapy. Although ACE inhibitors are the preferred antihypertensive medication in diabetic patients, they are not the first choice in this patient who presents with stroke (but an ACE inhibitor should be given after *starting* aspirin). Aspirin has been shown to prevent stroke recurrence and to improve mortality.

45) e.
Upper motor neurone signs are totally incompatible with idiopathic Parkinson's disease. They are common in other degenerative disease associated with parkinsonism (e.g. supranuclear palsy). In Parkinson's disease the signs are usually asymmetrical to start with, and then become bilateral after months or years. A symmetrical presentation should point to parkinsonism rather than Parkinson's disease. Jaw tremor interferes with eating. Head tremor or titubation is seen in essential tremor. Blepharospasm as well as blepharoclonus are seen. Depression is common and usually complicates the presentation and treatment options.

46) c.
Recurrent abscesses at an abnormal site and by an abnormal organism should prompt consideration of self-inflicted injury with deliberate contamination with faeces. Munchausen's syndrome, a form of factitious disorders, is named after the German Baron von Munchausen who was legendary for his inventive lying. The patient fabricates a highly typical and believable history and the presentation usually directs the inexperienced physician to proceed with complicated investigations and even highly invasive surgery. The treatment is notoriously ineffective, but recognition is vital to avoid invasive investigations and consumption of resources. Differentiation between somatization disorders, conversion disorders and factitious disorders are important examination themes.

47) c.
The description is typical of a dependent type of personality. The traits of personality disorder are exaggerations of characteristics that are recognized in many normal members of society. The aetiology is still unclear, but many individuals come from deprived families and may have been subjected to physical and psychological abuse during childhood. Personality changes are a common examination theme.

48) c.
Five to 10% of anorexia nervosa patients are male. Loss of sexual drive and interest replaces the female's amenorrhea as a diagnostic criterion. One of the most important features is the striking indifference to the weight loss and denial of problems.

49) c.
In bulimic patients there is metabolic alkalosis from continuous loss of acid in the vomitus. Metabolic acidosis would suggest another diagnosis

or a coexistent pathology. The low serum potassium may produce cardiac arrhythmia, muscle weakness and ileus. Normal weight can be seen in bulimic patients, unlike in anorexia nervosa patients. There is regular menses, while amenorrhea is the rule in anorexia nervosa. Erosion of dental enamel results from recurrent exposure to the decalcifying effect of gastric acid.

50) c.

Sudden and profound loss of self-identity and family details is highly characteristic of hysterical amnesia. The patient presents dramatically and the memory loss is patchy and inconsistent. Such a degree and mode of amnesia is rarely seen in organic brain diseases unless there is a coexistent gross dementia.

51) c.

This man fits the definition of agoraphobia. Explanation and reassurance is the mainstay in the management of all types of anxiety disorders. Medications have a limited role. Those who do not respond to reassurance should try relaxation techniques and treatment may be accompanied by gradual exposure or flooding under specialized supervision.

52) a.

This woman is likely to have a major depression. Electroconvulsive therapy (ECT) is usually safe and side effects are mild. Headache is the commonest complaint and some degree of anterograde and retrograde amnesia is frequent. Indications for ECT are depressive stupor, failure of medical therapy (or when antidepressants are contraindicated, unsafe or intolerable), severe malnutrition and attempted suicide. Up to 12 applications may be needed to produce an optimal result. The duration of the depressive illness per se is not an indication for ECT.

53) e.

Poor prognostic factors for schizophrenia are insidious onset of symptoms, no clear-cut precipitating factor, no affective symptoms, no catatonic features, positive family history of the same illness, schizoid premorbid personality, poor work and school record, and highly emotional family environment. Good prognostic factors are the opposite of these.

54) c.

Auditory hallucinations are part of the Schneider's first rank symptoms of schizophrenia, which are mainly seen during acute illness. Negative symptoms dominate chronic fluctuating cases and are usually more difficult to treat. The patient generally appears apathetic, avoids social interaction, and loses interest in himself and other people, and his mood is dull and monotonus and lacks the day–day variation. The patient's speech is sparse, and his/her answers are empty. Poverty of speech reflects poverty of thinking.

55) c.

Risk factors for committing suicide after a suicidal attempt are living alone, being divorced, widowed or recently separated, unemployment, male gender, having a chronic illness or cancer, illicit drug abuse, including alcohol abuse, age over 45 years, using a violent method (like hanging) and writing a suicide note, and previous attempts; marriage is protective!

56) d.

Affective symptoms appear by the third postnatal day in around 50% of women, peak on the fifth day, and gradually disappear within the next 10 days. They are distressing, and apart from careful reassurance and explanation, need no treatment. Postnatal blues do not predispose to major depression.

57) b.

Trans-sexualism is a form of gender identity disorder. The patient should be referred to specialized clinics and may receive hormonal therapy to develop secondary sexual characteristics of the opposite sex. Surgical reshaping of the external genitalia can be performed if the individual successfully adapts to the lifestyle of the opposite sex for at least 1 year. Transvestism is a sexual arousal brought about by wearing clothes of the opposite sex; paedophilia is sexual arousal with children; exhibitionism is genital exposure in public.

58) c.

The woman is preoccupied that she has a 'disease' infesting her body; note that she is not much concerned about the pruritis itself. This is hypochondriasis. Hypochondriasis is common in anxiety and depressive disorders but sometimes presents as a primary phenomenon with a long history. It is usually unresponsive to treatment.

59) a.

Somatization disorder is a chronic illness that is almost always seen in females, usually older than 30 years of age. Patients present with recurrent somatic complaints (symptoms, usually painful ones) in many organ systems, which require medical attention but are usually unresponsive to treatment. Somatization disorder is usually mistaken for hysterical conversion disorder.

60) c.

Korsakoff's syndrome (and Wernicke's encephalopathy) results from vitamin B_1 deficiency of any aetiology; usually alcoholism, malabsorption, hyperemesis gravidarum and malnutrition of malignancy, as well as the effect of chemotherapy and radiotherapy on appetite and bowel function. This patient denies his illness by reassuring the examining physician that nothing is wrong with him. Cases that follow one or more attacks of Wernicke's encephalopathy usually have minor nystagmus and gait ataxia as residual signs, and peripheral neuropathy (with lost ankles) can also be present.

61) d.

The question addresses the acute/subacute causes of lower limb weakness. Becker's muscular dystrophy is a slowly progressive process over many years. Rapidly progressive weakness may result from the muscle itself (as in acute polymyositis or rhabdomyolysis), motor endplate diseases (myasthenia gravis crisis, botulism), diseases of the peripheral nerves and roots (Guillain–Barré, disc prolapse with cauda equina compression, toxic neuropathy) and diseases of the spinal cord and brain (stroke, transverse myelitis).

62) d.

The duration of the illness and the distribution of the tremor are highly consistent with benign essential tremor. Such duration without further signs or progressive disability is against early-onset Parkinson's disease. Wilson's disease would have produced prominent neurological signs and hepatic dysfunction over this length of time. While head tremor and symmetrical presentation are against Parkinson's disease, jaw tremor and unilateral signs at presentation are highly consistent with it. Differentiation between Parkinson's disease and essential tremor is a common topic in the MRCP examination.

63) c.

Psychogenic syncope is a differential diagnosis of any transient loss of consciousness. It may occur as part of a somatoform disorder (somatization and conversion reaction), malingering or even in schizophrenics (catatonic type). Neurological examination during the period of unresponsiveness is normal with flexor plantar responses. Patients usually retain some degree of muscle tone in their eyelids during passive eye opening (unlike in organic causes, where there is incomplete and somewhat asymmetric eye closure after passive opening of the flaccid eyelids by the examiner).

64) d.

There are many potential sources of error when performing a visual field examination. Papilloedema would result in enlargement of the physiological blind spot and constriction of the peripheral field. Ptosis, even if mild, can result in suppression of the upper visual field. An uncorrected refractive error, even a 1D error, can result in significant reduction of central visual thresholds. Lens opacity has a profound effect on the visual field, especially when the pupil is also small. Miosis easily gives rise to visual field constriction; pupils < 3 mm should be dilated prior to formal perimetry examination.

65) b.

Age-related macular degeneration (ARMD) is the leading cause of severe irreversible visual loss in the western hemisphere in individuals older than

60 years. Drusen is the earliest clinically detectable feature of ARMD, with asymptomatic yellowish excrescences appearing beneath the retinal pigment epithelium and distributed symmetrically at both posterior poles. They are of four types: hard, soft, basal laminal and calcified drusen.

66) e.
Retinitis pigmentosa is progressive loss of photoreceptor and retinal pigment epithelial function. Although both cons and rods are involved, damage to the rod system is predominant. The autosomal dominant form is the commonest (45% of cases) and carries the best prognosis. The atypical forms usually have many systemic associations, like abetalipoproteinaemia, Laurence–Moon and Bardet–Biedl syndromes, and Friedreich's ataxia.

67) b.
Neovascular, or 100-day, glaucoma occurs around 3 months after central retinal vein occlusion in 50% of cases because of the diffuse retinal ischaemia and release of angiogenesis factors. This will result in rubeosis iridis and secondary glaucoma; the globe is blind and painful. CRVO is associated with chronic simple glaucoma on the one hand and results in secondary vascular glaucoma on the other.

68) b.
These Lisch nodules are pigmented iris hamartomas and they are neither premalignant nor predictors of the development of optic nerve glioma. They are part of the diagnostic criteria of neurofibromatosis type I (two or more in number); therefore, where this diagnosis is suspected (e.g. presence of axillary freckling), patients should have their eyes examined carefully for these lesions. Although they might be multiple, they almost never affect vision. In pale eyes, and especially when multiple, they can be seen with the aid of indirect ophthalmoscope. They can be detected in <10% of young children; this figure rises to at least 90% in adults.

69) e.
This boy has Marfan's syndrome, which has many abnormalities. The best known is upward lens dislocation. Other eye findings are flat cornea (or rarely keratoconus), blue sclera, hypoplasia of dilator papillae (this would make pupillary dilatation difficult), iris tremor (iridodenesis), spherical small lens and the susceptibility to rental detachment. Patients may develop glaucoma. Snow-flake cataract is characteristically seen in poorly controlled Type I diabetes mellitus.

70) c.
All diabetic patients should be referred to an ophthalmologist whenever there is sight-threatening retinopathy (i.e. proliferative retinopathy, pre-proliferative retinopathy and background retinopathy with macular involvement–as in this patient). Signs of the pre-proliferative stage are venous beads and loops and intraretinal microvascular abnormalities (IRMA), as well as multiple cotton wool (soft) exudates and blot

haemorrhages. Capillary tufts (on the disc or elsewhere) mark the proliferative stage and the patient should be referred urgently to an ophthalmologist. Note that diabetic patients have a higher risk of ocular infections, cataract formation, development of simple chronic glaucoma and central retinal artery and vein occlusions. Referral for pars plana vitrectomy would be totally unreasonable; complicated pars plana vitrectomy is used in advanced diabetic eye disease.

8. Rheumatology and diseases of bones and collagen: Questions

1) A 43-year-old woman with rheumatoid arthritis visits for a scheduled follow-up. Plain X-ray of the hands reveals marginal erosions at the metacarpal heads. Why are these erosions marginal?

   a. Random localization
   b. Plain X-rays fail to show central erosions
   c. Rotation of the film
   d. Marginal joint area is devoid of overlying cartilage
   e. Presence of sesamoid bones

2) A 61-year-old man with limited small cell lung cancer presents with diffuse bone pain. He is receiving chemotherapy and radiotherapy. His serum alkaline phosphatase is elevated with otherwise normal liver function testing. X-rays of many bony sites look normal. What would you do?

   a. Repeat skeletal survey using plain X-rays
   b. MRI of the entire spine
   c. Radioisotope bone scanning
   d. Do serum phosphate
   e. Brain CT scan

3) A 52-year-old woman with rheumatoid arthritis has normochromic anaemia, leucocytosis, thrombocytosis and raised ESR, with increased joint pain, stiffness, fever and anorexia. She has a flare-up of her disease. Which one of the following is *not* a positive acute phase reactant?

   a. Serum ceruloplasmin
   b. Serum iron
   c. Serum amyloid A
   d. α_1-Antitrypsin
   e. Serum complements

4) A 27-year-old woman with a history of two attacks of below-knee DVT presents because of recurrent abortion. She is not taking heparin. Her aPTT is 95 seconds and this does not correct following the addition of platelet-free plasma. Platelets count is 40×10^9/L. What is the cause of the abnormal aPTT test?

   a. β_2-Glycoprotein I antibodies
   b. ANA
   c. IgA anticardiolipin antibodies
   d. False-positive VDRL
   e. Lupus anticoagulant

5) A 34-year-old woman is given a diagnosis of primary antiphospho-lipid syndrome. Which one of the following is *not* consistent with that diagnosis?

a. Subungual splinter haemorrhages
b. Amaurosis fugax
c. Cushingoid habitus
d. Thrombocytopenia
e. Intrapulmonary haemorrhage

6) A 50-year-old woman is referred from the orthopaedic department for further evaluation. Following a minor fall to the ground, she sustained a bilateral Colle's fracture. Which one of the following is indicated?

a. DEXA scan
b. Myeloma screen
c. Plain X-rays of the pelvis
d. Bone scan
e. MRI of the femoral bones

7) A 61-year-old woman has undergone DEXA scanning because of right femoral neck fracture. The result suggests osteoporosis. What is her score?

a. T-score–2.0
b. Z-score–1.1
c. T-score–1.0
d. Z-score–2.3
e. T-score–2.7

8) A 13-year-old boy presents with an acutely painful, red, tender and swollen left knee joint. He denies local trauma and there is no notable history of bleeding tendency. What would you do?

a. Plain X-ray of the joint
b. MRI with contrast of the joint
c. Complete blood count
d. Blood culture
e. Joint aspiration

9) A 34-year-old man presents with a 4-month history of right knee joint swelling and pain. The joint is tender on movement. Which one of the following is *not* implicated as a cause of this joint problem?

   a. Crohn's disease
   b. Chronic fibrosing sarcoidosis
   c. Pyogenic arthritis
   d. Synovial sarcoma
   e. Rheumatoid arthritis

10) A 34-year-old man presents with pain in the lower lateral aspect of the arm. He states that the pain also radiates to the back of his forearm. You examine the patient and find that the pain is reproducible upon resisted active forearm extension. What does the man have?

    a. Golfer's elbow
    b. Bicipital tendinitis
    c. Colle's fracture
    d. Tennis elbow
    e. Olecranon bursitis

11) A male patient is referred from the general medical ward because of back pain. You interview and examine him and find that the pain is not a simple mechanical one. Which one of the following signs is *not* a 'red flag' in patients with back pain?

    a. Weight loss
    b. Dorsal spine pain
    c. Saddle anaesthesia
    d. Age 20–55 years
    e. Relentless pain unrelieved by rest

12) A 12-year-old boy presents with progressive kyphosis. The boy denies pain or systemic symptoms and his bloods are within their normal reference range. Plain X-rays of the thoracic vertebrae reveal irregular ossification of their endplates. There is no family history of note. Apart from kyphosis, his examination is unremarkable. The surgeon dismisses the idea of corrective surgery. What is the diagnosis?

    a. Tuberculous spondylitis
    b. Neurofibromatosis
    c. Osteoporosis
    d. Diffuse idiopathic skeletal hyperostosis
    e. Sheuermann's osteochondritis

13) A 45-year-old man with newly diagnosed rheumatoid arthritis presents with bilateral pitting leg oedema. His diagnosis was secured 9 months ago. He has taken penicillamine tablets since then to control the disease activity and he is doing well. His urine shows 4+ protein. Cardiac examination is unremarkable as is his chest X-ray. What is the likely cause of this man's current complaint?

a. Constrictive pericarditis
b. Secondary AA amyloidosis
c. UTI
d. Penicillamine-associated nephrotic syndrome
e. Renal vasculitis

14) A 53-year-old woman presents for a scheduled follow-up. She has rheumatoid arthritis for which gold injections have been prescribed for the past 8 months. Systemic review reveals morning joint pains, stiffness and painful movements involving both hands and feet; these symptoms have not changed since the last visit 3 months ago. What should you do?

a. Double the dose of gold injections
b. Halve the dose of gold injections
c. Stop gold injections
d. Add sulfasalazine
e. Do not change current regimen

15) A 34-year-old woman presents with flare-up of her rheumatoid arthritis in terms of joint stiffness, pain and swelling, during the second trimester of pregnancy. She takes no medications for the time being. What is the best treatment?

a. Methrotrexate
b. Cyclophosphamide
c. Prednisolone
d. Sulfasalazine
e. Hydroxychloroquine

16) A 62-year-old woman presents because of bilateral knee pain. She says that her pain is localized to the medial knee aspects and upper tibia, and going up- or down-stairs makes the pain worse and localizes it to the anterior knee. However, she has noticed that her posterior knee aspects are also painful. Plain knee X-ray confirms osteoarthritis. What is the cause of the back knee pain?

a. Osteophyte compression of the posterior tibial nerve
b. DVT
c. Baker's cyst
d. Lumbar canal stenosis
e. Adductor tendinitis

17) A 21-year old man presents to the rheumatology clinic with right knee pain and swelling. He is systemically well, he denies taking drugs or drinking alcohol and there is no family history of note. Plain X-ray of the area shows knee-joint space narrowing, marginal osteophytes and subchondral bony sclerosis. What is the likely cause for this young man's presentation?

a. Alkaptonuria
b. Haemochromatosis
c. Marfan's syndrome
d. Previous knee-joint trauma
e. Charcot's joint

18) A 54-year-old man presents with inflammatory polyarticular arthritis that is found to be due to rheumatoid arthritis. Which one of the following is true with respect to this disease?

a. It is a rare cause of inflammatory arthritis
b. More common in males
c. Atrophy of the synovial membrane is common
d. Rheumatoid nodules are not seen outside the skin area
e. No laboratory test is diagnostic

19) A 37-year-old female patient with rheumatoid arthritis attends for a follow-up. You examine the patient and arrange for blood and urine tests. The radiology department is going to X-ray her. Which one of the following is *not* an expected finding in this patient?

a. Dry eyes and tongue
b. Recurrent syncope
c. Spastic quadriparesis
d. Active urinary sediment
e. Bilateral Colle's fracture

20) A 54-year-old woman with seronegative rheumatoid arthritis is examined because of fatigue. She has anaemia and neutropenia. Her referring GP considers a diagnosis of Felty's syndrome. However, you reject this diagnosis because of which one of the following?

a. Generalized hyperpigmentaion
b. Abnormal liver function tests
c. Leg ulcers
d. Deforming disease
e. Negative rheumatoid factor

21) A 32-year-old man presents with a 6-month history of morning low back stiffness and pain that improves with activity. He has tenderness of both sacroiliac joints. His clinical features and X-rays are consistent with ankylosing spondylitis. Which one of the following is *not* an expected finding in patients with long-term ankylosing spondylitis?

a. Diastolic murmur down the left lower sternal border
b. Biapical lung crackles
c. Bilateral pitting led oedema
d. Visual blurring
e. Cervical lymphadenopathy

22) A 31-year-old patient with ankylosing spondylitis presents with chest pain. His description of the pain is consistent with pleuritic pain, and it is exacerbated by deep breathing. He is not taking his medications because of gastric upset, although his back pain and stiffness are unchanged. What is the cause of this chest pain?

a. Pulmonary tuberculosis
b. Rib fracture
c. Involvement of the costovertebral joints
d. Acute pericarditis
e. Occult chest trauma

23) A 32-year-old man presents with right knee and hip pain and swelling three weeks after having unprotected sex with a woman. He has hyperkeratotic lesions on both solar aspects of the feet, buccal ulcers and superficial erosions on the glans. Which one of the following is *not* seen in this disease?

a. Raised serum C-reactive protein
b. Seizures
c. Foot drop
d. Dropped beats
e. Diarrhoea

24) A 32-year-old man was given a diagnosis of ankylosing spondylitis 3 months ago because of low back pain and morning stiffness. He presents today for a general check-up. During examination you find something that refutes the diagnosis. Which one of the following have you found?

a. Limitation of the lumbar lordosis upon forward flexion
b. Tenderness of both sacroiliac joints
c. Distal interphalangeal joints arthritis
d. Anterior uveitis
e. Bradycardia

25) A GP refers a 49-year-old man to you for further evaluation of his raised serum uric acid. He takes many daily medications to control his diseases. Which one of the following is *not* a recognized cause of hyperuricaemia?

a. Ciclosporin
b. Pyrazinamide
c. Bendroflumethiazide
d. Low-dose aspirin
e. Losartan

26) A 63-year-old woman with long-standing hypertension presents with sudden painful swelling of the left knee joint. Joint aspiration reveals a cloudy fluid full of needle-shaped crystals which are negatively birefringent. What is the likely cause of this woman's monoarthritis?

a. *Staph. aureus*
b. Trauma
c. Hydrochlorothiazide
d. Calcium pyrophosphate dihydrate crystals
e. Rheumatoid arthritis

27) A 16-year-old girl presents with rapid onset of pain and redness over the first metatarsophalangeal joint of the left forefoot. She is reasonably well and healthy, and she denies taking drugs or drinking alcohol. She has never had sex. Her blood urea nitrogen and serum creatinine are within their normal reference range, but her serum uric acid is high. What is your reason for suspecting an enzymatic defect as a cause of this hyperuricaemia?

a. Site of the arthritis
b. Presence of tophi
c. Normal blood pressure
d. Patient's age
e. Rapidity of onset

28) A 66-year-old man with chronic renal failure presents with sudden painful swelling of his right ankle joint, aspiration of which confirms acute gouty arthritis. What is the best treatment?

a. Indometacin
b. Ciclosporin
c. Colchicine
d. Aspirin
e. Joint aspiration and intra-articular steroid injection

29) A 53-year-old uraemic woman has recurrent severe attacks of gouty arthritis and is being considered for receiving secondary prophylactic medication against these attacks. She has renal osteodystrophy for which she takes vitamin D metabolite and calcium, and her blood pressure is reasonably controlled with amlodipine and atenolol. Your senior house officer is considering probenecid but you do not support the use of this medication because of:

a. Gender of the patient
b. Her hypertension
c. Bone disease
d. Chronic renal failure
e. Oral calcium

30) A 29-year-old man presents with acute left ankle arthritis. Joint X-ray of that area is unremarkable. Aspiration of the left ankle reveals many rhomboid-shaped weakly positive birefringent crystals. He states that he is healthy, does not take drugs and his entire family is OK as far as he knows. He smokes five cigarettes a day and drinks alcohol at weekends. His past history reveals childhood supracondylar fracture of the right humerus. You are planning further investigations to explore his radiological finding because of:

a. His past fracture history
b. Smoking
c. Site of the fracture
d. Patient's age
e. His negative family history

31) A 31-year-old woman with SLE states that she feels well in terms of her hand pains but her facial rash is only slowly resolving. She denies chest pain or fever. Her ESR is raised as is her serum C-reactive protein (CRP). What does the result of the patient's CRP test imply?

a. Renal involvement
b. Risk of mononeuritis multiplex
c. Poor long-term prognosis
d. Coexistent infection
e. CNS complications

32) A 27-year-old woman with recently diagnosed SLE presents with a photosensitive rash and widespread arthralgia. What is best way to treat her complaints?

a. High-dose oral prednisolone
b. Azathioprine
c. Ciclosporin
d. Hydroxychloroquine
e. Diclofenac

33) A 51-year-old man presents with a 1-month history of bilateral hand and foot pain, and morning stiffness. There are many small non-tender nodules on the extensor surfaces of both forearms. Plain X-rays of the hands reveal periarticular osteoporosis and marginal erosions in the metacarpophalangeal and proximal interphalangeal joints. Testing for rheumatoid factor is positive. Which one of the following antibodies is useful to solidify the diagnosis of rheumatoid arthritis?

a. ANA
b. Anti-dsDNA
c. Anti-CCP
d. Anti-RNP
e. Antihistone

34) A 37-year-old woman with a 10-year history of well-controlled SLE presents with fatigue. She has difficulties with daily activities and she can no longer manage to do the shopping. Neurological examination is unremarkable. Her bloods are relatively normal. How would you improve her fatigue?

a. Increase dose of daily steroid
b. Add tacrolimus
c. Graded exercise therapy
d. Interferon-α
e. Refer her to a psychiatrist

35) A 55-year-old woman with diffuse systemic sclerosis presents for follow-up. Which one of the following is *not* an expected finding in this woman?

a. Recurrent upper GIT haemorrhage
b. Primary pulmonary hypertension
c. Flexor tenosynovitis
d. Renal impairment
e. Raynaud's phenomenon

36) A 52-year-old woman presents with extensive dental carries, dry mouth and a gritty sensation in both eyes with mucosal threads on the cornea, symptoms she has had for the past few years. Shirmer's test is positive. What is the mainstay of treatment?

a. Oral prednisolone
b. Pulse cyclophosphamide
c. Infliximab infusion
d. Plasma exchange
e. Artificial lubrication

37) A 63-year-old woman is referred to you for further evaluation of adult polymyositis. However, while examining the patient, you detect something that refutes this diagnosis. What have you detected?

a. Proximal weakness
b. Tender muscles
c. Fever
d. Intact deep tendon reflexes
e. Gottron's papules

38) A 65-year-old woman presents with fever, weight loss and proximal stiffness in the shoulder girdle, neck, and pelvic muscles. Her ESR is raised and there is normochromic anaemia, elevated serum alkaline phosphatase and raised serum creatine kinase. She responds to high-dose oral prednisolone. You suspect polymyalgia rheumatica. Which one of the following would suggest an alternative diagnosis?

a. Elevated serum alkaline phosphatase
b. The distribution of the stiffness
c. Age of the patient
d. Raised serum creatine kinase
e. Weight loss

39) A 63-year-old man presents with throbbing headache, fever, anorexia and weight loss. His ESR is 86 mm/hour. You are considering giant cell temporal arteritis. However, you find something that questions your provisional diagnosis. What have you found?

a. Pale swelling of the right optic nerve head
b. Jaw pain upon chewing
c. Intact knee reflexes
d. Altitudinal visual field defect in the left eye
e. Livedo reticularis over both thighs

40) A 7-year-old boy presents with features that are suggestive of Kawasaki disease. You conduct a through clinical examination and are about to confirm your provisional diagnosis. However, the presence of which one of the following would suggest an alternative diagnosis?

a. Polymorphous exanthema
b. Erythematous soles
c. Acute purulent axillary lymphadenopathy
d. Bilateral conjunctival congestion
e. Erythema of the tongue

41) A 50-year-old man presents with fever, weight loss, palpable purpura and livedo reticularis. There is hypertension and symmetrical sensorimotor peripheral neuropathy. How would you confirm your provisional diagnosis of polyarteritis nodosa?

a. Blood urea and electrolytes
b. Visceral angiography
c. cANCA testing
d. ANA
e. Neutrophil leucocytosis

42) A 64-year-old man presents with bloody nasal discharge, haemoptysis, right-sided proptosis, progressive loss of renal function and palpable purpura. There is leucocytosis and raised ESR. What is the likely diagnosis?

a. Microscopic polyangiitis
b. Wegener's granulomatosis
c. Churg–Straus syndrome
d. Henoch–Schönlein purpura
e. Classic polyarteritis nodosa

43) A 30-year-old Turkish immigrant presents with recurrent oral ulceration, scrotal erosions and erythema nodosum. He has had two attacks of anterior uveitis. Which one of the following is associated with this man's illness?

a. HLA-B27
b. HLA-DR4
c. HLA-A3
d. HLA-B51
e. HLA-B8/-DR3

44) A 67-year-old woman presents for a health check-up. Examination reveals an enlarged skull. Serum alkaline phosphatase is markedly raised with normal liver functions and serum calcium. What is the best option with respect to this woman's treatment?

a. Pamidronate
b. Calcitonin
c. Observation
d. Mitomycin-C
e. Radiotherapy

45) A 49-year-old woman with premature menopause comes to consult the rheumatologist because she read a brochure about osteoporosis. She is short and thin, smokes cigarettes, and drinks alcohol daily. Which one of the following does *not* decrease the risk of vertebral osteoporotic fractures?

a. Risedronate
b. Calcitonin
c. Hormonal replacement therapy
d. Tibolone
e. Raloxifene

46) A 9-year-old male patient is referred by his GP as a difficult to manage case of osteomalacia. He has not responded to high doses of parenteral vitamin D metabolites and calcium. His bloods show low serum calcium, high serum PTH, high serum 1,25(OH) D and raised alkaline phosphatase. What is the likely diagnosis?

a. Chronic renal failure
b. Vitamin D-dependent rickets type II
c. Hypophosphatasia
d. Aluminium toxicity
e. Long-term etidronate therapy

47) A 15-year-old girl is referred for further management of her osteomalacia. Her aunt has the same disease. She is found to have a mutation in the PHEX gene. Besides vitamin D metabolites, which one of the following would you add?

a. Oral calcium
b. Pamidronate
c. Oral phosphate
d. Parenteral calcium
e. Calcitriol

48) A 40-year-old woman presents with diffuse body pain, fatigue, headache, early morning stiffness and non-restorative sleep. Examination reveals many tender points that are consistent with fibromyalgia. Her investigations are normal. Besides graded aerobic exercises, what would you add as part of her treatment plan?

a. Pimoline
b. Amfetamine
c. Amitriptyline
d. Fluoxetine
e. Oestrogen

49) A 19-year-old man presents with poor exercise tolerance. Besides aortic regurgitation, his examination reveals a tall stature with arm span greater than his height, arachnodactyly, hypermobile joints and dorsal spine scoliosis of 30°, as well as upward dislocation of the ocular lens. What is the commonest gene to be mutated in this syndrome?

a. Fibrillin-1
b. Transforming growth factor beta receptor-2
c. Fibrillin-2
d. Transforming growth factor beta receptor-1
e. Marfanin

50) A 15-year-old boy with Ehlers–Danlos syndrome and a positive family history comes to see you. He has hypermobile joints, hyper-extensile skin, easy skin bruising, thin papyrceous skin scars and varicose vein. The overall picture is mild. Which one of the following is the basic defect responsible for type-X Ehlers–Danlos syndrome?

a. Type I collagen
b. Type III collagen
c. Type I procollagen
d. Lysyl hydroxylase
e. Fibronectin

Rheumatology and diseases of bones and collagen: Answers

1) d.

The intra-articular marginal area of the joint is the so-called bare area; the area is devoid of an overlying cartilage. The absence of overlying cartilage will directly expose the bone to the damaging effects of the inflammatory synovium and pannus. These erosions are not accompanied by periosteal reaction or new bone formation, resulting in atrophic non-proliferative bony erosions (unlike the proliferative ones in seronegative arthritides). Gradually, these erosions will march centrally to strip off the cartilage; joint space narrowing is therefore a late finding. The asymmetric marginal erosions of chronic tophaceous gout result from the pressure necrosis effect of intra- and extra-articular tophaceous deposits.

2) c.

The scenario is suggestive of skeletal metastases; however, his plain X-rays look normal. Isotope bone scanning using ^{99m}Tc-bisphosphonate will reveal clinically symptomatic as well as occult areas of bone secondaries, infection and inflammation, as well as pagetic areas (activity and extent). It would be an excellent option in this man.

3) b.

The serum concentration of many substances may increase or decrease in a variety of inflammatory and infectious disorders, trauma, tissue infarction and certain neoplasms. An acute phase response is defined as a change (increase or decrease) of at least 25% in the plasma concentration of a substance during an inflammatory disorder (or infection or trauma). This is thought to be a defensive/adaptive mechanism to injury. Such a response in seen in acute as well as chronic inflammatory disorders; the word 'acute' is therefore not that correct! The two well-known *negative* phase reactants are serum albumin and serum iron; their plasma concentration falls during such events.

4) e.

Lupus anticoagulant is not an antibody; it is the phenomenon of demonstrating failure of a prolonged phospholipid-dependent coagulation study to correct upon the addition of normal platelet-free plasma. Also, it is not an anticoagulant; it promotes thrombosis! β_2-glycoprotein I antibodies and anticardiolipin antibodies are antiphospholipid antibodies.

5) c.

The skin manifestations of primary antiphospholipid syndrome may include livedo reticularis, livedoid vasculopathy, skin necrosis and ulceration, digital gangrene, thrombophlebitis, pseudovasculitic nodules, atrophie blanche, malignant atrophic papulosis and splinter haemorrhages. Ocular manifestation can be in the form amaurosis fugax, retinal vein and arterial thromboses, and ischaemic anterior optic neuropathy. Bilateral adrenal haemorrhage is more common than bilateral adrenal vein thrombosis as a cause of Addison's disease (not Cushing's syndrome). Pulmonary microthrombi and emboli, intrapulmonary haemorrhage, ARDS and a fibrosing alveolitis-like picture can all be encountered. Thrombocytopenia, anaemia (which may be haemolytic), thrombotic thrombocytopenic purpura and HELLP syndrome are the usual haematological manifestations.

6) a.
This woman has a low trauma fracture; this calls for a DEXA scan to measure bone mineral density. The usual indications are previous history of low trauma fracture; clinical features of osteoporosis; family history of osteoporosis; early menopause (<45 years), thin body physique (BMI < 19); use of glucocorticoids (equivalent to at least 7.5 mg/day for >3 months); radiographic evidence of osteoporosis; certain diseases that increase the risk of osteoporosis (e.g. inflammatory bowel disease, celiac disease, prolonged hypogonadism in men); and as part of assessing disease response to antiosteoporosis medications.

7) e.
Osteoporosis is defined as a T-score <−2.5; a value between −1 and −2.5 is osteopenia. Note that the Z-score is not used in the definition, and some patients with a normal Z-score can have a highly abnormal T-score and osteoporosis.

8) e.
The presence of acute painful joint swelling always calls for joint fluid aspiration if there is no contraindication. The fluid is examined macroscopically and should be sent for biochemical and microbiological studies; if the facility is present, examination under polarized light microscopy is best. Note that the commonest causes of such a presentation in children are septic arthritis and juvenile idiopathic arthritis

9) c.
Pyogenic (septic) arthritis usually presents acutely; the presence of joint symptoms for >6 weeks should prompt a review of the list of causes of chronic monoarthritis. This man has chronic monoarticular arthritis. Tuberculosis and fungal infections can be implicated. Other causes are synovial chondromatosis, amyloidosis, pigmented villonodular synovitis and foreign bodies. Inflammatory arthritides may present as chronic monoarticular arthritis. The knee joint is the commonest one to be involved. The persistence of the clinical features beyond 6 months calls for synovial biopsy.

10) d.
The history clearly indicates tennis elbow; lateral epicondylitis. Medial epicondylitis is the golfer's elbow; pain occurs at the medial lower part of

the arm and radiates along the long flexors of the wrist and fingers, and can also be reproduced upon resisted active forearm flexion. Olecranon bursitis is characterized by a fluctuant painful and tender cystic swelling over the olecranon area. In bicipital tendinitis there is pain over the upper anterior arm. Colle's fracture occurs at the wrist!

11) d.

Back pain is a very common cause of visits to the outpatient clinic. The majority of cases are simple mechanical ones, occurring in otherwise healthy people between the ages of 20 and 55 years, with no systemic upset; a history of similar pain episodes may be elucidated. The pain is usually sudden, precipitated by lifting heavy objects, variable, usually relieved by rest, localized to the lower back and may radiate to the thighs (but never below knee). The majority of patients will have a good degree of recovery by 6 weeks. However, the presence of any of the following 'red flags' calls for further evaluation: patient's age <20 or >55 years; persistent severe pain unrelieved by rest; localization to the dorsal spine; radiation to below the knees; remarkable past medical history (e.g. TB, HIV, malignancy); neurological signs (e.g. saddle anaesthesia, radicular signs, sphincteric disturbance); and painful asymmetric spinal deformity.

12) e.

This brief scenario only fits Sheuermann's osteochondritis. This disease usually targets adolescent boys and is one of the causes of kyphosis. Despite the deformity, most patients do not require corrective surgery. All patients should be advised to avoid excessive activity and be educated to perform regular protective postural exercises. Diffuse idiopathic skeletal hyperostosis is defined as the presence of new bone formation along the anteriolateral surfaces of at least four contiguous vertebrae. There are no risk factors for osteoporosis is the scenario and also the radiographic findings are inconsistent with this diagnosis. Neurofibromatosis patients may have a severe form of scoliosis, but neither the history nor the clinical examination is compatible with this diagnosis. TB spondylitis usually has systemic manifestations and characteristic radiographic features, which are not mentioned in the question.

13) d.

Neither the disease's duration nor its current well-controlled activity puts the patient at risk of developing secondary AA amyloidosis or florid nephrotic syndrome. Penicillamine-associated nephritic syndrome would explain the clinical presentation and urinary finding; all patients taking penicillamine should have their blood count tested and their urine checked for protein 1–2 weeks after initiation of therapy and at a 4–6-week interval thereafter. Rheumatoid arthritis per se usually spares the kidneys and would not result in nephritis/nephrotic syndrome.

14) c.

Gold injections are prescribed in slowly escalating doses, and a clinical benefit is usually apparent after 2–3 months of starting treatment with weekly injections, after which the injections are given every month. Some patients may have breakthrough relapses which necessitate going back to weekly injections to control disease activity. However, if no benefit is noted after 6 months of carefully scheduled injections, the medication should be stopped and substituted with another slow-acting antirheumatic drug.

15) c.

The principal uses of glucocorticoids in rheumatoid arthritis are when rapid disease control is desirable, when disease activity is accompanied by systemic vasculitis or organ- or life-threatening features (so-called malignant rheumatoid arthritis), and it is the best option for the control of disease activity during pregnancy.

16) c.

This woman has the typical pain of knee osteoarthritis; the development of posterior knee pain should always suggest the presence of a Baker's cyst. Adductor tendinitis occurs in athletes and the pain and tenderness are localized to the site of the muscle insertion; the pain is reproduced with resisted thigh adduction.

17) d.

The commonest cause of early onset (<45 years) 'monoarticular' osteoarthritis is a prior joint trauma (with or without localized joint instability). Note that this man's right knee is his only abnormal joint. The causes of pauci- or poly-articular osteoarthritis in young individuals are prior joint disease (like juvenile idiopathic arthritis), ochronosis, haemachromatosis, epiphyseal dysplasia and joint hypermobility.

18) e.

Rheumatoid arthritis occurs in all ethnic groups and worldwide. It is the commonest cause of inflammatory arthritis. The disease is more common in females than males at all ages. The diagnosis is secured after proper history taking, careful examination and some blood tests to fulfil; no single laboratory test is diagnostic of the disease. Laboratory tests are conducted to monitor disease activity and to detect complications (including adverse effects of treatment). As well as the skin, rheumatoid nodules can be found in the lung, pleura, pericardium and sclera. The synovium is hypertrophied.

19) d.

The kidneys are usually immune from the direct inflammatory process and the finding of active urinary sediment should suggest an alternative diagnosis. Cardiac involvement may result in syncope. Sicca (secondary Sjögren's) syndrome is the commonest eye complication. Atlantoaxial subluxation or subluxation at subaxial levels in the neck may result in spastic quadriparesis. All patients should be tested for osteoporosis which is common and is due to the disease itself and its steroid therapy. Rheumatoid arthritis patients are at risk of falls and their consequences; a simple fall may fracture both distal radii.

20) e.

Felty's syndrome occurs in about 1% of patients with long-standing rheumatoid arthritis disease that is seropositive and deforming but inactive. This patient's negative rheumatoid factor should cast strong doubt upon the diagnosis of Felty's. Most patients are in their 50s and 60s and the disease is more common in females and Caucasians. Features include splenomegaly, lymphadenopathy, skin rheumatoid nodules and ulcers, weight loss, hyperpigmentation and recurrent infections. Bloods show neutropenia, normochromic normocytic anaemia, thrombocytopenia and abnormal liver functions.

21) e.

Prostatitis is seen in 80% of male patients with ankylosing spondylitis but is usually asymptomatic. Aortic regurgitation occurs in 5% of patients after many years. Biapical lung fibrocystic disease is rare. Secondary AA amyloidosis may result in bilateral leg oedema (nephrotic syndrome), as may cardiac decompensation because of aortic and mitral regurgitations. Anterior uveitis is the commonest extra-articular manifestation and can produce painful red eye with blurring of vision.

22) c.

A pleuritic type of chest pain is relatively common and results from involvement of the costovertebral joints; the patient is not taking his medications and the disease is active. Unlike in rheumatoid arthritis, acute pericarditis is not a recognized feature of ankylosing spondylitis. There are no clues to the other options.

23) e.

Reiter's syndrome can explain this patient's scenario. Peripheral neuritis may produce bilateral foot drop and hand weakness. Chest pain can be due to pleuritis and/or pericarditis. Cardiac involvement may result in conduction defects; aortic regurgitation may occur. Central nervous system involvement is uncommon but seizures and, rarely, meningoencephalitis do occur. Diarrhoea or urethritis may precede the syndrome, but by themselves they are not syndrome complications.

24) c.

Distal interphalangeal joint arthritis is characteristic of psoriatic arthritis and is seen in 15% of cases, usually associated with nail involvement. Its presence in a patient who has a diagnosis of ankylosing spondylitis should prompt review of this diagnosis. Bradycardia may occur in ankylosing spondylitis because of cardiac conduction defects.

25) e.
Losartan has a direct uricosuric effect and can inhibit the tubular reabsorption of urate. This medication is especially useful to counteract the hyperuricaemic effect of diuretics, e.g. in patients with heart failure or hypertension for whom they are prescribed.

26) c.
The joint fluid study confirms the presence of urate crystal in this woman with hypertension and for which she might well take a diuretic. Thiazides and loop diuretics are well-recognized causes of hyperuricaemia and secondary gout.

27) d.
Inherited enzymatic defects of purine synthesis are responsible for < 1% of all cases of primary gout, but should always be suspected in the presence of any one of the following: early onset gout before the age 25 years; strong family history of early-onset disease; and presentation with renal uric acid stones. The abnormalities are HGPRTase deficiency, PRPP synthetase overactivity and glucose-6-phosphatase deficiency.

28) e.
Joint aspiration in this man can give dramatic relief and is followed by intra-articular injection of a steroid; this is the best approach in uraemic and elderly patients. Ciclosporin is not used in the management of acute gouty arthritis. NSAIDs and colchicine are unsafe in uraemic patients.

29) d.
Probenecid is a uricosuric medication and a useful treatment for chronic hyperuricaemia. However, it is contraindicated in the presence of chronic renal impairment (its action is lost), renal urate stones (it increases stone formation) and in uric acid over-producers (urinary urate excretion is already high). In uraemic patients, cautious use of allopurinol 100mg/day is advised.

30) d.
The presence of any one of the following calls for further work-up to elucidate the cause of pseudogout: patient's age <55 years, recurrent acute attacks in the absence of chronic arthritis, polyarticular disease and evidence of an underlying predisposing disease. This young healthy-looking patient has calcium pyrophosphate dihydate crystal-induced arthritis (pseudgout) of the left ankle; he needs further work-up and evaluation to find out the reason. His past fracture history is unrelated (a distraction).

31) d.
Despite the florid inflammatory process and acute-phase reactant changes in SLE, the CRP serum level is usually immune to change; elevated serum levels usually indicate the presence of coexistent infection or

serositis. Checking serum levels of C_3, C_4, and CH_{50} is useful to monitor disease activity.

32) d.

Many patients with SLE have troublesome skin and joint symptoms without visceral or vital organ involvement; the best treatment option is hydroxychloroquine. Nephritis (and other vital organ involvement) is best treated with the combination of intravenous cyclophosphamide and oral (or intravenous) glucocorticoids rather than using either alone. Patients with thrombotic phenomena should receive long-term (and even life-long) anticoagulation. Patients on long-term steroid therapy should always be considered for receiving a steroid-sparing agent (azathioprine is a useful one).

33) c.

Testing for anti-CCP (anticitrulline-containing proteins) is especially helpful in differentiating early rheumatoid arthritis from primary Sjögren's syndrome and SLE; note this patient's disease duration is not >6 weeks. A positive test using ELISA has the same sensitivity as the latex test for IgM rheumatoid factor (RF), but its specificity is much higher (up to 96%; however, a positive test is also encountered in active tuberculosis and chronic hepatitis C infection). RF is positive in 70% patients with rheumatoid arthritis but is not diagnostic of the disease; a high titre implies a poor prognosis. RF is positive in 70% of cases of primary Sjögren's syndrome and around one-third of SLE patients. Anti-dsDNA is positive in 40–60% of 'active' SLE cases. Antihistone is especially useful in drug-induced SLE. Anti-RNP is mainly ordered in mixed connective tissue disease; a positive test can be seen in SLE, Raynaud's phenomenon, rheumatoid arthritis and scleroderma.

34) c.

A fibromyalgia-like picture is common in patients with long-term SLE and is not responsive to steroids. It should be managed in the usual way with a graded exercise programme, low-dose amitriptyline and cognitive behavioural therapy.

35) b.

Pulmonary fibrosis is the major cause of morbidity and mortality in patients with systemic sclerosis; mortality from scleroderma renal crisis has become uncommon following the introduction of ACE inhibitors. Pulmonary fibrosis is usually seen in the diffuse variety, especially in patients with positive anti-Scl_{70} antibodies. Primary pulmonary hypertension is a feature of the limited (CREST) variety and is usually rapidly progressive. Recurrent upper GIT bleeding, usually occult rather than gross, is a feature of watermelon stomach (seen in 20% of patients). Small bowel bacterial overgrowth may occur and may result in diarrhoea, steatorrhoea and malabsorption. Intestinal pseudo-obstruction may occur in autonomic neuropathy of small and large bowel. Low-grade myositis and flexor tenosynovitis with arthralgia are common but they are not that incapacitating; impaired hand function is usually due to skin thickening.

36) e.
This brief scenario illustrates the features of primary Sjögren's syndrome; there are no pointers to an underlying autoimmune disease. The treatment is largely symptomatic with artificial lubrication (artificial tears, artificial saliva and vaginal lubricants). Some extraglandular manifestations may respond to steroids, which should be used in small doses and for short periods if possible; however, in general, immune suppression should be avoided in these patients as they are at risk of developing lymphoma.

37) e.
The weakness pattern in polymyositis and dermatomyositis is proximal, tender in 50% of cases, has intact deep tendon reflexes (except in advanced long-term cases where the reflexes are lost) and is usually subacute/chronic. Systemic features like fever and weight loss are common. Skin signs are seen with dermatomyositis; Gottron's papules and the heliotrope eyelid rash often crop up in the MRCP examination. Gottron's papules are scaly reddish/violaceous papules (sometimes plaques) over the extensor surfaces of the DIP and PIP joints in the hands. In any suspected case of polymyositis, the skin should be examined carefully, as dermatomyositis is strongly associated with underlying malignant diseases.

38) d.
The history is typical of polymyalgia rheumatica (PMR); however, the elevated serum creatine kinase points towards polymyositis (an important differential diagnosis). All case of PMR should be carefully examined and a set of blood tests done. PMR patients respond to low-dose (and definitely to high dose) oral prednisolone. PMR patients with features of giant cell arteritis should receive high-, not low-, dose oral prednisolone. The ESR is usually raised (>50 mm/hour); however, rarely it has not had time to rise prominently and may be <40 mm/hour at presentation. In the latter situation, the serum CRP is usually elevated.

39) e.
The most feared complication of giant cell arteritis is the development of irreversible blindness due to arteritic anterior ischaemic optic neuropathy, resulting in pale swelling of the optic disc and altitudinal visual defect and then blindness. Once blindness occurs, the role of steroids is restricted to the prevention of involvement of the other eye, which usually follows within 2–3 months. Jaw claudication resulting from ischaemia of the masseters muscles is said to be characteristic of the disease. The afferent and efferent pathways as well as the quadriceps are intact so deep tendon knee reflexes are intact. Livedo reticularis is a deep skin venulitis that is not a feature of this disease; giant cell arteritis is a large vessel one.

40) c.

Acute non-purulent *cervical*, not axillary, lymphadenopathy is a feature of Kawasaki disease. Coronary artery thrombosis, transient dilatation, frank aneurysmal formation, myocarditis and pericarditis may occur. All patients should receive aspirin and intravenous immunoglobulin; steroids should be avoided as they promote the development of coronary artery dilatation. Patients have neutrophil leucocytosis, raised ESR and CRP, and positive testing for antiendothelial cell antibodies.

41) b.

Systemic upset in the form of fever, anorexia, weight loss, myalgia and arthralgia is commonly seen in many types of vasculitides, as is the presence of neutrophil leucocytosis, and raised ESR and CRP. Renal involvement in classical polyarteritis nodosa (PAN) is the result of renal infarctions rather than glomerulonephritis. PAN is RF negative, ANA negative and usually pANCA negative, i.e. there are no antibody markers for screening or monitoring disease activity. Tissue diagnosis (i.e. biopsy examination) and/or angiographic studies are required to secure the diagnosis of PAN. Chronic hepatitis B infection is coexistent in 50% of cases, and some patients may respond simply and dramatically to antiviral therapy. Otherwise, cyclophosphamide and prednisolone are the cornerstones in the management.

42) b.

The differential diagnosis in this man is between Wegener's granulo-matosis (WG) and Churg–Strauss syndrome (CSS). The presence of proptosis favours WG over CSS. Both may have nasal and paranasal sinus symptoms. cANCA test is positive in 90% of active WG and 40% of CSS.

43) d.

This patient's scenario fits Behçet's disease; HLA-B51 has a strong association. HLA-B27 has a strong association with seronegative spondylarthritides. HLA-A3 is associated with hereditary haemo-chromatosis and HLA-DR4 with rheumatoid arthritis. HLA-B8/DR3 is seen in Type 1 diabetes mellitus.

44) c.

This pagetic patient is not complaining of any symptoms and the question does not mention any neurological manifestations, persistent pain or development of sarcoma, the usual indications for anti-Pagetic medications (calcitonin is less potent than bisphosphonates). The best approach in this patient would be observation.

45) d.

Only bisphosphonates and hormonal replacement therapy have been shown to reduce the incidence of both vertebral (mainly dorsal spine) and non-vertebral (femoral neck and Colle's) osteoporotic fractures. Other antiostereoporosis medications have a variable effect on these sites. Tibolone has been shown to increase the overall bone mineral density, but its effect on the vertebral and non-vertebral fractures is less well-defined.

46) b.
The clinical scenario describes 'difficult' to manage osteomalacia using parental preparations (this rules out malabsorption). The most important differential diagnosis is between vitamin D-dependent rickets type II and hypophosphatasia. The latter would have 'low' serum alkaline phosphatase. The raised serum 1,25(OH)D is consistent with type II vitamin D-dependent rickets (type I has very low levels of that vitamin); serum levels of 25(OH)D are within their normal reference range in both types. Bisphosphonate-induced osteomalacia occurs in those receiving high doses of etidronate (usually for symptomatic Paget's disease of the bone). Aluminium toxicity occurs in uraemic patients taking aluminium hydroxide phosphate binders and in those on long-term haemodialysis; it is rare today.

47) c.
Mutation in the PHEX gene is responsible for X-linked dominant hypophosphataemic rickets; some mutations are transmitted in an autosomal dominant pattern and involve the *FGF23* gene. Rarely, renal phosphate loss is seen in tumours with ectopic synthesis and secretion of *FGF23*. The usual treatment is with active vitamin D metabolites and high doses of oral phosphate. Note that calcitrol is a vitamin D metabolite which the patient is already receiving.

48) c.
The management plan of fibromyalgia involves education, low-dose amitriptyline and supervised graded exercises. Fluoxetine may be added to amitriptyline but should not be used as the sole agent. The presence of abnormal lab tests (e.g. high ESR, anaemia, raised blood urea) calls for review of the diagnosis.

49) a.
Mutation of the fibrillin-1 gene on chromosome 15 is the commonest mutation identified in Marfan's syndrome. The product of this gene is important in elastic and non-elastic fibres within connective tissues and forms an essential component of microfibrils that are required for the normal process of elastic fibrillogenesis. Annuloaortic ectasia syndrome and the autosomal dominant ectopia lentis syndrome have also been linked to mutations in the fibrillin-1 genetic. Mutations in the fibrillin-2 gene (on chromosome 5) have been linked to the development of congenital contractural arachnodactyly. About 10% of cases of Marfan's syndrome have no detectable abnormality in the fibrillin-1 gene; instead, they demonstrate a mutation in the transforming growth factor beta receptor 1 and 2. There is no marfanin gene—this is a distraction. Note that the skin in Marfan's syndrome is normal (neither hyperextensile nor fragile); however, abdominal wall and incisional hernia may occur, striae

may be seen over the shoulders, and characteristic skin papules may develop over the nape.

50) e.

Ehlers–Danlos syndrome (EDS) is a heterogenous group of diseases characterized by variable defects in collagen and related fibres. The inheritance is variable; the majority have an autosomal dominant inheritance, some are autosomal recessive (like type X and some cases of type VI) and one type (type V) is X-linked recessive. Most have a defect in collagen fibres (e.g. type I collagen in type II disease and type III procollagen in type IV disease); however, type VI disease (oculo-scoliotic) has deficiency of the enzyme lysyl hydroxylase and type X disease has a defect in fibronectin. The MRCP part I usually asks about the inheritance or type of defect in EDS types rather than specifically enquiring about features of the syndrome (which are diverse).

9. Tropical medicine, infections and sexually transmitted diseases: Questions

1) A 28-year-man presents with a 1-week history of fever, headache, malaise, limb aching and constipation. Examination reveals a pulse rate of 80 beats/minute and high fever. His fever is gradually rising in a stepladder fashion. The anti-O and anti-H titres are high in the Widal test. Which one of the following is *uncommon* during the second week of this man's illness?

   a. Cough
   b. Diarrhoea
   c. Erythematous spots on the upper abdomen
   d. Melaena
   e. Splenomegaly

2) A 51-year-old woman visits for a scheduled follow-up. She was treated successfully with antibiotics for enteric fever of typhoid and she is now symptom-free. You carry out some investigations which confirmed that this woman has become a chronic carrier. She has gallstones but declines their surgical removal. How would you eradicate the infectious organism?

   a. Laparoscopic gallbladder removal
   b. Ciprofloxacin for 4 weeks
   c. High-dose ampicillin for 1 week
   d. Gallbladder radiotherapy
   e. Cefotaxime for 2 weeks

3) Two days after returning from Kenya, a 43-year-old British man has a painful swelling at his mid-forearm with regional lymph node enlargement. He remembers that he was bitten by an insect 10 days ago. Four weeks later he presents with coma. His work-up reveals myocarditis, pleural effusion and hepatitis. What is the likely diagnosis is this man?

   a. Leptospirosis
   b. Falciparum malaria
   c. African trypanosomiasis
   d. Yellow fever
   e. Acute HIV seroconversion illness

4) A 54-year-old man develops bouts of fever while visiting Nigeria. The fever is accompanied by rigor for half an hour, followed by flushing. The patient states that after several hours he develops severe sweating with resolution of the fever. These bouts are repeated every few days. How would you confirm your clinical diagnosis?

a. Thick blood film
b. Blood cultures
c. Urine culture
d. HIV serology
e. Thin blood film

5) A 32-year-old male tourist recently arrived from Uganda has drowsiness and seizures. Thin and thick blood film confirms the presence of falciparum malaria. What level of blood parasitaemia would you expect?

a. >50%
b. >10%
c. <1%
d. >2%
e. 20%

6) A 25-year-old woman is about to visit Papua New Guinea. She asks about the risk of malaria infection and how to protect herself. The country she plans to visit is endemic with highly chloroquine-resistant strains of *P. falciparum*. Which one of the following would you choose for malaria chemoprophylaxis in this woman?

a. High-dose chloroquine
b. Proguanil
c. Chloroquine with proguanil
d. Quinine
e. Mefloquine

7) A 19-year-old man develops mild watery diarrhoea with cramping abdominal pains one week after visiting Malaysia. He denies blood in his stool. Stool examination does not show pus cells, red blood cells or any pathogenic organism. How would treat him?

a. Tetracycline
b. Ampicillin
c. Oral rehydration
d. Ciprofloxacin
e. Metronidazole

8) A 46-year-old man presents with a 4-day history of bloody diarrhoea. His bowel opens six times a day with cramping abdominal pains and nausea. Which one of the following is not a potential cause of this man's presentation?

a. *Vibrio parahaemolyticus*
b. *Clostridium difficile*
c. Non-typhoidal salmonella
d. Enterotoxigenic *E. coli*
e. Enteroinvasive *E. coli*

9) A 28-year-old man develops flushing, sweating, abdominal colic, chest tightness and wheezes, nausea, vomiting and hypotension a few minutes after ingesting tuna in a local restaurant. He has widespread pruritic urticaria. What is the cause of this man's presentation?

a. *Staph. aureus* food poisoning
b. Chinese-restaurant syndrome
c. Scombrotoxic fish poisoning
d. Paralytic shellfish toxin poisoning
e. Ciguatera fish poisoning

10) A 32-year-old pregnant woman visits the infectious diseases out-patient clinic because she is concerned that she was in close contact accidentally with her neighbour's child who has severe chickenpox. Her past records indicate that she had chickenpox when she was 10 years old. What is your reaction?

a. Aciclovir
b. VZV immunoglobulin
c. Check her VZV antibody titre
d. Reassure and discharge
e. Ribavirin

11) A 17-year-old girl presents with high fever, vomiting, limb ache, headache and diffuse erythematous skin rash. Blood urea and serum creatinine are raised, as is the serum creatine kinase. Her sister states that the patient uses vaginal tampons. Which one of the following is *not* true with respect to this girl's illness?

a. Antistaphylococcus antibiotics are given
b. Blood culture is useful to check the organism's sensitivity to antibiotics
c. Resuscitation with fluids and electrolytes in all cases
d. Skin rash will desquamate after 1 week
e. Disease produces poor immunity

12) A 32-year-old sewage worker presents with a 1-week history of fever, jaundice, skin bruises and renal impairment. He has raised ESR and CRP with neutrophilic leucocytosis and thrombocytopenia. What is the likely diagnosis?

a. Q-fever
b. Crimean-Congo haemorrhagic fever
c. Dengue haemorrhagic fever
d. Leptospirosis
e. Fulminant hepatitis B infection

13) A 14-year-old girl who has just arrived in the UK from Thailand presents with saddle-back fever, prostration, headache, bone pain, myalgia and vomiting. She has morbilliform skin rash. A few days later she develops haematemesis and skin ecchymosis. She has leucopenia and low platelets count. What is the likely diagnosis in this girl?

a. Dengue haemorrhagic fever
b. Falciparum malaria
c. Pneumococcal bacteraemia
d. Yellow fever
e. Brucellosis

14) A 43-year-old man presents with fever, frontal headache, haemorrhagic skin rash, myalgia, arthralgia, anorexia, dry cough and conjunctival suffusion. There is a four-fold rise in Weil–Felix test titre. What is the vector of this epidemic typhus?

a. Trombicula mite
b. Ixodes tick
c. Body louse
d. Flea
e. Reduviid bug

15) A 15-year-old boy presents with fever and weight loss. He has pallor, facial hyperpigmentation and splenomegaly. Sodium stibogluconate is given and he makes a remarkable improvement. Later, he reports that his face has developed a nodular eruption. What is the reason for this current complaint?

a. Erythema nodosum leprosum
b. Skin metastases
c. Lupus vulgaris
d. Post-kala azar dermal leishmaniasis
e. Lepromatous leprosy

16) A 29-year-old woman presents with drowsiness, diarrhoea, diffuse abdominal distension, cough and chest tightness 4 weeks after starting high-dose oral prednisolone for hand arthropathy. Her blood culture reveals Gram-negative enteric bacteria and her stool shows motile larvae. What is the likely diagnosis?

   a. Malignant rheumatoid arthritis
   b. Disseminated tuberculosis
   c. Ascaris infection
   d. Strongyloides hyperinfestation syndrome
   e. *Salmonella typhi* septicaemia

17) A 26-year-old immigrant from Yemen is referred from the dermatology department. He has diffuse shin thickening with pruritis and hyperpigmentation. His inguinal lymph nodes are enlarged and there is gross scrotal swelling, as well as many skin nodules of about 1 cm in diameter. Which one of the following is the most serious complication of this man's illness?

   a. Scrotal cancer
   b. Cardiomyopathy
   c. Blindness
   d. Spastic paraparesis
   e. Bladder squamous cell cancer

18) A 45-year-old man presents with seizures. His brain CT scan reveals many calcified nodules. Examination reveals many pea-sized skin nodules. X-ray of both arms shows many calcified spots. Which one of the following would *not* be used in the treatment of this man?

   a. Praziquantel
   b. Albendazole
   c. Carbamazepine
   d. Prednisolone
   e. Ivermectin

19) A 32-year-old tourist in Brazil visits the hotel's doctor, who detects many linear serpiginous itchy skin rash over both feet and elbows. The man says that these linear lesions lengthen at a rate of 2–3 cm/day. What is the diagnosis?

   a. Strongyloides autoinfection
   b. Oriental sore
   c. Ascaris
   d. Cutaneous larva migrans
   e. Yaws

20) A 33-year-old man is diagnosed with paucibacillary tuberculoid leprosy. Besides daily dapsone, which one of the following would you add?

a. Daily clofazimine
b. Monthly clofazimine
c. Monthly rifampicin
d. Biweekly rifampicin
e. Weekly clofazimine and rifampicin

21) A 53-year-old man with lepromatous leprosy is given medical treatment for his disease. One week after starting his medications, he develops fever, painful lymph node enlargement, dactylitis, red eyes and tender nerves. What is the cause of this deterioration?

a. Lepra reaction type 1
b. Re-infection
c. Coexistent disseminated tuberculosis
d. Acute HIV seroconversion illness
e. Lepra reaction type 2

22) A 32-year-old woman from Tanzania presents with progressive pallor, left hypochondrial heaviness and early satiety. Examination reveals massive splenomegaly. Serum IgM antibodies against plasmodia is very high. Her bloods show minor plasmodia parasitaemia. What is the diagnosis?

a. Tropical eosinophilia
b. Kala azar
c. Disseminated tuberculosis
d. Tropical splenomegaly syndrome
e. Schistosomal liver cirrhosis

23) A 43-year-old man presents with a single painless ulcer on the glans 2 weeks after having unprotected sex with a prostitute. His inguinal lymph glands are enlarged but they are neither painful nor tender. His VDRL test is negative. What is the likely reason for VDRL negativity in this case of primary syphilis?

a. Wrong diagnosis
b. Test ordered too early
c. Coexistent HIV infection
d. Technical error
e. Patient's sample is wrongly labelled

24) A 43-year-old man develops fear of impending death and hallucinations immediately following the start of treatment for secondary syphilis. What is the reason?

a. Jarisch–Herxheimer reaction
b. Syphilitic meningitis
c. General paresis of insane
d. Procaine reaction
e. Malingering

25) A 32-year-old pregnant woman presents with burning micturition and frequency. She states that her husband has been treated for gonorrhoea. Examination of her urethral discharge shows many intracellular Gram-negative diplococci. How would treat her?

a. Single injection of 250 mg ceftriaxone
b. Doxycyclin 2 g single dose
c. Ciprofloxacin 250 mg single dose
d. Intramuscular injections of spectinomycin 2 g/day for 1 week
e. Intravenous infusion of cefotaxime 1 g every other day for three doses

26) A 43-year-old man presents with infrequent attacks of genital herpes in the form of a few vesicles and erosions. He is not that bothered by these attacks. What is the best medical advice?

a. Aciclovir 200 mg twice a day for 1 month
b. Normal saline washes during recurrences
c. Famciclovir 250 mg five times a day for 6 months
d. Ribavirin 1000 mg/day for 2 years
e. Valaciclovir 500 mg/day for 3 months

27) A 34-year-old man is referred to receive the hepatitis B vaccine because he is at risk of acquiring this infection. Which one of the following is *not* a risk factor for hepatitis B viral infection?

a. Intravenous drug abuser
b. Regular sexual partner of a chronic carrier
c. Uraemic patient on haemodialysis
d. Intensive care unit nursing staff
e. Heterosexual female

28) A 45-year-old surgeon injures himself many times with the needle while stitching the skin wound of a patient with chronic hepatitis C infection. He asks if there is any way the acquisition of hepatitis C viral infection can be prevented. Which one of the following is correct with respect to prevention of this infection in this man?

a. Ribavirin for 1 week
b. Zalcitabin for 28 days
c. There is no preventive method
d. Hepatitis C vaccine
e. Hepatitis C immunoglobulin

29) A 32-year-old Indian immigrant is undergoing a Heaf test as part of a routine pre-employment examination. His test result is reported as 'confluent papules forming a ring'. Which Heaf grade does this represent?

a. Grade 1
b. Grade 2
c. Grade 3
d. Grade 4
e. Grade 5

30) A 41-year-old man has a tuberculin skin test of 7 mm induration. His GP considers this to be a strongly positive test because the patient has certain risk factors. To which one of the following categories does this patient belong?

a. HIV-positive individual
b. Secondary school teacher
c. Intravenous drug abuser
d. Laboratory personnel
e. Prisoner

31) A 29-year-old homosexual man presents with fever, headache, myalgia and sore throat 3 weeks after having sex with a stranger. Examination reveals mouth ulcers, maculopapular rash over the trunk and cervical lymph node enlargement. What is the likely diagnosis?

a. Secondary syphilis
b. Eczema herpeticum
c. Acute HIV seroconversion illness
d. Disseminated CMV infection
e. Disseminated gonococcal infection

32) A 46-year-old HIV-positive man on examination and work-up is found to have something that indicates a CD4$^+$ cell count <50 cells/ml^3. Which one of the following has been found?

a. Oesophageal candidiasis
b. Skin Kaposi's sarcoma
c. Primary CNS lymphoma
d. CMV retinitis
e. Persistent generalized lymphadenopathy

33) A 32-year-old HIV-positive man presents to A&E with a 4-week history of watery diarrhoea and cramping abdominal pains. He says that his daily stool volume is large and is not lessened by antibiotics. He denies fever or blood in stool. His current CD4$^+$ count is 150/ml^3. Routine general stool examination does not show any pathogenic organism. What would you do next?

a. Give ciprofloxacin
b. Prescribe loperamide
c. Repeat stool examination using modified acid-fast stain
d. Do colonic biopsy
e. Order abdominal CT scan

34) A 51-year-old intravenous drug abuser presents to A&E with a 3-week history of fever, breathlessness and malaise. Examination reveals oropharyngeal candidiasis, multiple bluish skin macules and nodules, widespread wet crackles and O$_2$ desaturation upon exercise. Chest X-ray shows bilateral perihilar ground-glass shadowing. Serum LHD is raised and serum albumin is low. What is the diagnosis?

a. Miliary tuberculosis
b. Acute pulmonary histoplasmosis
c. *Pneumocystis carinii* pneumonia
d. Pulmonary Kaposi's sarcoma
e. *Mycoplasma* pneumonia

35) A 31-year-old HIV-positive man presents with severe *Pneumocystis carinii* pneumonia despite taking primary chemoprophylaxis. His past records reveal severe skin reactions to sulpha drugs, oesophageal candidiasis, and skin and oral Kaposi's sarcoma. What is the treatment?

a. High dose co-trimoxazole
b. Clindamycin plus primaquine
c. Prednisolone
d. Inhaled pentamidine
e. Atovaquone

36) A 49-year-old woman presents with fever, confusion and right-sided hemiparesis. Her CD4$^+$ cell count is 80/ml^3. Brain CT scan reveals multiple ring enhancing lesions in both cerebral hemispheres. She is not taking any medication for the time being. What would you do?

a. Trial of antitoxoplasma therapy
b. Stereotactic brain biopsy
c. Ceftriaxone and vancomycin
d. Whole brain irradiation
e. Aciclovir infusion

37) A 32-year-old homosexual man presents for a follow-up. He has not been seen for the past 1 year. Apart from infrequent oral candidiasis and fatigue, he reports no other problems. He declines to be examined. His up-to-date CD4$^+$ cell count is 180/ml^3. What is the next best step?

a. Advise regular follow-ups
b. Skin biopsy
c. Oral nystatin lozenges
d. Start highly active antiretroviral therapy
e. Co-trimoxazole

38) A 21-year-old woman is brought to A&E after being brutally raped by an HIV-positive heroine addict. She is crying, yelling at the medical staff and is declining any form of examination. What would you do?

a. Order HIV serology
b. Give hepatitis B immunoglobulin
c. Start zidovudine, lamivudine and indinavir for 28 days
d. Refer for plasma PCR for HIV RNA
e. Advise a future visit

39) A 32-year-old HIV-positive man is found to have a tuberculin skin induration of 13 mm as part of his HIV work-up. He denies cough or chest tightness and his chest X-ray is unremarkable. What is your response to this testing?

a. Repeat the test after 6 months
b. Sputum acid-fast staining
c. Urine culture
d. CSF analysis
e. Rifampicin and isoniazid

40) An obstetrician calls you about one of your HIV-positive patients who is 24-years-old and is not taking any anti-HIV medication. She is about to undergo induction of labour. The obstetrician asks if you have anything to suggest. What is your reply?

a. Avoid general anaesthesia
b. Use forceps delivery
c. Start intravenous infusion of zidovudine
d. Advise oral ritonavir for 16 weeks after labour
e. Nothing to add

41) The medical SHO is asking your advice about a 32-year-old HIV-positive patient with respect to his immunization status. He is planning to immunize the patient but he is not sure about which vaccines to avoid. The patient's current CD4$^+$ count is 260/ml^3. Which one of the following vaccines is *not* to be given to this patient?

a. Varicella
b. Yellow fever
c. MMR
d. Hepatitis B
e. Influenza

42) A 65-year-old healthy-looking man who received 23-polyvalent pneumococcal vaccine 3 years ago, asks about the timing of revaccination. He is reasonably well and neither smokes nor drinks alcohol. Examination is unremarkable. What is your reply?

a. No need for revaccination
b. Revaccinate after 12 years
c. Vaccinate today using the 14-valent pneumococcal vaccine
d. Revaccinate after 3 years
e. Revaccinate after 6 years

43) An 11-year-old child is brought by his mother to consult you. The child showed first symptoms of mumps 14 days ago and the mother asks if he is still infectious to others. He has mild non-tender parotid glands enlargement. You tell her that:

a. He should receive aciclovir
b. He should not go to school for another 2 weeks
c. His saliva should be cultured
d. He is not infectious any more
e. His testes should be examined

44) A 21-year-old man visits his GP because of a certain infection. His history discloses an incubation period of <1 week. Which of the following infections is this man *unlikely* to have?

a. Gonorrhoea
b. Anthrax
c. Scarlet fever
d. Typhus
e. Diphtheria

45) A 32-year-old man presents with a 3-day history of fever, drowsiness and vomiting. Examination reveals neck stiffness and a positive Kernig sign. His past records are unremarkable. CSF analysis shows neutrophilic pleocytosis, sugar 20 mg/dl (blood sugar 120 mg/dl) and protein 200 mg/dl. How would you treat him?

a. Aciclovir
b. Ampicillin
c. Piperacillin
d. Cefotaxime and vancomycin
e. Isoniazid, rifampicin, pyrazinamide and ethambutol

46) A 32-year-old man has been treated successfully with cefotaxime for pyogenic meningitis due to *Neisseria meningitides*. His household close contacts have been given rifampicin for 2 days. What would you do before discharging him?

a. Rifampicin 600 mg twice a day for 2 days
b. Cefuroxime for 10 days
c. Dexamethasone for 4 days
d. Blood culture
e. Throat swab

47) A 43-year-old man is brought to A&E after being bitten by a stray dog in what he reports was an unprovoked attack. The bite is to the left lateral calf. The wound is being cleaned with soap and water as well as disinfectants. You are arranging a rabies vaccination schedule for him. What else would you do?

a. Culture the wound
b. Check the blood count
c. Rabies immunoglobulin
d. Serology for tetanus
e. HIV status

48) A 54-year-old man is referred to you from the ENT department because of frontal headache and vomiting. He had severe frontal sinusitis 3 weeks ago. Brain CT scan reveals a frontal lobe ring-enhancing lesion of 3×5 cm with massive surrounding oedema. What organism is likely to cause this brain abscess?

a. *Staph. aureus*
b. Streptococci
c. *E. coli*
d. Pseudomonas
e. Nocardia

49) A 68-year-old man is evaluated further for suspected cryptic miliary tuberculosis because of unexplained weight loss and hepatospleno-megaly. Which one of the following is *not* true with respect to this form of tuberculosis?

a. May present as pyrexia of unknown origin
b. Tuberculin skin testing is always positive
c. Chest plain films can be normal
d. Leukaemoid reaction is encountered
e. Diagnosed histologically

50) A 32-year-old man develops fever, cough, tachypnoea and chest tightness one week after being hospitalized for severe diarrhoea. Chest X-ray shows bilateral bronchopneumonic shadowing. What is the treatment?

a. Co-amoxiclav
b. Clarithromycin
c. Cefotaxime plus gentamicin
d. Vancomycin
e. Doxycyclin

Tropical medicine, infections and sexually transmitted diseases: Answers

1) d.
The history is consistent with typhoid fever. During the second week, the spleen becomes palpable, rose spots appear on the upper abdomen (which fade on pressure), diarrhoea replaces constipation, bronchitis with dry cough may appear and epistaxis is sometimes seen. Disease complications usually become evident by the third week (or sometimes at the end of the second week) in the form of delirium and coma (usually absent in those who were exposed to antibiotics which would modify the clinical scenario), ileal ulceration, lower GIT haemorrhage, meningitis, cholecystitis, osteomyelitis, arthritis and myocarditis.

2) b.
Ciprofloxacin for 4 weeks is an effective mode of eradicating the organism from her gallbladder. Cefotaxime for 2 weeks is the usual therapeutic regimen when the organism's susceptibility to ciprofloxacin is questioned. This patient does not wish to consider surgical therapy, so laparoscopic gallbladder removal is an unreasonable option.

3) c.
Only African trypanosomiasis can explain this man's clinical manifestations: a painful swelling (trypanosomal chancre) and regional lymph node enlargement (Winterbottom sign), followed by gradual invasion of the bloodstream resulting in hepatitis, myocarditis, pleural effusion, and finally coma. The man has recently returned from East Africa where *Trypanosoma rhodesiense* is endemic. *T. gambiense* is endemic in West and Central Africa. He was bitten by a tsetse fly. Gambiense infections are generally less severe and have a slower course (which might fluctuate) over months or even years.

4) a.
The overall picture is highly suggestive of malaria. A thick blood film is used for rapid diagnosis of malaria infection; a larger blood sample is used than for thin blood film, red blood cells undergo haemolysis and release any organisms. The so-called thin blood film is used to confirm the diagnosis, identify the species of the organism and to measure the level of parasitaemia.

5) d.
'Severe' falciparum malaria is present when >2% of the RBCs are infected with the organism in non-immune individuals. A level >10% in non-immune individuals is 'hyperparasitaemia'; this calls for exchange transfusion. The question describes CNS involvement in someone with falciparum malaria; his blood parasitaemia must be >2%.

6) e.
When chloroquine resistance is high, mefloquine, malarone (atovaquone plus proguanil) or doxycyclin can be used for chemoprophylaxis against *P. falciparum*. When no resistance is present to chloroquine, chloroquine *or* proguanil are the usual options. When the organism is moderately resistant to chloroquine, weekly chloroquine *with* daily proguanil is prescribed. The usual contraindications to mefloquine are pregnancy and lactation, seizure disorders, mental illness and cardiac conduction defects. Patients should be advised to start taking their tablets 1 week before visiting the malarious area and the medication should be continued for at least 4 week after leaving it. Insect repellents, mosquito nets and other physical measures to prevent insect bites should not be forgotten.

7) c.
This man has mild travellers' diarrhoea. All that is required is advise that he increases intake of oral fluids with salts. If the diarrhoea is severe or bloody, ciprofloxacin can be added (which decreases the duration of the illness).

8) d.
Enterotoxigenic *E. coli* is the commonest cause of travellers' diarrhoea, which is a toxin-mediated small bowel diarrhoea where the organism's toxin is neither invasive nor produces epithelial necrosis and mucosal sloughing. Causes of non-infectious bloody diarrhoea should never be overlooked in the appropriate clinical settings (e.g. inflammatory bowel disease and ischaemic colitis).

9) c.
Under improper storage conditions the histidine content of scombroid fish (e.g. tuna and skipjack) will be converted by bacteria into histamine as well as other chemical compounds. After ingestion of this fish meat, patients develop histaminergic features *within a few minutes* (scombrotoxic fish poisoning). Paralytic shellfish poisoning results from the saxitoxin content of shellfish and induces nausea and vomiting, followed within half an hour by respiratory paralysis and failure. The ciguatoxin of coral reef fish induces nausea, vomiting and diarrhoea 1–6 hours after ingestion, followed by paraesthesia of limbs and lips and finally flaccid areflexic paralysis. Chinese-restaurant syndrome occurs within 1–4 hours of ingestion of a preformed toxin of *Bacillus cereus* with nausea and prominent vomiting and resembles *Staph. aureus* food poisoning.

10) c.
There is a history of past exposure to the wild virus; this will produce some degree of immunity. If there is any doubt about this woman's current immunity the best approach is to check her VZV antibody status. If there is good degree of immunity, there is no need for immunoglobulin administration. Give VZV immunoglobulin if the immunity has waned.

11) b.

Staphylococcus toxic shock syndrome is a toxin-mediated disease and the organism per se does not invade the blood; blood cultures are of no value in diagnosis. Cases associated with the use of vaginal tampons should be advised not to use tampons for at least 1 year. As with other toxin-mediated diseases, immunity is poor and recurrence may occur upon re-exposure. The mainstay in the treatment is fluid and electrolyte resuscitation, the use of antistaphylococcal antibiotics and removal of the tampon if present. The TSST1 toxin may act as a super-antigen which stimulates $CD4^+$ T-helper cell response with secondary neutrophil activation.

12) d.

The patient's occupation puts him at risk of leptospirosis, and his neutrophilic leucocytosis is consistent with this. The other viral infections would produce leucopenia. Q-fever may produce atypical pneumonia, granulomatous hepatitis and endocarditis.

13) a.

The overall scenario and the girl's origin are consistent with dengue haemorrhagic fever. The fever can be continuous or saddle-back. The dengue virus is a flavivirus which is inoculated into the victim via the bite of *Aedes albopticus*; the incubation period is 2–7 days. Yellow fever is present in certain parts of Africa and South America.

14) c.

Rickettsia prowazekii is transmitted via body lice and causes epidemic typhus. Mite-born typhus is the scrub typhus and is caused by *R. tsutsugamushi*. The endemic (murine) typhus is flea-borne and the organism responsible is *R. mooseri*. Rocky Mountain spotted fever is tick-borne and caused by infection with *R. rickettssi*. Reduviid bug is the vector of *Trypanosoma cruzi* (Chagas' disease).

15) d.

The clinical scenario points to someone with visceral leishmaniasis who is recovering from that disease after receiving the proper treatment. However, at this stage, some patients may go on to develop post-kala azar dermal leishmaniasis. The disease is transmitted via the bite of the sand fly and is caused by *Leishmania donovani*. Definitive diagnosis is by demonstrating the presence of the organism after careful examination of aspirates obtained from the bone marrow, lymph nodes, liver and sometimes the spleen. The organism is usually scanty when skin biopsies are examined for the amastigotes forms of the parasites in cases of post-kala azar dermal leishmaniasis.

16) d.

Systemic strongyloidosis occurs when the immune system is compromised. The larvae will migrate through the GIT and enter many organ systems, causing severe systemic manifestations and even death.

This is commonly accompanied by Gram-negative bacteraemia. Treatment is with repeated doses of ivermectin.

17) c.
Onchocerciasis (river blindness) is transmitted by the Simulum fly. Dead microfilariae of *Onchocerca volvulus* incite an intense inflammatory reaction which may result in sclerosing keratitis, choroiditis, retinitis, glaucoma and even optic neuritis. Histopathological examination of the cornea reveals the characteristic snowflake deposits at its edges.

18) e.
This man has taeniasis solium which has presented with neurocysticercosis. Albendazole is the treatment of choice of neurocysticercosis. Praziquantel is an alternative. Prednisolone can be added during the first 2 weeks of albendazole or praziquantel therapy. Niclosamide can be used to kill the intestinal worm. Antiepileptics are prescribed to control this man's seizures. Ivermectin has no place.

19) d.
The picture is typical of cutaneous larva migrans. The most important differential diagnosis is strongyloides autoinfection (larva currens); the skin lesions in the latter appear more quickly, are usually transient and are mainly seen around the buttocks. Oral albendazole or topical tiabendazole can be curative.

20) c.
Paucibacillary leprosy identifies patients who have two to five skin lesions. The WHO recommends daily dapsone and monthly rifampicin. Multibacillary patients should receive daily dapsone and clofazimine as well as monthly supervised rifampicin and clofazimine.

21) e.
Erythema nodosum leprosum, or lepra reaction type 2, is an immune complex disease that is mainly seen in lepromatous leprosy and borderline lepromatous leprosy due to pre-existent antibodies with a high antigenic load of the organism. Red eyes may be due to anterior uveitis or episcleritis. Some patients run a chronic intermittent course. Mild reactions can be controlled with aspirin; severe ones should receive prednisolone or thalidomide. A type 1, or reversal, reaction generally occurs in borderline leprosies; the relatively intact cell-mediated immunity combined with arthus reaction causes painful enlargement of peripheral nerves with new skin lesion development. Fever is rare.

22) d.
Over-production of IgM antibodies against the malaria parasite results in their aggregation and phagocytosis by the spleen and the liver (to a lesser extent), resulting in gradual splenomegaly (which may be huge).

The malaria infection per se seems to be mild. Life-long proguanil is required to shrink the spleen and for anaemia resolution.

23) b.

Positivity of non-treponemal tests (VDRL and rapid plasma reagin) becomes apparent about 4 weeks after the primary infection; this patient's 2-week history makes the test unreliable for the time being. Patients with congenital syphilis are positive at birth. Acute false-positive VDRL (up to 6 months) testing can be obtained in pregnancy, chickenpox and other infections. Positivity beyond 6 months marks a false-positive test as being chronic; this is seen especially in autoimmune diseases. A false-negative VDRL test may occur in secondary syphilis because of the so-called prozone phenomenon.

24) d.

Accidental injection of procaine penicillin into a vein may result in seizures and hallucinations. Many patients have 'impending fear of death' and physical restraint may be required to control their agitation. Jarisch–Herxheimer reaction develops after starting antisyphilitic therapy and involves fever, headache and malaise that usually lasts <1 day. It is more common in early syphilis than in late syphilis. Patients with CNS symptoms or laryngeal gummata may be given prednisolone for 1 day before starting antisyphilitic therapy to prevent flare-up at these sites.

25) a.

Ciprofloxacin is best avoided in pregnancy and doxycyclin is contraindicated in pregnancy. During pregnancy, a single dose of intramuscular ceftriaxone (250 mg) or intramuscular spectinomycin (2 g), or a single dose of 3 g oral ampicillin *plus* 1 g oral probenecid are the usual options.

26) b.

After a primary genital herpes simplex infection, some patients may develop recurrences. Mild and infrequent attacks may require no more than local saline washes; there is no need for long-term suppressive therapy. Severe recurrences require active treatment (like aciclovir 200 mg five times a day for 5 days); patients with troublesome, frequent recurrences should be advised about suppressive therapy (like aciclovir 400 mg twice a day for 12 months).

27) e.

Heterosexual females are not an at-risk group for acquiring hepatitis B unless they have multiple sexual partners (e.g. prostitution). Recombinant hepatitis B vaccine produces immunity in at least 95% of recipients. Those who are exposed accidentally to the virus (e.g. accidental needle stick injury, skin cut exposure to infected blood) should receive intramuscular injections of hyperimmune serum globulin within 24 hours of exposure. Some patients may receive active–passive immunization following this high-risk exposure (hyperimmune serum globulin plus recombinant hepatitis B vaccine). Note that the best way to prevent hepatitis B infection is by preventing hepatitis B infection in the first place.

28) c.

Unfortunately, there is neither an active nor a passive method of preventing hepatitis C infection following a high-risk exposure, and there is no chemoprophylaxis against this virus either.

29) b.

Heaf skin testing uses purified protein derivative and a multi-puncture method. The result is read after 3–7 days. Grade 1 is the presence of 4–6 papules, while the presence of confluent papules forming a ring is grade 2. Grade 3 has central induration but if the diameter of the induration is >10 mm, this is grade 4. There is no grade 5!

30) a.

Tuberculin skin testing for latent tuberculosis is read according to the following: (1)≥5-mm induration is considered positive in HIV-positive individuals, close contacts with smear-positive pulmonary TB, chest X-ray showing fibrotic changes of old TB, organ transplant recipients and those on immune suppressants (equivalent to 15 mg/day prednisolone for at least a month); (2)≥10-mm induration is positive in recent (within 5 years) immigrants from highly endemic areas, intravenous drug abusers, mycobacterial laboratory personnel, employees and residents of certain institutions (prisons, nursing care homes, homeless shelters), certain at-risk groups (uraemia, leukaemia, silicosis, gastrectomy) and children younger than 4 years of age; (3)≥15-mm induration is considered positive in low-risk individuals. Therefore, a test≥5-mm induration in an HIV-positive individual is considered positive. In intravenous drug abusers, laboratory personnel and prisoners,≥10-mm induration is the cut-off for a positive text. Secondary school teachers have a low risk of developing TB and therefore, an induration≥15 mm is considered positive in them.

31) c.

The interval after sexual exposure, the patient's homosexuality and the clinical features all are consistent with acute HIV seroconversion illness. This occurs 2–4 weeks after exposure in up to 80% of patients. Most patients recover by 1–2 weeks. The diagnosis is secured by finding the viral RNA in plasma (by PCR) or by doing an immunoblot assay for early anti-HIV antibodies.

32) d.

CMV retinitis (and gastrointestinal disease) and disseminated *Mycobacterium avium intracellulare* infection occur when the patient's $CD4^+$ cell count falls below 50 cells/ml^3 (but the miliary/extrapulmonary tuberculosis is encountered when the cell count is below 200/ml^3). Oropharyngeal candidiasis is seen with a $CD4^+$ cell count between 200 and 500/ml^3, while candidiasis of the oesophagus occurs when that cell count falls below 200/ml^3. A cell count <100/ml^3 puts the patient at risk of primary CNS lymphoma, non-Hodgkin's lymphoma, brain toxoplasmosis, cryptococcal meningitis and HIV-dementia complex. Persistent generalized lymphadenopathy (and recurrent vaginal candidiasis in females) occurs with a CD4$^+$ count >500/ml^3. Kaposi's sarcoma, HIV-associated ITP and oral hairy leucoplakia manifest when the cell count is between 200 and 500/ml^3.

33) c.

The history is suggestive of chronic small bowel diarrhoea in this HIV-positive man with a low CD4$^+$ cell count; *Cryptosporidium* is responsible for up to 20% of HIV diarrhoea and should be looked for in this man. Stool examination using modified acid-fast stain or immunofluorescence staining will detect the organism in 90% of cases; sometimes the organism is shed intermittently in stool and a duodenal biopsy examination will reveal the oocyst in the duodenal wall. The diarrhoea can be eradicated successfully by using highly active antiretroviral therapy (HAART) to increase the CD4$^+$ cell count above 100/ml^3; azithromycin and paramomycin may be tried to control the infection.

34) c.

The oropharyngeal candidiasis and the skin lesions (?Kaposi's sarcoma) in this intravenous drug abuser point towards HIV infection. All options mentioned in the question feature in the list of differential diagnoses, but *Pneumocystis carinii* pneumonia ranks top and fits with all the clinical and laboratory features. This man should be treated against this infection and counselled about undergoing an HIV infection screen.

35) b.

Inhaled pentamidine and atovaquone are used in mild cases. Steroids have been shown to reduce mortality in severe cases when given as an adjunct; they should not be used alone. High-dose co-trimoxazole is contraindicated because of the patient's previous skin reaction. Severe pulmonary infections in sulpha-allergic patients can be treated with a combination of clindamycin and primaquine.

36) a.

This woman's advanced HIV infection with this presentation has two differential diagnoses; cerebral toxoplasmosis and primary CNS lymphoma. No single clinical or imaging feature can discriminate between them with certainty. The patient's toxoplasma serology status is not given; if it was positive, this would favour toxoplasmosis over lymphoma. The best step for the time being is a trial of antitoxoplasma therapy. If there is no response to this therapeutic trial after 1–2 weeks (in terms of clinical and imaging features), brain stereotactic biopsy is indicated, as it is in patients with a completely negative toxoplasma serology or an atypical clinical presentation.

37) d.

The indications for using highly active antiretroviral therapy (HAART) are the presence of symptoms attributed to HIV infection (regardless of the $CD4^+$ count) or a $CD4^+$ count $<200/ml^3$. Patients with acute HIV seroconversion illness should be considered for HAART. The higher the plasma viral load, the earlier the treatment should be considered. The other options seem reasonable and applicable in this patient, but starting HAART is the next most important step.

38) c.

The rapist's hepatitis status is not given but he is known to be HIV-positive. This form of non-occupational exposure to HIV should be managed exactly as the occupational one. All individuals exposed to the virus should be given postexposure prophylaxis within a few hours of exposure in the form of zidovudine, lamivudine and indinavir for 28 days. Side effects are common and this is the major cause for non-compliance; only 40% finish their recommended course.

39) e.

Primary prophylaxis against certain infections in HIV-positive patients is part of their overall management and has been shown to decrease the incidence of many infections responsible for the bulk of their morbidity and mortality. A tuberculin skin induration $\geq 5\,mm$ is considered positive in this man. The brief scenario indicates the presence of latent TB; rifampicin and isoniazid should be prescribed. Co-trimoxazole is the first-line agent in primary chemoprophylaxis against cerebral toxoplasmosis ($CD4^+$ count $<100/ml^3$) and *Pneumocystis carinii* infections ($CD4^+$ count $<200/ml^3$). Note that prophylaxis against latent TB is not governed by the $CD4^+$ cell count.

40) c.

Perinatal reduction in the risk of transmission of HIV can be achieved in several ways. One is starting anti-HIV medications at the 16th week of gestation and continuing them in the neonate for 6 weeks postpartum. Caesarean section, avoiding the use of fetal scalp electrodes and preventing prolonged rupture of membranes and chorioamnionitis are advised. The use of perinatal anti-HIV medications, like intravenous zidovudine, at the onset of labour and then treating the neonate with zidovudine for 6 weeks is a well-established regimen.

41) a.

This vaccine concept (i.e. vaccination in HIV-positive individuals) covers live-attenuated ones. Note the following: (1) Patients with $CD4^+$ count $>200/ml^3$ who are planning to travel to an endemic area with yellow fever, can be *safely* given yellow fever vaccine but only 35% of them will achieve seroconversion (many MRCP BOF books consider this vaccine to be a contraindication!). (2) Varicella vaccine is *not* recommended in children or adults who are HIV positive, regardless of the $CD4^+$ cell count. (3) Because of its unknown efficacy and its risk of disseminated tuberculosis (even after many years), BCG vaccination is *not* recommended in HIV-positive individuals.

42) d.

Pneumococcal vaccination is recommended for all healthy individuals over the age of 50 years, and re-vaccination is done after 6 or more years. Patients at risk of pneumococcal disease (e.g. asplenia, sickle cell disease, alcoholics, nephrotic syndrome) should receive pneumococcal vaccine and their revaccination schedule follow specific guidelines.

43) d.

The period of infectivity in mumps is from 4 days before salivary gland(s) enlargement to 7 days after the appearance of the enlarged gland(s). In measles, it starts with the prodromal stage and extends up to 4 days after the appearance of the skin rash. For German measles the period of infectivity is from 7 days before the appearance of the rash to 4 days after its appearance.

44) d.

Typhus fever has an incubation period of 1–2 weeks, while that of typhoid fever is 1–3 weeks. Diseases with possible incubation periods of years are leprosy, filariasis, *Trypanosoma gambiense* and tuberculosis.

45) d.

The patient's overall clinical picture and CSF analysis are consistent with community-acquired pyogenic meningitis. The commonest organisms are pneumococci, *N. meningitides* and *H. influenza*; cefotaxime (or ceftriaxone) will cover these agents, but given the increasing resistance to penicillins, vancomycin (or rifampicin) is added against penicillin-resistant pneumococci. The CSF analysis is not consistent with aseptic (viral) meningitis, and the temporal profile does not support tuberculosis (subacute/chronic; it rarely presents with an acute pyogenic meningitis-like picture). High dose ampicillin (2 g 4 hourly) is added when the history is suggestive of *L. monocytogenes* (e.g. alcoholism, immune suppression, prominent brainstem signs).

46) a.

Except patients who have received ceftriaxone (which achieves good tissue penetration of the nasopharynx and sterilizes it), all patients with meningococcal meningitis should be given rifampicin 600 mg twice a day for 2 days to kill the organism in the nasopharynx. All 'close' household contacts should receive a similar therapy for chemoprophylaxis.

47) c.

Postexposure prophylaxis against rabies involves thorough cleansing of the wound, rabies immunoglobulin and a scheduled rabies vaccination. The other options are not relevant.

48) b.

Frontal lobe abscesses are usually the result of local extension from the paranasal sinuses or teeth; therefore, the expected organisms are streptococci and anaerobes. Temporal lobe abscesses result from middle ear diseases, and *Enterobacteria* and streptococci are the responsible organisms, while cerebellar abscesses are usually associated with sphenoid sinus infection with *Pseudomonas* and anaerobes. The presence of multiple brain abscesses in multiple lobes points towards metastasis from a distant site of infection with streptococci and anaerobes.

49) b.

Cryptic miliary tuberculosis is a rare form of tuberculosis which usually presents non-specifically with intermittent fever, malaise and unintentional weight loss. Hepatosplenomegaly is seen in 25% of cases. A low or high white cell count may be seen and the chest X-ray can be totally unremarkable. Tuberculin skin testing may be negative. Bone marrow or liver biopsy examination is the diagnostic method of choice by showing the presence of caseating granuloma and/or acid-fast bacilli.

50) c.

This patient has hospital-acquired pneumonia. Gram negatives, anaerobes and meticillin-resistant *Staph. aureus* are the usual organisms causing this type of pneumonia. A third-generation cephalosporin *plus* an aminoglycoside, or imipenem, or a monolactam *plus* flucloxacillin are the recommended regimens. Patients with aspiration pneumonia can be treated with co-amoxiclav *with* metronidozaole. Monotherapy with clarithromycin can be used in uncomplicated community-acquired pneumonia.

10. Dermatology: Questions

1) A 52-year-old man presents with diffuse erythematous skin rash involving almost his entire body. Which one of the following is an *unexpected* finding in this man with erythroderma?

   a. Axillary and inguinal lymph node enlargement
   b. Leg oedema
   c. Hypertension
   d. Tachycardia
   e. Shivering

2) A 27-year-old woman presents with urticarial rash. She states that the individual urticarial spots last about 2 days and they are painful rather than itchy. What is the likely diagnosis?

   a. Pressure urticaria
   b. Food allergy
   c. Systemic lupus erythematosus
   d. Contact with animal saliva
   e. Ascaris infestation

3) A 31-year old schizophrenic patient states that he develops a terrible sunburn whenever he goes to the beach, and that the sunburn appears within a few minutes of sun exposure and involves mainly light-exposed areas. What is the diagnosis?

   a. Solar urticaria
   b. Polymorphic light eruption
   c. Phototoxic drug eruption
   d. Pellagra
   e. Photoallergic drug eruption

4) A 63-year-old woman presents with widespread flaccid blisters and erosions. Her mouth has many ulcers. Immunofluorescence study of a skin biopsy reveals IgG and C_3 deposition between the dermis keratinocytes. What is the target skin antigen in this bullous skin disease?

   a. Desmoglein-3
   b. Type VII collagen
   c. Type XVII collagen
   d. BP-220
   e. Desmoglein-100

5) A 41-year-old woman presents with diffuse hair thinning. Examination shows areas of scalp scarring. Which one of the following does this woman have?

a. Hyperthyroidism
b. Postpartum alopecia
c. Alopecia areata
d. Telogen effluvium
e. Folliculitis decalvans

6) A 32-year-old woman presents with a well-circumscribed area of hair loss in the scalp. There are no signs of inflammation or trauma. Many exclamation sign hairs are seen. During examination of the patient's nails, which one of the following could be seen?

a. Subungual hyperkeratosis
b. Black discoloration
c. Paronychia
d. Longitudinal wrinkling
e. Periungual fibroma

7) A 5-year-old girl is referred from the dermatology department. Her mother has noticed the growth of excessive hair over her limbs and face. What action should you take?

a. Use of depilatory creams
b. Brain CT scan
c. Full endocrinology investigations
d. Oestrogen replacement
e. Genetic analysis

8) A 12-year-old boy presents with an itchy hyperpigmented skin rash with lichenification over the back of the knees and ankles and the anterior surfaces of the wrists and elbows. He is taking salbutamol and beclometasone inhalers. What is the dermatological diagnosis?

a. Seborrhoeic dermatitis
b. Allergic contact dermatitis
c. Atopic dermatitis
d. Lichen planus
e. Scabies

9) A 21-year-old man presents with a small rounded papulo-vesicular rash with itching just below the umbilicus. He is otherwise healthy and has no chronic illnesses. What is the likely diagnosis?

a. Kaposi's sarcoma
b. Skin secondary tumour
c. Atopic dermatitis
d. Allergic contact eczema
e. Dermatitis artifacta

10) A 19-year-old man has been diagnosed with chronic plaque psoriasis and is to receive treatment for it. Which one of the following is true with respect to this man's disease?

a. HLA-Cw6 may be positive
b. No family history of the same illness
c. Skin parakeratosis is not consistent with the diagnosis
d. Nail changes are rare
e. The guttate variety follows *Staph. aureus* skin infections

11) A 34-year-old woman presents to the dermatologist. She has a chronic skin disease which is diagnosed as psoriasis. The skin lesions are bilateral and symmetrical, red and shiny, but lack scaling. Where do you think the lesions lie?

a. Extensor elbow
b. Anterior surfaces of the knees
c. Scalp
d. Submammary
e. Volar wrist

12) A 49-year-old woman with chronic plaque psoriasis with well-demarcated oval erythematosus plaques that have silvery white scales presents with peripheral asymmetrical oligoarthritis. Which of the following would be your choice of treatment?

a. Tar
b. Calcipotriol
c. PUVA
d. Methotrexate
e. Dithranol

13) A 19-year-old college student presents with a 2-year history of severe nodulo-scarring acne that involves the face, upper neck and upper back. What is the best treatment for this woman?

a. Topical clindamycin
b. Oral erythromycin
c. Topical benzoyl peroxide
d. Oral isotretinoin
e. Topical tretinoin

14) A 53-year-old man visits his GP because of facial erythema and pustules. Examination reveals telangiectasia on the cheeks but there are no comedones. The patient says that the disease started with episodic facial flushing. Which one of the following is *not* a well-recognized precipitant of this episodic facial reaction in this man?

a. Alcohol
b. Spicy food
c. Cold weather
d. Emotional stress
e. Toothbrushing

15) A 43-year-old man presents with skin rash over the volar aspects of both forearms. He says that he has been diagnosed with lichen planus. You review the diagnosis because you have found something that is not consistent with this diagnosis. Which one of the following points towards an alternative diagnosis?

a. Polygonal papules
b. Scarring alopecia
c. Nail dystrophy
d. No itching
e. Mouth buccal lace-like lesions

16) A 62-year-old man presents with rapidly enlarging, fungating mass over the dorsal aspect of his left hand, biopsy of which reveals well-differentiated squamous cell cancer. Which one of the following is *not* a risk factor for this type of non-melanoma skin cancer?

a. Immune suppression
b. Ultraviolet light exposure
c. Chronic arsenic poisoning
d. Chronic skin ulcers
e. Cigarette smoking

17) A 54-year-old Australian woman has a semi-rounded pigmented lesion on her left shin. The lesion is 13 mm in maximum diameter and has irregular border and variegate appearance. Local regional lymph nodes are enlarged. Biopsy of the skin lesion is consistent with malignant melanoma. The surgeon excises the lesion. Which one of the following is true regarding this woman's cancer?

a. Family history is not significant
b. Males fare better than females
c. Inguinal lymph nodes should be surgically excised
d. Interferon-α is used mainly in stage I disease
e. 70% of tumours have no superficial radial growth

18) A 32-year-old man with inflammatory bowel disease has developed a necrotic skin lesion with bluish undermined edges over the upper right thigh. Which one of the following is true regarding this man's skin problem?

a. There is no diagnostic histological finding
b. Rheumatoid arthritis is not a risk for it
c. The lesion is painless
d. Dapsone is contraindicated
e. There is no recurrence

19) A 56-year-old man presents with unintentional weight loss. He has hyperpigmented velvety skin thickening in the axillae which are itchy. What is the likely diagnosis?

a. Insulin resistance
b. Gastric cancer
c. Candidiasis
d. Lichen planus
e. Drug eruption

20) A 51-year-old homosexual man with widespread bluish skin macules, nodules and plaques is referred to you by the dermatology department for further evaluation. He has many similar oral lesions. Testing for HIV infection is positive with a $CD4^+$ cell count of 120/ml^3. What is the treatment of this skin lesion?

a. Radiotherapy
b. Systemic chemotherapy
c. Laser therapy
d. Intralesional chemotherapy
e. Cryotherapy

21) A 43-year-old intravenous drug abuser is referred by his GP because of rapid progression of seborrhoeic dermatitis. The condition is severe and extensive and involves the head, neck, chest, axillae and groin. It is not responding to conventional treatment. What is the overall diagnosis in this man?

a. Tinea capitis
b. SLE
c. HIV infection
d. Atopic eczema
e. Ichthyosis

22) A 19-year-old man who was in prison consults his GP about his skin. The GP diagnoses scabies. Which one of the following is true with respect to scabies?

a. Itching is usually absent
b. Involvement of the face is rare
c. Topical treatment is useless
d. Atopic eczema may complicate it
e. Caused by body louse

23) A 21-year-old woman complains that her lower left anterior abdominal wall skin rash has worsened after using a topical treatment prescribed by her GP. To start with, the rash was oval, 2×1 cm in area, red, scaly and itchy, with a central area of pallor. Now it is 4×6 cm in area, more itchy and redder. What is the current diagnosis?

a. Tinea corporis
b. Candidiasis
c. Erythema multiforme
d. Psoriasis
e. Tinea incognito

24) While examining a 32-year-old man you found splinter haemorrhages of the nails. What is the commonest cause of this nail sign?

a. Infective endocarditis
b. Psoriasis
c. Trauma
d. Lichen planus
e. Atopic eczema

25) A 59-year-old man presents with a skin lesion. The lesion grew rapidly as a nodule with a central crater that was then filled by a plug. However, after several months, the lesion started to get smaller and smaller until it disappeared leaving an ugly scar on his upper back. What is the most important differential diagnosis of this lesion?

a. Malignant melanoma
b. Basal cell carcinoma
c. Squamous cell cancer
d. Actinic keratosis
e. Skin secondary tumour

1) c.
Erythroderma is defined as the presence of an erythematous skin rash, with or without scaling, that involves most of the body surface (>80% body surface). The usual causes are psoriasis, lichen planus, eczema, drug reactions, cutaneous T-cell lymphoma, certain forms of ichthyosis and pityriasis rubra pillaris. Impairment of skin temperature control occurs, and fever and shivering may follow. Low plasma albumin combined with high output cardiac failure can result in leg oedema. Lymph node enlargement is usually part of the reaction to skin inflammation; however, exclusion of lymphoma should always be considered. *Hypotension is a risk.*

2) c.
The presence of painful rather than itchy urticaria with individual lesions lasting >24 hours should always prompt a search for vasculitis (urticarial vasculitis). Urticaria that is present for >6 months is chronic.

3) c.
This patient is schizophrenic and he may well be taking a phenothiazine. Phenothiazines can result in phototoxic or photoallergic drug skin eruptions. The former presents as severe sunburn involving light-exposed areas *within a few minutes* of sun exposure, while the latter has a dermatitis-like picture that takes at least *24 hours* to develop. Solar urticaria presents as itchy urticarial skin lesions that appear after 1 hour of sun exposure. Polymorphic light eruption is the development of an itchy papulo-vesicular skin rash within a few hours of sun exposure. Solar urticaria, polymorphic light eruption and chronic actinic dermatitis are the so-called idiopathic photosensitive dermatoses.

4) a.
Type VII collagen is the target antigen in bullous SLE and epidermolysis bullosa acquisita. IgG (and C_3) targets the basement membrane zone's BP-220 (which is part of hemi-desmosomes) in bullous pemphigoid. Type XVII collagen is the target in pemphigoid gestationis. Although coarse granular IgA deposition in the dermal papillae is found in dermatitis herpetiformis, the target antigen is still unknown. The clinical features and skin biopsy study are consistent with pemphigus vulgaris; desmoglein-3 is the target skin antigen.

5) e.
The usual diseases responsible for diffuse 'scarring' alopecia are discoid lupus, radiotherapy, lichen planopillaris and folliculitis decalvans. The other options are causes of generalized non-scarring alopecia.

6) d.

Longitudinal wrinkling, pitting and whitish discoloration of the nail plate are the usual nail signs in alopecia areata. Subungual hyperkeratosis is seen in psoriasis, and periungual fibroma is a sign of tuberous sclerosis.

7) c.

Excessive growth of hair should always be taken seriously if it has rapid onset and progression, there are signs of virilization (e.g. clitoromegaly and breast atrophy) or menstrual irregularities, or it occurs in children. The first step should be full endocrinology investigations.

8) c.

The distribution of the rash and its characteristics point towards atopic eczema in this asthmatic child. During infancy and adulthood, the rash involves the face and the trunk. Patients have an increased risk of food allergy, secondary bacterial infections (secondary impetigo, molluscum contagiosum, herpes simplex and eczema herpeticum), secondary irritant eczema, sleep disturbances and behavioural changes.

9) d.

Nickel in jean studs is a well-known allergen of this allergic contact eczema; note the site and characteristics. Other allergens are epoxy resin in resin adhesives, colophony in sticking plaster and Balsam of Peru in perfumes.

10) a.

Psoriasis is generally seen in two groups: young patients with a family history of the disease and who are positive for HLA-Cw6, and elderly patients with no family history of the disease and who are negative for HLA-Cw6. The guttate variety is usually precipitated by streptococcal throat infections in young individuals. Nail changes are common in the form of coarse pitting, onycholysis and subungual hyperkeratosis. Histologically, there are epidermal hyperkeratosis and microabscesses, together with irregular epidermal thickening and dermal T-cell infiltration.

11) d.

The description of the psoriatic skin lesions in this woman suggests flexural lesions; axillary folds, natal clefts and submammary areas are the usual sites. The localized palmoplantar pustulosis is more common than the generalized pustular form. The guttate variety usually follows streptococcal pharyngitis and is mainly seen in children and adolescents; the majority of patients will pass into the chronic plaque variety in adulthood. The generalized erythrodermic form usually follows improper use of phototherapy or topical tar.

12) d.

This patient has psoriatic arthritis as well as chronic skin plaques; the best method to treat both is to use a systemic therapy like methotrexate or ciclosporin. Mild chronic plaque psoriasis can be well-controlled with topical steroids and emollients. Flexural psoriasis usually responds to topical steroids or topical tacrolimus; if it is severe and unresponsive, use systemic therapy. Extensive disease or disease unresponsiveness to topical measures, or the presence of arthritis, should call for systemic therapy.

13) d.

The disease's severity warrants the use of the oral vitamin A preparation isotretinoin. The woman's acne has been severe for the last 2 years and she may well have tried many oral and topical preparations. Mild disease can be treated with topical agents. Acne with minor symptoms may require no intervention.

14) e.

Toothbrushing is a precipitant of lancinating pain in trigeminal neuralgia! This man has rosacea. The precipitation of facial flushing by alcohol ingestion does not necessarily imply the patient is a heavy drinker. Facial flushing is precipitated by many stimuli; fixed erythema gradually follows. Ocular manifestations are gritty and foreign body sensation in the eyes, blepharitis, keratitis, conjunctivitis, meibomian gland dysfunction and irregularity of the lid margin. Rhinophyma is a late sign. The skin rash generally resembles that of acne vulgaris (papules, pustules and even nodules) but comedones are characteristically absent.

15) d.

The lesions of lichen planus are characteristically intensely itchy; absence of itching should cast strong doubt upon the diagnosis. Oral lesions are usually lace-like and resemble the Wickham skin striae; these may undergo atrophy or hypertrophy or even form erosions. Erosive or ulcerative skin lesions become painful.

16) e.

Ultraviolet light exposure, excessive PUVA therapy, chronic skin irritation by sinuses or ulcers, immune suppression (especially following organ or bone marrow transplantation) and scarring genetic skin diseases (like dystrophic epidermolysis bullosa) are the usual risk factors. Cigarette smoking has many adverse effects on the skin, but it is not a risk factor for the development of non-melanoma skin cancer.

17) c.

Family history is positive in 10% of cases. Females fare better than males, and tumours of the lower legs generally have a better prognosis than upper extremity ones. Stage II disease patients (with regional lymph node involvement) should have their regional lymph nodes resected en bloc. Patients with metastatic disease (or those at high risk of systemic metastasis) may receive interferon-α therapy. Around 70% of tumours have a gradual superficial and radial growth phase, except the nodular variety.

18) a.

Pyoderma gangrenosum has many morphological varieties but the diagnosis is purely clinical as there are no diagnostic histopathological features. It is associated with inflammatory bowel disease, rheumatoid arthritis, HIV infection and leukaemia. With pain control and local measures with antiseptics and dressings, systemic steroids can be useful to control disease activity; alternatives are dapsone, minocyclin, ciclosporin and sulfasalazine. The lesions are painful, and even after proper control and healing, recurrences may occur.

19) b.

The description of the skin lesions is consistent with acanthosis nigricans. Obesity is the commonest cause and insulin resistance is commonly associated. However, rapid development of acanthosis nigricans, especially if pruritic, in 'thin' patients should always prompt a search for underlying malignancy; gastric cancer is the commonest associated cancer.

20) b.

The skin lesions of Kaposi's sarcoma in this patient are widespread and oral lesions are predictive of the presence of gastrointestinal and pulmonary Kaposi's sarcoma. This man's Kaposi's sarcoma cannot be controlled with local or topical measures; systemic chemotherapy as well as highly active antiretroviral therapy is the usual management plan.

21) c.

The rapid onset of severe and extensive seborrhoeic dermatitis always calls for HIV testing. Both the incidence and severity rise as the CD4$^+$ cell count falls. This skin disease can be encountered in up to 80% of AIDS patients.

22) b.

Scabies is caused by the mite *Sarcoptes scabii*. The disease is intensely itchy and itching may persist even after successful eradication of the infection. The face and scalp are characteristically spared (except in overwhelming infections in infants). Secondary eczema may occur but it is not atopic. Topical therapy is the usual form of therapy, is usually successful and should always include other (asymptomatic) members of the family. Systemic ivermectin is given to immune compromised patients, those with extensive infection and when poor compliance with topical therapy is present.

23) e.

The rash is that of tinea corporis. Later, after the application of a topical (steroid) preparation, the inflammatory signs worsened and this defines tinea incognito. The site is atypical for chronic plaque psoriasis and topical steroids would produce some degree of improvement; a flare-up may occur following sudden withdrawal of that topical agent.

24) c.

Though classically described in infective endocarditis, trauma is in fact the commonest cause of splinter haemorrhages. They are seen as thin longitudinal brown lines.

25) c.

The most important differential diagnosis of keratoacanthoma, clinically and histologically, is primary squamous cell skin cancer. The latter has a slower pace of progression and has no spontaneous involution. Actinic keratoses are focal skin areas of partial dysplasia which appear macroscopically as small, red and scaly macules on sun exposed skin; they may progress to squamous cell cancer.

11. Clinical pharmacology, therapeutics and toxicology: Questions

1) A 45-year-old man with renal impairment has been referred to you. He has renovascular hypertension, hyperlipidaemia, congestive heart failure and chronic stable angina. His GP has found it difficult to manage him because of this constellation of co-morbidities. All of the following medications should be avoided in severe renal impairment, except:

   a. Potassium salts
   b. Aspirin
   c. Simvastatin
   d. Metformin
   e. Telmisartan

2) A 43-year-old man with a sallow colouration of skin presents to A&E with nausea, vomiting, confusion and myoclonic jerks. He has a long history of renal stone disease and gradual deterioration in his renal function. The SHO considers the possible medications that can be used in this man. Which one of the following *cannot* be used in patients with advanced chronic renal failure?

   a. Gabapentin
   b. Cefotaxime
   c. Atenolol
   d. Tetracycline
   e. Clopidogrel

3) A gynaecologist consults you about a patient who is planning to conceive. The woman takes many medications because of multiple illnesses which are reasonably controlled. Her gynaecologist asks if any of these medications will impart a harmful effect on the future fetus. Which one of the following can be safely used in pregnant women?

   a. Carbamazepine
   b. Heparin
   c. Candesartan
   d. Danazole
   e. Ciprofloxacin

4) A 31-year-old woman presents with headache, nausea, vomiting and flu. She has generalized epilepsy, hypertension and Type 1 diabetes mellitus. She gave birth to a full-term baby last week. The baby was 3.1 kg and is breast-fed. Which one of the following is contra-indicated in this nursing mother?

a. Domperidone
b. Oral contraceptives
c. Insulin
d. Lamotrigine
e. Enalapril

5) A 48-year-old woman with liver cirrhosis comes for a scheduled visit after being successfully treated for moderate hepatic encephalopathy. You give her a list of medications that can be safely used in liver disease. Which one of following is on your list?

a. Aspirin
b. Morphine
c. Omeprazole
d. Chlorpromazine
e. Oestrogen

6) A 50-year-old man with low-grade cerebral glioma has focal motor fits for which he takes daily phenytoin. He presents to A&E with con-fusion, tremor and vomiting a few days after the introduction of a medication to his daily regimen. All of the following medications enhance phenytoin toxicity, except:

a. Aspirin
b. Fluconazole
c. Amiodarone
d. Ciclosporin
e. Tolbutamide

7) A 65-year-old man visited the cardiology clinic with rapid palpita-tions. ECG revealed rapid atrial fibrillation. Rate control and anti-coagulation were instituted and he was discharged home. He was doing well until 1 week ago when he developed a diarrhoeal illness and flu for which his GP has prescribed many medications. Today he presents with gum and nose bleed, ecchymosis and bloody vomitus. Which one of the following is *not* implicated as a cause of this deterioration?

a. Propafenone
b. Carbamazepine
c. Simvastatin
d. Itraconazole
e. Aspirin

8) A 32-year-old woman with major depression presents to A&E with confusion, dry flushed skin, tachycardia, hypotension and three generalized seizures. ECG reveals QRS complex duration of 170 ms with sinus tachycardia. You resuscitate her. Which one of the following should have priority in your management plan?

a. Digoxin
b. Sodium bicarbonate
c. Activated charcoal
d. Phenytoin
e. Haemodialysis

9) A 5-year-old girl is referred from a rural hospital because of limited resources in managing intoxications. The girl's father states that she ingested 15 g of paracetamol tablets 12 hours ago but the referring hospital has not checked the serum level of the medication. She is being resuscitated in A&E. What is the best management option?

a. Give normal saline
b. Haemodialysis
c. N-acetyl cysteine
d. Fresh frozen plasma
e. Refer for liver transplantation

10) A 20-year-old woman is brought to A&E after a suicide attempt. Her flatmate states that the patient has ingested many paracetamol tablets after breaking up with her boyfriend. Which one of the following does not impose an increased risk of developing hepatotoxicity following this ingestion?

a. Concomitant alcohol ingestion
b. Anorexia nervosa
c. Co-ingestion of carbamazepine
d. Cancer
e. AIDS

11) A 31-year-old man is being considered for liver transplantation following massive paracetamol ingestion. He was treated appropriately but he developed something that has called for this surgical therapy. The development of which one of the following indicates a poor prognosis in paracetamol-related acute liver failure?

a. Serum creatinine 200 μmol/L
b. Serum bilirubin >300 μmol/L
c. Serum pH 7.1, 24 hours following ingestion
d. Patient's age >50 years
e. Grade 2 hepatic encephalopathy

12) A 17-year-old secondary school girl is brought to A&E. Her mother reports that she ingested 'many adult aspirin tablets', and adds that 'she failed her recent exams'. The patient has tachypnoea and serum bicarbonate 12 mEq/L, with increased anion gap. Which one of the following is *not* an indication for haemodialysis in this girl?

a. Coma
b. Generalized seizures
c. Renal impairment
d. Serum aspirin 100 mg/dl
e. Pulmonary oedema

13) A 36-year-old man with bipolar disorder presents to A&E. 'He got tired with his disease and he decided to ingest as many lithium tablets as he could,' his sister states. This happened an hour ago. While you are examining him, you order the management plan. Which one of the following is of *no* value in this man?

a. Rehydration
b. Activated charcoal
c. Whole bowel irrigation
d. Haemodialysis
e. Avoidance of diuretics

14) A 34-year-old man with mania presents with coarse irregular tremor, unstable stance and gait, muscle twitching and vomiting. He has sinus bradycardia and leucocytosis. His blood pressure was found to be high by his GP who prescribed a medication to control it 1 week ago. Which medication is responsible for this man's presentation?

a. Lisinopril
b. Atenolol
c. Amlodipine
d. Hydralazine
e. Prazosin

15) A 7-year-old child ingests many cardiac tablets which belong to his grandfather. He has bradycardia and hypotension, and his 12-lead ECG reveals prolongation of the PR interval, long QT interval and ventricular dysrhythmia. Apart from resuscitation, what antidote will you *not* give to this beta-blocker intoxication?

a. Glucagon
b. Calcium
c. Isoproterenol
d. Glucose and insulin
e. Diltiazem

16) A 65-year-old man with chronic atrial fibrillation presents with headache, dizziness, nausea, vomiting, diarrhoea and abdominal pain 6 days after taking a new medication added by his GP. His 12-lead ECG reveals accelerated junctional rhythm. What is the likely cause of this man's presentation?

a. Infective diarrhoea
b. Small bowel embolization
c. Digoxin toxicity
d. Hypokalaemic ileus
e. Verapamil intoxication

17) A 63-year-old man develops nausea, vomiting, confusion, blurred vision and altered colour perception. He is being treated for congestive heart failure. He has hyperkalaemia and sinus bradycardia with frequent ventricular ectopics. Serum digoxin is raised. Which one of the following is *not* used in the treatment of digoxin toxicity?

a. Calcium gluconate
b. Repeated doses of activated charcoal
c. Digoxin-specific Fab fragment
d. Atropine
e. Intubation and oxygen

18) A 54-year-old woman is referred to you with digoxin toxicity. The referring physician reports that 'the patient should be treated with digoxin-specific Fab fragment which we do not have'. Which one of the following is an indication for the use of this form of therapy in digoxin intoxication?

a. Xanthochropsia
b. Severe nausea and vomiting
c. Haemodynamic collapse
d. Serum potassium 3.0 mEq/L
e. Ingestion of 5 mg of digoxin in adults

19) A 45-year-old man is recovering from digoxin toxicity after being managed appropriately in A&E 5 days ago. His GP today asks you to check his plasma digoxin level but you decline to do this. Why?

a. Serum digoxin will remain high for a long period
b. No need for the time being
c. Digoxin-specific Fab fragments interfere with the test
d. The test is costly
e. The test will add nothing

20) A 21-year-old man presents to A&E with severe reduction in visual acuity. He admits to having ingested an antifreeze solution because he had run out of whisky. Fundoscopy reveals bilateral optic nerve head swelling. The consequences of this toxic ingestion are due to?

a. Methanol
b. Formic acid
c. Lactic acid
d. Glycolate
e. Sulphuric acid

21) A 32-year-old woman presents with rapid and deep breathing, obtundation and seizures twelve hours after accidental ingestion of an antifreeze solution containing ethylene glycol. Which one of the following is *not* seen in this form of poisoning?

a. Tetany
b. Haematuria
c. Hypotension
d. Normal anion gap metabolic acidosis
e. Oliguric renal failure

22) A 19-year-old man with seizures, coma and acidotic breathing is given a diagnosis of antifreeze poisoning after the presence of metabolic acidosis with high osmolar and anion gaps is confirmed. Which one of the following is ineffective at treating this form of poisoning?

a. Activated charcoal
b. Haemodialysis
c. Sodium bicarbonate
d. Fomepizole
e. Ethanol infusion

23) A 9-year-old child accidentally ingested 20 iron tablets. Plain radiographs of his abdomen confirmed the presence of multiple opacities that are highly suggestive of iron pills. He was resuscitated in A&E because of nausea, vomiting, haematemesis and melaena with shock. Six weeks later he presents with persistent vomiting. What has the boy developed?

a. Oesophageal ulceration
b. School phobia
c. Erratic iron ingestion
d. Hepatotoxicity
e. Gastric outlet obstruction

24) A 34-year-old man presents with abdominal colic, constipation, muscle pain and difficulty in concentration. His serum lead is increased. Which one of the following would cast doubt upon the diagnosis of lead poisoning?

a. Basophilic stippling of red blood cells
b. High stepping gait
c. Renal impairment
d. Reduced sperm count
e. Low free erythrocyte protoporphyrin

25) A 29-year-old man is brought to A&E with headache, malaise and vomiting. He was found on the ground in his backyard behind his car. How would you confirm the diagnosis of carbon monoxide poisoning in this man?

a. Pulse oximetry
b. Haemoglobin electrophoresis
c. Carboxyhaemoglobin level
d. Exhaled breath CO level
e. Blood PO_2

26) A 43-year-old woman presents to A&E with coma, hypoventilation and hypotension after ingesting 18 tablets of lorazepam. Her sister states that the patient takes daily lorazepam because of insomnia, but she does not know the reason for this deliberate massive ingestion. You resuscitate the patient with the ABC and consider the use of flumazenil. This antidote has a risk of:

a. Precipitating further hypotension
b. Pseudoallergic reaction
c. Precipitating withdrawal syndrome
d. Hypercoagulable state
e. Bleeding tendency

27) A 10-year-old child has accidentally been exposed to a solution. He presents to A&E with burns on the lips, buccal ulceration and nose bleed. He has retrosternal pain and oesophagoscopy reveals multiple oesophageal ulcers. Two days later the child develops renal failure. What is the likely cause of this child's grave presentation?

a. HCl
b. Methanol
c. Mercury
d. Paraquat
e. Thallium

28) A 31-year-old patient is referred to you for further evaluation because of chronic arsenic exposure. He is asking about the risk of developing malignant diseases. Chronic arsenic poisoning is associated with the development of all of the following types of malignancies, except:

a. Squamous cell skin cancer
b. Liver angiosarcoma
c. Lung cancer
d. Urinary bladder cancer
e. Colonic cancer

29) A 22-year-old man presents to A&E with clouded consciousness. His friend states that the patient drinks a quarter of a bottle of whisky each night, but today he seems to be abnormal. Investigations reveal an increased osmolar gap with a serum bicarbonate of 10 mEq/L. Which one of the following explains this man's presentation?

a. Co-ingestion of methanol
b. Hypoglycaemia
c. Subdural haematoma
d. Hepatic encephalopathy
e. Meningitis

30) A 51-year-old woman with recurrent lower limb DVT presents with headache, vomiting and diplopia. Her current complaints are found to be due to superior sagittal-sinus thrombosis-associated pseudotumour cerebri. She is taking daily warfarin and her current INR is 1.1. She admits to taking many medications. Which one of the following is *not* a cause of this anticoagulation failure?

a. Phenytoin
b. Carbamazepine
c. Secobarbital
d. Rifapentine
e. Clarithromycin

31) A 54-year-old man presents to A&E with repetitive generalized seizures. His friend states that the patient was reasonably well until 1 week ago, when he had mild flu for which he took an antibiotic, and that his GP has told him that his renal graft is working well. What is the likely cause of this man's presentation?

a. Pyogenic meningitis
b. Ciclosporin toxicity
c. Renal graft rejection
d. Brain secondary tumour
e. Acute renal failure

32) A 43-year-old woman is admitted after ingesting a potentially toxic dose of a drug. Your SHO asks you about the use of whole gut irrigation with polyethylene glycol. You respond that it can be used in all of the following intoxications, except:

a. Lithium
b. Iron
c. Theophylline
d. Drug body packets
e. Methanol

33) A 3-year-old child is brought to A&E following the ingestion of a substance. His mother does not know what he ingested 1 hour ago. You order activated charcoal as part of his treatment plan. Repeated, rather than single, doses of activated charcoal can be used in the intoxication of the following substances, except:

a. Carbamazepine
b. Theophylline
c. Aspirin
d. Dapsone
e. Quinine

34) A 4-year-old boy is brought to A&E 1 hour after accidentally ingesting many tablets of a medication. As a mode of bowel decontamination, the SHO orders activated charcoal. You disagree because you think that this charcoal will be ineffective. Why?

a. Ingested substance is small
b. Charcoal has expired
c. Patient is young
d. Patient had ingested lithium
e. Large doses of charcoal are required

35) A young mother rushes into A&E with her 10-year-old boy who has ingested many of her oral contraceptive pills 30 minutes ago. You reassure the mother and discharge the boy. All of the following have a low toxicity profile even when ingested in large amount, except:

a. Omeprazole
b. Silica gel
c. Zinc oxide cream
d. Washing-up liquid
e. Isoniazid

36) A 21-year-old man is brought to A&E with severe retrosternal chest pain. His records show that he is a drug addict. He admits to having snorted a large amount of cocaine in the last hour. ECG reveals ST-segment elevation in leads V_1–V_4. He has hypertension and tachycardia. Which one of the following is true with respect to this man's presentation?

a. Metoprolol is useful
b. Thrombolytics are useless
c. Hypotension never occurs
d. Hypothermia is expected
e. Liver transplantation is life-saving

37) A 17-year-old girl presents to A&E two hours following a deliberate ingestion of ecstacy tablets. She is resuscitated. Which one of the following would cast doubt upon amfetamine intoxication?

a. Small pupils
b. Hyponatraemia
c. Trismus
d. Hepatocellular necrosis
e. Adult respiratory distress syndrome

38) A 20-year-old man was caught by airport security. He admits to hiding many cocaine-filled condoms in his rectum. The officer asks you about how to remove these condoms from his body. Your response is:

a. Remove them with a colonoscope
b. Remove them manually
c. Use polyethylene glycol whole gut irrigation
d. Paraffin-containing laxatives
e. Wait until they rupture

39) A 39-year-old man presents to A&E after accidental exposure to a large amount of an organophosphorus insecticide. His soiled clothes are removed and his skin is washed. He responds to intravenous atropine. Following the administration of intravenous pralidoxim, he develops many side effects. Which one of the following is *not* an adverse effect of pralidoxim?

a. Laryngospasm
b. Tachycardia
c. Muscle rigidity
d. Hypotension
e. Neuromuscular blockade

40) A 31-year-old HIV-positive man is being considered for highly active antiretroviral therapy (HAART). He has surfed the net and found that these medications can have a multitude of adverse effects. All of the following can be encountered when using protease inhibitors, except:

a. Potentiated bleeding tendency in haemophiliacs
b. Fat redistribution
c. Hyperglycaemia
d. Vivid dreams
e. Raised serum levels of liver enzymes

41) A 46-year-old homosexual man after receiving anti-HIV medications presents because he has noticed that his finger nails are pigmented. Which one of the following is responsible for this nail pigmentation?

a. Zidovudine
b. Stavudine
c. Zalcitabine
d. Didanosine
e. Lamivudine

42) A 32-year-old homosexual man presents for follow-up. He has developed hypocalcaemia and hypokalaemia, which are attributed to foscarnet therapy given as part of secondary prevention of CMV retinitis. All of the following are true with respect to this medication, except:

a. Can result in hypomagnesaemia
b. Ineffective in thymidine kinase-deficient herpes viruses
c. Given only via the intravenous route
d. Nephrotoxic
e. Inhibits the herpes viral DNA polymerase

43) A 30-year-old man is being treated in the hospital for a serious infection. The SHO asks you about the antibiotic he is being given which belongs to a class called streptogramins. Which one of the following is true about these antibiotics?

a. Are effective when given orally
b. Weak against meticillin-resistant Staphylococcus aureus
c. They do not cross the blood–brain barrier
d. Can result in eosinopenia
e. Cause local numbness when given intravenously

44) A 43-year-old patient with congestive heart failure presents with a 4-day history decompensation. His GP has introduced a new medication and you think that this is the cause of his current presentation. Which one of the following has *not* been prescribed by the GP?

a. Atenolol
b. Propafenone
c. Disopyramide
d. Verapamil
e. Amiodarone

45) A 61-year-old man with mild congestive heart failure and atrial fibrillation is taking digoxin, captopril and furosemide. According to the modified Vaughan–Williams classification of antiarrhythmics, digoxin belongs to:

a. Class Ia
b. Class III
c. Class II
d. Unclassified
e. Class IV

46) A 59-year-old man with cardiac dysrhythmia presents with bilateral red painful eyes with blurred vision and vomiting. Examination reveals a cloudy cornea and elevated intraocular pressure. His GP introduced an antiarrhythmic medication 3 days ago. Which one of the following medications is responsible for this man's current complaints?

a. Amiodarone
b. Propafenone
c. Verapamil
d. Disopyramide
e. Mexiletine

47) A 63-year-old man is referred from the cardiology clinic because of progressive exertional dyspnoea. The referring physician states that the patient's heart condition is stable and well-controlled. Examination reveals bibasal crackles and a plain chest X-ray shows lower zone reticular interstitial infiltrates. Which one of the following has resulted in this man's current dyspnoea?

a. Bisprolol
b. Ibutilide
c. Amiodarone
d. Lidocaine
e. Enalapril

48) A 34-year-old man with chronic persistent asthma presents with palpitations. ECG reveals supraventricular tachycardia. His blood pressure is 120/75 mmHg. Vagal manoeuvres fail to terminate the tachyarrhythmia. Which one of the following medications is useful in terminating this rhythm?

a. Adenosine
b. Propranolol
c. Atenolol
d. Atropine
e. Verapamil

49) A 56-year-old man presents because of shortness of breath and leg oedema. He has poorly controlled Type 2 diabetes for which he takes glibenclamide and metformin. His current presentation is attributed to congestive heart failure. Which one of the following is true with respect to this man's illnesses?

a. Furosemide produces hypoglycaemia
b. Ramipril is contraindicated
c. Metformin should be stopped
d. No need to increase the daily dose of glibenclamide
e. Insulin is not effective

50) A 50-year-old man with polyuria and polydipsia is given the diagnosis of Type 2 diabetes. He is being treated for congestive heart failure which is well-controlled these days. He has a history of TIA and gallbladder surgical removal. All of the following antidiabetic medications can be used in this man, except:

a. Glyburide
b. Insulin
c. Repaglinide
d. Rosiglitazone
e. Acarbose

51) A 48-year-old taxi driver presents for follow-up. He was given a diagnosis of Type 2 diabetes 2 years ago and is taking glibenclamide tablets. He works 16 hours/day. He says that he develops 'frequent hypos'. How would you respond?

a. Increase the dose of glibenclamide
b. Split the doses of glibenclamide
c. Use intermediate-acting insulin
d. Stop glibenclamide and give repaglinide
e. Stop glibenclamide and give glyburide

52) A 16-year-old secondary school girl with recently diagnosed Type 1 diabetes comes with her parents to your office. The girl states that she developed bilateral ankle oedema for 2 weeks but that this disappeared gradually without any intervention. Her fasting plasma glucose is 6 mmol/L. What is the likely reason for this observation?

a. Cyclical leg oedema
b. Pioglitazone therapy
c. Bilateral DVT
d. Insulin therapy
e. Precipitation of heart failure

53) A 28-year-old woman presents with palpitation, anxiety, tremor and weight loss. She has goitre with bruit and lid lag, and her TSH, free T_4 and T_3 are typical of hyperthyroidism. You start carbimazole in the hope of achieving a euthyroid state. Which one of the following is true with respect to carbimazole?

a. Skin rash is a very common adverse effect
b. Patients hypersensitive to it are also hypersensitive to propylthiouracil
c. There is no place for regular blood count checking
d. Does not lower serum thyroid receptor antibodies (TRAb)
e. Usually given for 6 months

54) A 27-year-old who is one of your patients gave birth to a full-term healthy-looking baby yesterday. She phones you to ask whether her current carbimazole therapy can be continued or not. She is planning to breastfeed her baby girl. What is your response?

a. Continue carbimazole with the same daily doses
b. Increase the daily carbimazole by two 5 mg tablets
c. Stop carbimazole and start propylthiouracil
d. Stop carbimazole and take propranolol
e. Stop carbimazole

55) A 43-year-old man with chronic fistulating Crohn's disease presents with a 1-month history of productive cough and haemoptysis. His sputum is full of acid-fast bacilli. What is the reason for developing this chest problem?

a. Crohn's extraintestinal manifestation
b. HIV positivity
c. Infliximab therapy
d. Silicosis
e. His occupation

56) A 6-year-old child presents to A&E with his parents with rapidly progressive pallor, jaundice and dark urine. His mother states that her son had had tonsillitis for which he was given an antibiotic. 'My younger brother has a genetic disease affecting his blood', she adds. Which one of the following medications is unsafe in this genetic disease?

a. Ceftriaxone
b. Azithromycin
c. Nalidixic acid
d. Procaine penicillin
e. Ampicillin

57) A 56-year-old man presents with malaise, sweating, weight loss and left hypochondrial heaviness. His blood count points to chronic myeloid leukaemia (CML). Bone marrow study confirms this and his Philadelphia chromosome is negative. He asks about imatinib mesylate therapy for his new diagnosis. Which one of the following is true with respect to imatinib in this man's treatment?

a. Can be given in this newly diagnosed CML
b. Should be reserved for the accelerated phase
c. Should be used in the blastic crisis
d. Should be given when there is resistance to interferon-α
e. Has no place in this patient

58) A 65-year-old man with hairy cell leukaemia is receiving interferon-$\alpha 2_b$ as part of his management plan. He develops flu-like symptoms every time he injects himself with the medication. All of the following can result from interferon-$\alpha 2_b$ injections, except:

a. Hypoglycaemia
b. Anaemia
c. Raised serum ALT
d. Neutropenia
e. Hypocalcaemia

59) A 22-year-old sexually-active woman consults you about the pros and cons of taking the combined oral contraceptive pill. These pills can produce which one of the following effects?

a. Decrease the risk of ovarian cancer
b. Reduce serum HDL
c. Potentiate oral hypoglycaemics
d. Decrease the risk of developing venous thromboembolism
e. Protect against ischaemic stroke

60) A 32-year-old woman seeks your advice. She has idiopathic general-ized epilepsy for which she takes an antiepileptic. She is married but is not planning a pregnancy and she has started to take the conventional combined oral contraceptive pill. She read a newspaper article about contraceptive failure and the use of antiepileptic medications. Which one of the following antiepileptics can safely be prescribed in this woman?

a. Topiramate
b. Phenytoin
c. Carbamazepine
d. Lamotrigine
e. Primidone

Clinical pharmacology, therapeutics and toxicology: Answers

1) c.

The following should be remembered with regard to medications in patients with renal impairment: (1) The elimination of a medication (or drug or substance) and/or its metabolite(s) may be impaired in renal failure; therefore, toxicity can ensue rapidly; (2) Many renal failure patients are sensitive to some medications even if the excretion of that medication is not that impaired; (3) In general, renal failure patients tolerate adverse effects of drugs and medications poorly; (4) Some medications and drugs are not that effective when renal impairment is present, regardless of the severity of the impairment. Statins are generally safe in chronic renal failure; even in severe renal impairment; 10 – 20 mg/day of simvastatin can be given safely and higher doses can be used with close monitoring.

2) d.

In renal failure patients, adjustment of the daily dose/frequency of a medication is usually required, even for 'safe' medications, if there is no alternative that can be used. For example, in end-stage renal disease, atenolol can be given as 25 mg/day or as a single tablet of 100 mg every 4 days. If there is any doubt about the safety of the medication, avoid its use from the outset and use a safer one. Tetracycline is unsafe even in mild renal impairment; doxycyclin is safe, but avoid using large doses of minocyclin. Cefotaxime can be used in severe renal impairment as a 1 g loading dose to be followed by half the normal dose. Clopidogrel can be used with caution if the patient needs an antiplatelet; half the optimal daily dose is used in renal impairment.

3) b.

Any sexually-active woman of child-bearing age should be asked specifically about her periods (? pregnancy). Medications and drugs can have a teratogenic effect when given in the first trimester (usually between 3 and 11 weeks of gestation), while those given in the second and third trimesters can be toxic and interfere with the development and growth of fetal tissues and organs. ACE inhibitors and angiotensin receptor blockers are contraindicated during pregnancy (fetal renal agenesis). Carbamazepine and valproic acid are risks for neural tube defects. Quinolones interfere with bone and cartilage development. Danazole exerts an androgenic effect.

4) b.

Some medications and drugs are excreted in breast milk in pharmacologically significant amounts and some attain a higher concentration in the breast milk than in the mother's blood. These can be toxic to the breastfed baby. ACE inhibitors, domperidone, lamotrigine and insulin are excreted in amounts that are too small to have a significant clinical effect on the baby. Oral contraceptive pills (e.g. given for treatment of hirsutism) should be avoided until the baby is weaned (or at least 6 months after birth) because of their adverse effects on lactation itself.

5) c.

The liver is the major organ involved in drug and toxin metabolism and elimination. It is not surprising therefore that a diseased liver can have a multitude of effects on drug metabolism. Some medications, like rifampicin, are excreted unchanged in bile and accumulate rapidly in obstructive jaundice. Impaired clotting factor synthesis puts patients at risk of generalized bleeding tendency and this will potentiate the effect of anticoagulants. Medications with salt and water retention actions can exacerbate ascites and oedema formation. Centrally acting depressants can easily produce/exacerbate cerebral dysfunction in hepatic encephalopathy. Many medications are tightly protein-bound and the presence of a low serum albumin will increase the free fraction of the medication and clinical toxicity can rapidly evolve. Omeprazole is safe in liver disease patients.

6) d.

Ciclosporin increases the metabolism and elimination of phenytoin and reduces its antiepileptic action. The other options increase plasma phenytoin concentration and enhance clinical toxicity.

7) b.

Carbamazepine enhances the metabolism of warfarin and reduces its anticoagulant effect. Itraconazole and fluconazole potentiate warfarin but griseofulvin reduces its effect. Frequent monitoring of INR is indicated whenever a medication is introduced/withdrawn, or the patient has liver disease or a concurrent illness.

8) b.

Tricyclic antidepressant (TCA) use is common and toxicity usually presents in the form confusion, seizures, cardiac conduction abnormalities and anticholinergic manifestations. Obtundation (due to central antihistamine effect) is more common than delirium (due to central anticholinergic effect). Examination may reveal confusion, myoclonic jerks and seizures, hyperactive reflexes and even extensor plantars. This woman's depression puts her at risk of suicide. Such patients usually use their own medication (TCA) in their suicide attempt; therefore, all patients should have a limited supply only of their TCA. The 12-lead ECG is the most valuable method of assessing intoxication; QRS complex duration >100 ms carries a 25% risk of ventricular dysrhythmia and seizures, a figure that jumps to >50% if the QRS duration exceeds 160 ms. Phenytoin is notoriously ineffective with respect to treating toxin-mediated seizures. TACs are highly protein-bound and non-dialyzable (a common mistake in the MRCP examination is to choose dialysis as the treatment option). Lines of management are: resuscitation, bowel decontamination, and the use of sodium bicarbonate if the QRS is

>100 ms or there is ventricular dysrhythmia, seizures and/or hypotension; sodium bicarbonate has been shown to narrow the QRS complex, tackle dysrhythmia, treat seizures and to improve blood pressure. Bowel decontamination with activated charcoal is useful if the patient presents within 1–2 hours; as the picture is florid in this patient and indicates an established TCA poisoning, sodium bicarbonate is more appropriate.

9) c.

Paracetamol intoxication is one of the commonest causes of intentional poisoning and ranks at the top of the list of causes of toxin-related deaths in the West. The scenario does not mention the patient's clinical features (such a 'mode' of questioning is very common in the MRCP examination). You should be able to guess that the question concerns the indications for N-acetylcysteine use in paracetamol poisoning, which are: (1) Serum level of paracetamol is above the possible hepatic toxicity line on the Rumack–Matthew nomogram following acute ingestion; (2) Patients who have ingested >7.5 g (or >150 mg/kg in children) of paracetamol by history and in whom the serum level of the medication is not checked within 8 hours of the ingestion; (3) Any patient with laboratory evidence of hepatoxicity (raised ALT, prolonged PT) and history of excessive paracetamol ingestion; (4) Patients with unknown 'timing' of the ingestion with a serum level of paracetamol >10 μg /ml; (5) Patients with repeated ingestion of large amounts (by history), who are at risk of hepatoxicity (e.g. alcoholics, malnutrition, AIDS), and who have a serum level of the medication >10 μg/ml. N-acetylcysteine is a glutathione precursor and is the antidote of choice in treating paracetamol poisoning. Significant hepatic damage and death are rare if it is used within 8–10 hours of ingestion, regardless of the paracetamol blood level. Liver transplantation is used in fulminant hepatic failure (this patient's clinical status is not given). Note that haemodialysis and haemoperfusion can remove paracetamol from the blood but they do not prevent hepatotoxicity; their 'regular' use in paracetamol poisoning should be discouraged.

10) a.

Acute alcohol ingestion does not increase the risk of developing liver damage from paracetamol intoxication. On the contrary, it seems to be protective by acutely inhibiting liver enzymes and competing with paracetamol for the CYP2E1 system; the net result is reduction in the formation of toxic paracetamol metabolites (N-acetyl-p-benzoquinoneimine). Patients who co-ingest enzyme-inducing drugs (e.g. carbamazepine, phenytoin, which enhances the formation of toxic metabolites), pre-existent chronic alcoholism, malnutrition (e.g. HIV, anorexia nervosa, malabsorption, because of already depleted glutathione stores) are likely to show hepatotoxicity following paracetamol ingestion.

11) c.

The poor prognostic indicators in paracetamol-related fulminant hepatic failure are: (1) blood pH <7.3 at or beyond 24 hours of ingestion; *or*

(2) Grade 3 or 4 hepatic encephalopathy, PT prolongation >100 s and serum creatinine >300 μmol/L. Note that serum bilirubin, AST and ALT are not prognostic indicators.

12) d.

The mainstay in the treatment of aspirin poisoning is resuscitation, bowel decontamination (to reduce the systemic absorption of the drug) and alkalization of serum and urine (using sodium bicarbonate, reaching a serum pH target of 7.4–7.5). The presence of any one of the following calls for haemodialysis: coma, seizures, renal impairment, refractory acidosis (this would increase the passage of aspirin across the blood–brain barrier), pulmonary oedema and serum levels >400 mg/dl in adults (or >300 mg/dl in the elderly). Patients who deteriorate continuously despite appropriate medical therapy should receive haemodialysis.

13) b.

The mainstay in the management of lithium poisoning is proper hydration, avoidance of diuretics, whole gut irrigation and (in severe cases) haemodialysis. Activated charcoal does not bind lithium.

14) a.

ACE inhibitors (e.g. lisinopril), angiotensin receptor blockers and diuretics increase serum lithium concentration and enhance its toxicity. Calcium channel blockers (diltiazem and verapamil, but not amlodipine) and alpha methyldopa can cause clinical neurotoxicity without increasing lithium plasma concentration. Volume loss (as in diarrhoeal illnesses) can easily cause a clinical syndrome of lithium intoxication. The indications for haemodialysis are serum lithium concentration >4 mEq/L regardless of the clinical status of the patient, and patients with serum lithium >2.5 mEq/L who are having a factor that limits renal handling and excretion of lithium (renal failure, congestive heart failure and cirrhosis).

15) e.

Beta-blocker intoxication is not that common, is usually mild and is most clinically significant when the agent has a membrane stabilizing action (MSA). The prolonged QT interval in this patient points to sotalol. The usual treatment plan in symptomatic patients is to resuscitate and to give glucagon and atropine; more severely affected patients can be treated with phosphodiesterase inhibitors (like milrinon), calcium infusion, insulin and glucose and catecholamine (like isoproterenol). Haemodialysis has a minimal role and is usually effective with hydrophilic minimally protein-bound agents, like atenolol and sotalol; propranolol and metoprolol are not dialyzable. Seizures and ventricular dysrhythmia usually occur when hypotension is severe; however, they can be encountered in minimally symptomatic patients, especially with sotalol.

16) c.

This patient has chronic atrial fibrillation, and digoxin is probably one of his daily medications. The introduction of a new medication by his GP may well enhance digoxin toxicity, as suggested by the patient's clinical features. Digoxin toxicity can be acute or chronic. All patients should be asked specifically about any change in the daily dose of digoxin (or acute ingestion) and if any medication has been added recently (which could enhance its toxicity, like verapamil, amiodarone, quinidine, ciclosporin, paroxetine, tetracycline and erythromycin). These medications cause clinical toxicity mainly by increasing serum level of digoxin. The removal of an enzyme-inducing agent, like rifampicin, will slow digoxin metabolism and toxicity may result from drug accumulation. The earliest ECG sign is ventricular ectopy. The presence of accelerated junctional rhythm and bidirectional ventricular tachycardia is somewhat specific for digoxin toxicity and should suggest the condition until proved otherwise. Note that any form of cardiac rhythm (with the exception of supraventricular tachycardia with 1:1 conduction) can be seen in digoxin toxicity.

17) a.

Hyperkalaemia in digoxin toxicity should be treated in the conventional way; one exception is that calcium infusion is contraindicated. This would increase the intracellular calcium, which is one of the fundamental derangements in digoxin intoxication. Moribund patients should be intubated and receive oxygen, although this is rare in clinical practice. Haemodialysis can be useful in tackling hyperkalaemia and volume overload in those with coexistent renal failure; however, it should not be used for removal of digoxin per se. Bradycardia can be treated with atropine (although this is somewhat ineffective in chronic cases); isoproterenol and transvenous pacing have been shown to increase the risk of ventricular dysrhythmia.

18) c.

Eighty per cent of patients who receive digoxin-specific Fab fragments will have complete resolution of signs and symptoms of digoxin toxicity, and a further 10% will improve, while 10% will not show any improvement. Failure to improve has been attributed to the presence of the underlying cardiac disease (for which digoxin has been prescribed), using a low dose of the Fab and treating moribund patients. The indications for this Fab infusion are: (1) haemodynamic collapse (due to intoxication); (2) life-threatening arrhythmia (due to intoxication); (3) severe bradycardia, even in those who have responded well to atropine (this would prevent recurrence following wearing off of the effect of atropine); (4) serum potassium >5.0 mEq/L, irrespective of the clinical and ECG features; (5) ingestion of >10 mg digoxin in adults and 4 mg in children; and (6) plasma digoxin level >10 ng/ml, irrespective of the clinical and ECG features.

19) c.

Digoxin-specific Fab antibody fragments are purified from sheep but idiosyncratic and allergic reactions are rare (<1%). Their infusion can result in rapid development of hypokalaemia; all patients should be monitored by measuring their serum potassium. They can exacerbate congestive heart failure and may increase the ventricular response rate in patients with atrial fibrillation. The antibody fragments interfere with the plasma digoxin assay and results will be unreliable if is done within 1–2 weeks of administration of antibody fragments.

20) b.

Methanol itself is non-toxic and mainly produces central sedative action; its metabolite, formic acid, is highly toxic to the optic nerve, presumably by damaging the intracellular mitochondria. Methanol and ethylene glycol are found in many antifreeze solutions, windshield wiper fluids, cleaners, fuels and solvents. Ingestion of >1 g of the parent alcohol is lethal. Visual blurring and blindness are suggestive of methanol poisoning, while presentation with loin pain and haematuria is indicative of poisoning with ethylene glycol.

21) d.

This poisoning is due to the toxic effects of ethylene glycol metabolites (glycolic acid, glyoxalic acid and oxalate), which in turn increase the blood anion gap as well as the blood osmolar one. Tetany can result from oxalate-induced hypocacaemia. Bilateral loin pain and development of haematuria result from oxalate renal stone formation; oliguric or anuric renal failure can ensue rapidly. The development of coma, seizures and hypotension is indicative of severe intoxication.

22) a.

Activated charcoal, syrup of ipecac, gastric lavage and peritoneal dialysis are ineffective at treating this form of poisoning; the parent alcohol is rapidly absorbed and remaining in the stomach does not bind to charcoal, and the peritoneal route is inefficient at removing the toxic metabolites. Oral or intravenous infusion of ethanol is used when fomepizole is not available.

23) e.

The first phase of iron intoxication (within 30 minutes to 6 hours after ingestion) involves direct damage to the gastric mucosa, resulting in vomiting, haematemesis and melaena. A latent phase of 'apparent' recovery ensues within 6–24 hours (which may not be seen in severe intoxication); however, some degree of hypovolaemia, metabolic acidosis and oliguria may be detected after careful evaluation. After that, cardiovascular toxicity, metabolic acidosis and prolongation of PT (from the direct effect of iron on the PT) can occur. Within 2 days, hepatotoxicity may appear from direct liver cell damage because of increased iron absorption via the portal system. Three to 8 weeks later, bowel obstruction results from GIT fibrosis caused by the toxic effect of iron; gastric outlet obstruction is the commonest one and presents with repeated vomiting. In the acute setting, plain X-ray of the abdomen may show the pills; however, many liquid iron preparations and chewable vitamins with iron do not impart an opacity (or minor opacities may be seen), although ingestion may still be significant. The desferrioxamine challenge test is no longer indicated as a confirmatory test for toxic ingestion. Iron is not well bound to activated charcoal.

24) e.
Most exposures to lead occur in the workplace. 'Blue lines on gums' (due to interaction between lead and dental plaques) is not a sensitive sign. Renal interstitial fibrosis and renal impairment is common. Men may have decreased libido, decreased sperm count and increased abnormal sperm morphology. Anaemia is common and may be hypochromic microcytic, normochromic or even haemolytic. Free red cell protoprophyrin and zinc protoporphyrin are *increased*, as well as serum lead. Motor nerve axonal degeneration may be seen as wrist/foot drop. 'Lead lines' in the bone metaphysis are seen in children. Oral DMSA is an effective method of chelating lead in adults and children. Vitamin C is a promising adjunct in treating mild cases. Removing the patient from the source of exposure is the first key step in the management.

25) c.
The diagnosis of acute CO poisoning is usually made from the combination of a compatible history, clinical features and measurement of carboxyhaemoglobin blood level (using co-oximetry of the blood gas sample). The diagnosis of chronic poisoning is notoriously difficult. Up to 40% of patients who recover from the acute presentation will go on to develop delayed neuropsychiatric manifestations in the form cognitive dysfunction, parkinsonism, involuntary movements, vague personality disorders and even focal neurological deficits. The clue in the acute setting is the presence of profound hypoxaemia with normal pulse oximetry (because the latter does not differentiate between oxyhaemoglobin and carboxyhaemoglobin).

26) c.
Patients with acute benzodiazepine poisoning following the chronic ingestion of a benzodiazepine (especially a short-acting one) may develop florid withdrawal syndrome if they are given the antidote flumazenil; this should always be kept in mind when administering this antidote in the appropriate clinical setting. Flumazenil neither produces bleeding tendency nor a hypercoagulable state. It improves hypoventilation and hypotension.

27) d.
The weed killer paraquat has a local caustic effect and systemic manifestations following its absorption. The presence of multiple burns on the face, lips and mouth together with oesophageal ulceration is highly suggestive of paraquat poisoning. Reversible renal impairment occurs within 2 days following the toxic exposure. Inhalation may result in adult respiratory distress syndrome within 2 days, and this may progress to diffuse fibrosis in survivors. Forced diuresis to remove paraquat is not effective.

28) e.

Chronic arsenic intoxication has been linked to the development of cancers of the skin (squamous and basal cell), lung, kidney, liver, urinary bladder, nose and prostate. Chronic exposure also may produce peripheral sensorimotor neuropathy, hypertension, Type 2 diabetes and Bowen's disease of the skin. Do not forget Mees lines as a sign of chronic arsenic intoxication.

29) a.

This chronic alcoholic patient has developed impaired consciousness, for which the options listed are all differential diagnoses. The development of such deterioration with 'severe' metabolic acidosis and a high osmolar gap in a chronic alcoholic should always prompt a search for co-ingestion of methanol and/or ethylene glycol. Hypoglycaemia is a risk in this patient. All patients should receive parenteral thiamine to prevent or treat a possible associated Wernicke's encephalopathy.

30) e.

Reduction in/potentiation of the effect of warfarin is a common theme in the MRCP examination. The first four options are enzyme inducers, which lessen the anticoagulant effect of warfarin. Clarithromycin, as well as ketoconazole, tolbutamide, fluconazole, nicardipine, delavirdine and sulphonamides, are enzyme inhibitors which may cause warfarin clinical toxicity and bleeding tendency.

31) b.

Questions about ciclosporin toxicity (e.g. seizures and renal impairment) or ciclosporin failure (graft rejection) are common in the MRCP examination. The scenario always addresses the addition/withdrawal of a medication. Here, the antibiotic that is given is likely to be an enzyme inhibitor, which will elevate the serum concentration of ciclosporin, causing a clinical toxicity that presents as seizures. There is no clue to any of the other options.

32) e.

Methanol and ethylene glycol are rapidly absorbed from the upper GIT and whole gut irrigation with polyethylene glycol as a mode of bowel decontamination is usually ineffective. It is useful in the first four options. The patient should be asked to drink 1 L of polyethylene glycol solution hourly until his/her rectal fluid becomes clear. The main contraindications are GIT haemorrhage and obstruction.

33) c.

All patients with a history of ingestion of a potentially toxic amount of a medication/drug should receive activated charcoal if they are eligible. A single dose usually suffices; however, multiple doses (50 g every 4 hours) are best for all the options mentioned other than aspirin.

34) d.

Activated charcoal does not bind to acids, alkalis, iron, lithium, methanol, ethanol and ethylene glycol. Age per se is not a contraindication to its use, and the scenario does not mention the toxin or the amount ingested.

35) e.

Generally, any substance can be toxic if ingested in a high enough dose. However, some substances are usually safe, even when ingested in large amounts, like oral contraceptives. Antibiotics are safe, except anti-TB medications and tetracycline. Other relatively safe substances are the antiulcer H_2 blockers and PPIs, wallpaper paste (and paper glues), chalk, emollients, 'lead' pencils and household plants. Note that washing-up liquids are generally safe, but dishwasher tablets are highly corrosive.

36) b.

Cocaine-induced myocardial ischaemia is due to coronary artery spasm in this young man. Beta-blockers are contraindicated as the unopposed alpha-adrenoceptor stimulation will increase the spasm. The spasm, not an intraluminal thrombus, is the cause of the coronary ischaemia; therefore, thrombolytics have no role. Coronary artery spasm in this clinical setting can be tackled with oral or intravenous nitrates. Massive myocardial infarction may follow and may produce hypotension and cyanosis. Features of severe intoxication are hyperthermia, rhabdomyolysis, DIC and acute renal failure. Severe hypertension and stroke may occur. Cocaine-induced supraventricular tachyarrhythmia should be treated with intravenous verapamil (beta-blockers are contraindicated because the unopposed alpha stimulation would induce severe hypertension).

37) a.

Dilated, not small, pupils are seen in amfetamine intoxication. Cardiac dysrhythmia is common and is one of the causes of death. Rhabdomyolysis, acute renal shutdown, DIC, liver failure and coma with seizures can all be encountered. Hyponatraemia results from dehydration, excessive water drinking and SIADH.

38) b.

Bodypacks in the rectum or vagina should be removed manually. Those in the small or large bowel (seen on plain X-ray) can be removed using either a laxative or polyethylene glycol whole gut irrigation to speed their exit; paraffin laxatives can cause rupture (which may be fatal as large quantities of drugs are carried) and should always be avoided. Bodypacks in the stomach can be removed carefully using an upper GIT endoscope.

39) d.

Cholinesterase re-activators, like obidoxim and pralidoxim, are useful if they are given early. They should be given to all symptomatic patients as a slow intravenous injection and a clinical response is usually seen within

30 minutes of administration. Repeated or large doses may cause many adverse effects; *hyper*tension is one of them.

40) **d.**

Neuropsychiatric manifestations are often seen with the non-nucleoside reverse transcriptase inhibitor nevirapine. Fat redistribution syndrome is seen in one-third of patients within 2 years of protease inhibitors (PIs) administration. Asymptomatic insulin resistance occurs in two-thirds and impaired glucose tolerance in one-third of cases, while frank diabetes complicates around 10% of patients. Dyslipidaemia occurs in up to 50% of patients and may explain the increased prevalence of premature coronary artery disease in them. PIs are powerful CYP3A4 inhibitors, and this is responsible for a variety of drug interactions in AIDS patients.

41) **a.**

Zidovudine can produce anaemia, neutropenia, cardiomyopathy and myopathy. Nucleoside reverse transcriptase inhibitors may cause pancreatitis, peripheral neuropathy, lactic acidosis and hepatic steatosis. Mouth and oesophageal ulcerations are commonly seen with zalcitabine, and hypersensitivity reactions (which might be fatal upon re-challenge) occur mainly with abacavir.

42) **b.**

Foscarnet inhibits the herpes viral DNA polymerase and is especially effective in thymidine kinase-deficient or mutated strains of the virus that are resistant to aciclovir. The medication is nephrotoxic in up to 20% of patients and may cause electrolyte disturbances (hypokalaemia, hypocalcaemia and hypomagnesaemia); these may induce cardiac dysrhythmia.

43) **c.**

Quinupristin/dalfopristin are streptogramins; these antibiotics are reserved for meticillin-resistant *Staph. aureus* and vancomycin-resistant *Enterococcus faecium* (not *faecalis*) infections. They are given only via the intravenous route; local pain and thrombophlebitis are very common. Anaemia, eosinophilia, and raised serum creatinine are well-recognized adverse effects. They reach tissues in a good concentration but they do not cross the placenta or the blood–brain barrier.

44) **e.**

Many cardiac medications, like flecainide, may have a myocardial depressant effect. Amiodarone is safe in congestive heart failure. This should be kept in mind when treating cardiac dysrhythmia in patients with frank or borderline congestive heart failure.

45) **d.**

Digoxin and adenosine have no place in the modified Vaughan–Williams classification. Class Ia (quinidine and disopyramide): block the fast sodium channels and prolong the action potentials (seen as a prolonged QT interval). Class Ib (lidocaine and mexiletine): block fast sodium channels but shorten the action potentials. Class Ic (flecainide and propafenone: block fast sodium channels and have no effect on action potential duration. Class II (metoprolol, bisprolol, atenolol): beta-blockers. Class III (amiodarone, ibutilide, dofetilide, azimilide and D-sotalol): block potassium channels and prolong action potential (seen as prolonged QT interval). Class IV (verapamil and diltiazem): slow calcium channel blockers.

46) d.

This man has developed bilateral acute angle closure glaucoma; the antiarrhythmic medication must have an anticholinergic property. Disopyramide can precipitate acute glaucoma and urinary retention in prostatism because of its anticholinergic action.

47) c.

The picture is suggestive of pulmonary interstitial fibrosis. Amiodarone can result in a multitude of adverse effects; pulmonary fibrosis, corneal deposits, thyroid dysfunction, liver toxicity, prolongation of QT-interval (and torsades de pointes VT) and skin photosensitisation are seen in around 30% of cases. It potentiates the effect of digoxin and warfarin.

48) e.

Adenosine can cause chest pain, chest tightness and bronchospasm; it should not be used in asthmatics. Its effect is lessened by concomitant use of xanthines and is potentiated by dipyridamole. Non-selective beta-blockers (like propranolol) can also precipitate severe bronchospasm in asthmatics. Cardioselective beta-blockers (like atenolol) lose their 'selectivity' when given in high doses and are also unsafe. Atropine produces tachycardia and obviously is inappropriate here. The rate-limiting calcium channel blockers are excellent options in those with bronchial hyperresponsiveness.

49) c.

Metformin is contraindicated in heart and liver failures and in chronic alcoholics because of the risk of lactic acidosis. The medication should be temporarily withheld in any acute illness with hypoxaemia or shock. This man's diabetes can be controlled by adding insulin and/or increasing the dose of glibenclamide (the question does not mention the daily dose) or by the addition of another oral antidiabetic agent. Diuretics impair glycaemic control. ACE inhibitors are useful agents in diabetics with hypertension or heart failure; this man has no contraindication to their use.

50) d.

Diabetic patient with heart failure should not be given metformin (risk of lactic acidosis) or thiazolidinediones. The latter group promotes fluid retention, oedema and may precipitate heart failure and increase body weight.

51) d.

The MRCP scenarios will always give at least one clue. The patient is a taxi driver and works long hours; he will definitely have difficulty scheduling his meals and snacks, which puts him at risk of hypoglycaemia. Such patients benefit from insulin sensitizers (metformin and TZDs) but this option is not listed. Repaglinide is a non-sulphonylurea direct insulin secretagogue and therefore should be taken immediately before meals, making it suitable for those who frequently skip meals and consume irregular snacks (like this patient). Even if you have not thought along these lines, you should have excluded the other options because they will maintain or increase the risk of hypoglycaemia!

52) d.

This patient has been recently diagnosed with Type I diabetes; her treatment must be insulin injections. Pioglitazone is not used in Type I diabetes (although TZDs, like pioglitazone, can also result in leg oedema and weight gain). Cyclical leg oedema is only diagnosed if there is a history of this complaint. No clue is given to suggest congestive heart failure or thrombophilia. Insulin injections can result in salt and water retention in the short-term, which may manifest as leg oedema; this would fit this girl.

53) c.

The antithyroid medication carbimazole inhibits the intrathyroidal iodination of tyrosine resulting in reduced synthesis (and thus release) of thyroid hormones. It also has an immune-suppressant effect and lowers the serum concentration of TRAb (although this has no practical importance). The hypersensitivity is not class-specific and there is no cross-sensitivity to methimazole or propylthiouracil; patients hypersensitive to carbimazole can safely be given another antithyroid medication. Skin rash is seen in only 2% of patients who are taking carbimazole, while agranulocytosis occurs in about 0.2%. As the latter is completely unpredictable there is no place for ordering CBC as a mode of screening to detect it early. Rather, the most important predictor is the development of sore throat and/or anal pain; all patients should be educated to report these symptoms as soon as possible. Therapy should be continued for 18–24 months in the hope of inducing remission; unfortunately, 50% of patient will relapse.

54) c.

It can be concluded that this woman had hyperthyroidism during (and maybe preceding) pregnancy and she has been taking carbimazole. This should have been stopped at least 4 weeks before the expected date of delivery to allow maximum development of fetal brain tissue (the question does not mention this latter point but directs your attention to the use of antithyroid medication in nursing mothers). Propylthiouracil is excreted to a much lower extent than carbimazole in breast milk;

therefore, stopping carbimazole and starting propylthiouracil is the reasonable option.

55) c.

You can deduce that a patient with severe 'fistulating' Crohn's may be receiving infliximab therapy to heal his fistulae and to induce remission. This form of therapy predisposes to TB infection and his presentation fits with infliximab as the cause of bloody sputum and cough. The question does not mention any risk factors for HIV acquisition and his occupation is not given!

56) c.

The scenario obviously points towards G6PD deficiency (note the X-linked inheritance). Nalidixic acid, dapsone, niridazole, nitrofurantoin, sulfamethoxazole and primaquine are unsafe in class I, II, and III G6PD deficiency. Streptomycin, quinolones, isoniazid, pyrimethamine, chloroquine, chloramphenicol and trimethoprim are unsafe in class I deficiency only (they are relatively *safe* in class II and III).

57) e.

This patient lacks Philadelphia (Ph) chromosome; this renders imatinib therapy virtually useless. In Ph-positive patients, imatinib can be used in the newly diagnosed chronic phase, chronic-phase resistance to interferon-α therapy, accelerated phase and in blastic crisis. Other uses are in Ph-positive acute lymphoblastic leukaemia (refractory or relapsed), *c-kit* (CD117)-positive gastrointestinal stromal tumours (unresectable and/or metastatic), dermatofibrosarcoma protuberance (unresectable, recurrent or metastatic), aggressive systemic mastocytosis (*c-kit* mutation status unknown or negative), chronic eosinophilic leukaemia and myelodysplastic syndromes with platelet-derived growth factor receptor gene rearrangement.

58) a.

Interferon-$\alpha2_b$ therapy can result in *hyper*glycaemia, raised serum levels of AST (as well as ALT and alkaline phosphatase), anaemia, thrombocytopenia and neutropenia. Flu-like symptoms are seen within 1 hour in up to 90%. Contraindications to this form of therapy are decompensated chronic liver disease (Child–Pugh B or C), autoimmune hepatitis and hypersensitivity to interferon-α (or to benzyl alcohol). The usual precautions are diabetes, thyroid dysfunction and psychiatric disorder. Treatment should be discontinued if neutrophil count falls below 0.5×10^9/L, platelet count falls below 25×10^9/L or there are persistent (or worsening) neuropsychiatric manifestations.

59) a.

Conventional combined oral contraceptive pills decrease the risk of ovarian and endometrial cancers and increase the risk of cervical cancer; the risks for breast cancer are conflicting, while the impact on skin melanoma is unclear. These pills impair glycaemic control and raise serum

HDL, LDL, and triglyceride. There is a small but statistically significant increase in the risk of ischaemic stroke, while there is a two-fold increase in the risk of thromboembolic phenomena.

60) d.

The contraceptive failure rate is 0.7/100 women-years, a figure that rises to 3.1/100 women-years in those who co-ingest antiepileptics (AEPs). The majority of AEPs are either enzyme inducers or interfere with blood concentration of the pills. Lamotrigine, felbamate and valproic acid are generally safe in women taking oral contraceptive pills. Increasing the oestrogen dose of the pill to at least 50 μg is safer than changing the AEP. Otherwise, using an alternative form of contraception is also advised.

12. Clinical sciences: Questions

1) A 28-year-old patient with SLE has glomerulonephritis with impaired renal function and active urinary sediment. Her serum complements are low. Which one of the following is *not* part of the classical complement pathway?

 a. C_1q
 b. C_4
 c. C_5
 d. C_1r
 e. C_2

2) An 18-year-old man presents with recurrent meningococcal meningitis. A search for anatomical defect was fruitless. However, he is subsequently diagnosed as having deficiency of one of the complement system proteins that is inherited in an X-linked recessive pattern. Which one of the following complement proteins is deficient in this man?

 a. C_1q
 b. C_6
 c. Properdin
 d. C_9
 e. C_1q inhibitor

3) A 41-year-old man with rheumatoid arthritis has been found to have a deficiency in mannan-binding lectin (MBL). This lectin pathway protein generally resembles which one of the following?

 a. C_3b
 b. C_5a
 c. C_1q
 d. Factor D
 e. C_4

4) A 32-year-old patient with aplastic anaemia developed Budd–Chiari syndrome with tender hepatomegaly and ascites. His final diagnosis is paroxysmal nocturnal haemoglobinuria. Flow cytometry will detect an abnormality in which one of the following?

 a. CD25
 b. CD3
 c. CD55
 d. CD20
 e. CD8

5) A 24-year-old patient with SLE has a flare-up of her disease. You are planning to check her complement serum levels as a marker of disease activity. Besides serum C_3 and C_4, which of the following is measured in this woman?

a. C_6
b. C_1 inhibitor
c. CH_{50}
d. C_3bBb
e. C_2

6) A young physician is researching genetic diseases in the community. Which one of the following has the highest carrier rate in the western European population?

a. Hereditary haemochromatosis
b. Duchenne muscular dystrophy
c. Gaucher's disease
d. Cystic fibrosis
e. Friedreich's ataxia

7) A 27-year-old man presents with neurological signs and symptoms. Some of his family members have the same disease. Genetic testing reveals trinucleotide CAG repeats expansion. Which one of the following does this man *not* have?

a. Huntington's disease
b. Myotonia dystrophica
c. Spinocerebellar ataxia type I
d. Spinomuscular atrophy of Kennedy
e. Dendatorubral-pallidoluysian atrophy

8) A healthy-looking 34-year-old woman is concerned that many of her family members have developed cancer because they have a genetic disease. Which one of the following does *not* increase the risk of cancer development?

a. Li–Fraumeni syndrome
b. von Hippel–Lindau syndrome
c. Peutz–Jeghers syndrome
d. Kearns–Sayre syndrome
e. Retinoblastoma

9) You have recently diagnosed a genetic syndrome caused by chromosomal microdeletion. Which one of the following have you *not* diagnosed?

a. Williams' syndrome
b. Prader–Willi syndrome
c. Machado–Joseph disease
d. DiGeorge syndrome
e. Angelman's syndrome

10) A 34-year-old woman with common variable immune deficiency syndrome is pregnant with twins. She is afraid that the disease could be been transferred to her babies. Your reply is:

a. Only one of the twins will carry the mutated gene
b. Both babies will manifest the disease
c. One baby will be a carrier and one will manifest the disease
d. Both babies will be carriers
e. Neither twin will carry or manifest the disease

11) A 63-year-old woman has hard and knobbly hepatomegaly. Ultrasound examination of the abdomen shows many target lesions in the liver. Immunohistochemistry study of these lesions reveals high S-100. Which one of the following is the likely cause of these liver secondaries?

a. Small cell lung cancer
b. Malignant melanoma
c. Ovarian epithelial cancer
d. Breast lobular carcinoma
e. Colonic cancer

12) A 5-year-old boy has been diagnosed with Burkitt's lymphoma because of an abdominal mass. Which one of the following is likely to be abnormal in this malignant disease?

a. c-*myc*
b. *bcl-2*
c. *K-ras*
d. Telomerase
e. *p53*

13) A 43-year-old woman with breast cancer is being considered for receiving systemic chemotherapy. The oncologist suggests the addition of trastuzumab. What is the reason for this addition?

a. Mutation in *BRCA1*
b. Duplication in *p53*
c. Mutation in *BRCA2*
d. Over-expression of HER-2
e. Tumour is CD20 positive

14) A 21-year-old man is referred to you for further evaluation of immunoglobulin deficiency state. His disease has resulted in repeated chest infections and malabsorption. Which one of the following is the commonest cause of inherited immunoglobulin deficiency?

a. Common variable immune deficiency syndrome
b. Selective IgA deficiency
c. X-linked agammaglobulinaemia
d. Hyper-IgM syndrome
e. Severe combined immune deficiency syndrome

15) You are investigating a 12-year-old girl with a mutation in the *INF-γR1* gene. The patient's macrophages fail to produce IFN-α in response to IFN-γ. This patient is at risk of:

a. Disseminated *Neisseria* infections
b. Disseminated mycobacterial infections
c. Sprue-like malabsorption
d. CMV retinitis
e. Recurrent mouth ulceration

16) An 11-month-old infant has recurrent sinusitis, otitis media and tonsillitis. His serum levels of IgG and IgA are very low while that of IgM is prominently elevated and polyclonal. You suspect hyper-IgM syndrome. Which basic defect is responsible for the clinical features of this syndrome?

a. Defective CD154
b. Adenosine deaminase deficiency
c. Janus kinase 3 deficiency
d. Deficient CD18
e. IL-2Rα

17) A 17-year-old boy presents with polyuria and polydipsia. There is a strong family history of diabetes in many young members in an autosomal dominant fashion. Mutations in which one of the following cause the commonest type of maturity onset diabetes of the young (MODY)?

a. Hepatic nuclear factor 4α
b. Glucokinase
c. Insulin promoter factor I
d. Hepatic nuclear factor Iα
e. Hepatic nuclear factor Iβ

18) An 11-month-old male infant presents with recurrent infections, atopic eczema and skin petechiae. Investigations reveal low serum IgM, raised serum IgA and IgE, and low platelet count. What is the likely diagnosis?

a. Ataxia telangiectasia
b. Chédiak–Higashi disease
c. Wiskott–Aldrich syndrome
d. HIV infection
e. Severe combined immune deficiency syndrome

19) A 7-year-old boy is referred to you for further evaluation of recurrent chest infections with staphylococci with recurrent abscess formation in the lung, skin and bone. The patient has pruritic eczema-like rash. You suspect hyper-IgE syndrome. Which one of the following would suggest an alternative diagnosis?

a. Low serum IgG
b. Sputum eosinophilia
c. Absence of pulmonary allergic symptoms
d. Many pneumatoceles on plain chest X-rays
e. Normal blood B-cell count

20) A 16-year-old girl presents with rapidly progressive asphyxiation for which a laryngostomy is created. Examination reveals gross swelling of the face, lips and tongue. Her mother states that her daughter has had recurrent abdominal pain with no apparent cause. No history of insect bite or drug ingestion is elucidated. You suspect hereditary angioedema. Which of the following regarding this disease is true?

a. Attack frequencies are lessened by emotional stress
b. During attacks, serum level of C_3 is normal
c. C_1 inhibitor is usually qualitatively abnormal
d. Fresh frozen plasma prevents further attacks
e. Danazol is contraindicated

21) You are reading a recent review article about the function of white blood cells. Which one of the following is true regarding T lymphocytes?

a. CD_3 is present on the surface of B and T cells
b. T cells form about 15% of the while cell pool
c. T_H1 cells recognize antigens on the surface of B cells
d. $CD8^+$ cells constitute about one-third of the T-cell population
e. $CD4^+$ cells recognize antigens in association with MHC class I

22) You are skimming an article about the cellular mechanisms behind the synthesis and secretion of TNF-α. Which one of the following is *not* true with respect to this cytokine?

a. Is secreted by macrophages
b. Is part of T_H2 responses
c. Induces the secretion of interleukin-6
d. Activates T-cells
e. Enhances angiogenesis

23) You conduct research into the effect of a novel medication on preventing cerebral vasospasm following non-traumatic subarachnoid haemorrhage. You find that 11% of patients who received this medication had no such vasospasm while 7% of patients on placebo achieved the same vascular target. How many patients do you need to treat actively to prevent one vasospasm event?

a. 15
b. 35
c. 25
d. 10
e. 5

24) Your colleague researched the clinical application of a new test in the screening of SLE. The results are as follows:

	Number with SLE	Number with no SLE
Positive result	95	15
Negative result	5	85

What is the positive predictive value of this new test?

a. 99%
b. 80%
c. 53%
d. 77%
e. 86%

25) You read an original article in a medical journal about the role of a new test, 'Testin', in screening for ischaemic heart disease (IHD). You review the sensitivity and specificity of this novel test by examining the following data:

	Number with IHD	Number with no IHD
Positive testing	98	20
Negative testing	2	80

What is Tentin's sensitivity?

a. 100%
b. 98%
c. 80%
d. 82%
e. 22%

26) After finishing a study about the long-term effect of a novel medication on relapse rate in multiple sclerosis, you notice that there is a type I error in the calculation of the P value (>0.04). What does this error type imply?

a. The null hypothesis is truly rejected
b. The null hypothesis is not applicable
c. The null hypothesis is wrongly rejected
d. The P-value is statistically non-significant
e. The P-value is clinically significant

27) One of your colleagues is about to calculate the results of his study. His data are normally distributed and you suggest the use of a parametric test for the study analysis. Which one of the following do you suggest?

a. Wilcoxon rank sum test
b. Mann–Whitney U-test
c. Chi-square test
d. Spearman's rank correlation test
e. Student's t-test

28) You are asked by the local health authority to check the incidence of a disease in your population. You are about to conduct research for this purpose. Which one of the following types of research study would you choose?

a. Case-control
b. Cohort
c. Interventional
d. Cross-over
e. Cross-sectional

29) You are conducting research into the effect of a novel therapy for non-small cell lung cancer mortality and you find the following:

	Number who survive	Number who die
With medication	49	50
With no medication	41	42

Which is the best test with which to analyse these data?

a. Weber's test
b. Kendall's W-test
c. Student's *t*-test
d. Kendall's tau
e. Chi-square test

30) Your friend asks you to help him choose the correct test when analysing height in 100 men and women in your population. Which one would you choose?

a. Kuiper's test
b. Student *t*-test
c. Chi-square test
d. Paired Student *t*-test
e. Anderson–Darling test

31) A blood sample is taken from a patient who attends the outpatient clinic and this is sent to the laboratory. You order testing for leucocyte alkaline phosphatase (LAP) score. The result is high. Which one of the following is *not* associated with increased LAP score?

a. Chronic myeloid leukaemia blastic crisis
b. Polycythemia vera
c. Leukaemoid reaction
d. Paroxysmal nocturnal haemoglobinuria
e. Pregnancy

32) The local laboratory haematologist is using brilliant cresyl blue to stain a blood sample taken from a patient with haemolytic anaemia. This will stain which one of the following?

a. Platelets
b. Eosinophils
c. Reticulocytes
d. Band cells
e. Erythroid progenitors in the bone marrow

33) An 8-year-old child presents with recurrent bacterial and fungal infections that he has had since infancy. He is diagnosed with chronic granulomatous disease of childhood. Which one of the following diagnostic tests has been used?

a. Bone marrow Prussian blue stain
b. Supravital stain on lymph node biopsy
c. Haematoxylin/eosin on peripheral blood film
d. Nitroblue tetrazolium test on blood sample
e. Non-specific esterase on bone marrow aspirate

34) A 44-year-old man presents with pallor and generalized bleeding. His bone marrow aspirate study report states undifferentiated acute leukaemia. The haematologist is considering the use of immunophenotyping to differentiate between lymphoid and myeloid leukaemia. Which one of the following is a myeloid antigen?

a. CD3
b. CD20
c. CD117
d. CD5
e. CD22

35) A 68-year-old man with colonic cancer is found to have a mutation in a tumour suppressor gene. Which one of the following is a tumour suppressor gene?

a. c-myc
b. c-fos
c. c-jun
d. p53
e. K-ras

36) You are preparing a lecture about the liver to be given to undergraduate medical students. Which one of the following is true about the liver?

a. 90% of liver cells are hepatocytes
b. Ito cells are storage cells for ferritin
c. Kupffer cells are located in the space of Disse
d. The portal vein supplies 90% of the liver blood
e. Normal portal tracts never contain inflammatory cells

37) A 34-year-old man presents with precordial chest pain and palpitation 1 month after his father's death from sustained massive myocardial infarction. His final diagnosis is cardiac neurosis. You reassure him that his heart is normal. Which one of the following is true regarding the normal heart?

    a. Pericardial fluid is 300 ml
    b. AV node lies just below the orifice of the coronary sinus
    c. Z-line separates the sarcomeres
    d. Free wall of the right ventricle measures 14 mm
    e. Apex is formed by the right ventricle

38) A 43-year-old male patient develops severe thunder-clap headache followed by coma. Brain CT scan reveals massive subarachnoid blood and four-vessel cerebral angiography shows an aneurysm of the anterior communicating artery. Which one of the following is true with respect to the cerebral vasculature?

    a. Posterior cerebral arteries originate from the carotid siphon
    b. Basilar artery is located at the posterior surface of the pons
    c. Middle cerebral artery supplies the inferiomedial temporal lobes
    d. Anterior communicating artery connects the middle cerebral arteries
    e. Vertebral arteries unite to form the basilar artery

39) A 22-year-old woman presents for a health check-up. She is healthy-looking and denies any symptoms. However, she is short and she states that 'she dislikes her short bones'. Which one of the following is incorrect with respect to normal adult bones?

    a. Woven bone is found in the mid-femur
    b. Osteoclasts are multinucleated
    c. 65% of the bone is composed of inorganic material
    d. Plasma osteocalcin is produced by osteoblasts
    e. Intramembranous bone formation is responsible for the formation of skull bones

40) A 47-year-old man has generalized itching. His skin looks normal apart from excoriation marks. Which one of the following is correct regarding normal skin?

    a. The epidermis and dermis have no clear-cut boundary
    b. Melanocytes are found mainly in the upper epidermis
    c. Langerhans' cells are antigen-presenting cells in the epidermis
    d. The reticular dermis is the upper part of the dermis
    e. The colour of the skin is determined by the number of melanocytes

41) You are reviewing the kidneys because you are to give lectures on this subject. Which one of the following is an incorrect statement?

a. Each kidney has one million nephrons
b. Each day, the kidneys filtrate 170 L of fluid
c. Macula densa is part of the juxtaglomerular apparatus
d. Mesangial cells are found within the central portion of the Bowman's capsule
e. Vasa recta supply the renal cortices

42) An undergraduate medical student asks you about cell surface receptors. Specifically he wants to know about a blood substance that binds to a cell surface receptor which has tyrosine kinase activity. Which one of the following substances is the student referring to?

a. Norepinephrine (noradrenaline)
b. TSH
c. Insulin
d. Acetylcholine
e. Cortisol

43) A 29-year-old woman presents with anxiety, palpitations, sweating and weight loss. She has goitre with audible bruit. You suspect hyperthyroidism and arrange for some blood tests. Which one of the following has the highest affinity for T_4 hormone?

a. Prealbumin
b. Thyroid-binding globulin
c. Albumin
d. Ceruloplasmin
e. Transferrin

44) Your SHO discusses the cause of ventricular fibrillation (VF) in one of your patients. He reports that an extrasystole occurred during the vulnerable period of the cardiac cycle and that this is the likely precipitant of this VF. Where does this vulnerable period lie?

a. Peak of R wave
b. Nadir of S wave
c. Upstroke of R wave
d. End of Q wave
e. Mid-portion of T wave

45) A 16-year-old boy with congenital adrenal hyperplasia presents for a follow-up. He has deficiency of the adrenal enzyme 21β-hydroxylase. This enzyme acts on progesterone and results in the formation of which one of the following?

a. Dehydroepiandrosterone
b. 11-Deoxycorticosterone
c. Oestrodiol
d. Pregnenolone
e. Aldosterone

46) Following a road traffic accident, a 51-year-old man says that food tastes differently and many things smell similarly. You review his brain CT scan and suspect damage to the olfactory bulbs. Where does this smell-related structure lie?

a. Parasellar
b. Beneath the amygdala
c. Above the entorhinal cortex
d. On the cribriform plate of ethmoid bone
e. Behind the calcarine cortex

47) A healthy-looking 30-year-old man is enrolled in a trial involving a novel medication that is supposed to act on cholecystokinin-pancreozymin (CCK-PZ). Out of curiosity, he asks about the physiology of this gut hormone. Which one of the following is true with respect to CCK-PZ?

a. Causes relaxation of the gallbladder
b. Inhibits pancreatic secretion
c. Inhibits gastric emptying
d. Reduces the secretion of enterokinase
e. Inhibits glucagon secretion

48) You attend a symposium about the Krebs cycle and its implementation in clinical medicine. Which one of the following is the first event in this cycle?

a. Combination of acetyl-CoA with oxaloacetic acid
b. Conversion of α-ketoglutarate to succinate
c. Conversion of oxaloacetate to pyruvate
d. Release of ATP, H^+ and CO_2
e. Formation of NAD^+

49) Your colleague is preparing a paper about the fear reaction. He says that this reaction can be consciously produced by stimulating a certain area of the brain. Which area is he referring to?

a. Broca's area
b. Hypothalamus and amygdala
c. Dorsal thalami
d. Peri-acquiductal grey mater
e. Frontal eye field 8

50) You and a colleague are discussing the general condition of a patient in the intensive care unit. The patient's oxyhaemoglobin dissociation curve is shifted to the right. Which one of the following would produce a rightward shift in the oxyhaemoglobin dissociation curve?

a. Stored blood
b. Hypothermia
c. Chronic renal failure
d. Enalapril therapy
e. Fetal haemoglobin

Clinical sciences: Answers

1) **c.**
C_1q, C_1r, C_1s, C_2 and C_4 are parts of the classical complement pathway which is activated by IgG, IgM and C-reactive protein. This activation leads to the formation of C_3 convertase which then forms C_5 convertase, ending in the formation of membrane attack complex (MAC). Although IgA may activate the alternative pathway, generally this pathway does not require an antibody for activation; there is continuous autoactivation of C_3 so that when this fragment encounters a microbe it will stick to its surface and activate the alternative pathway.

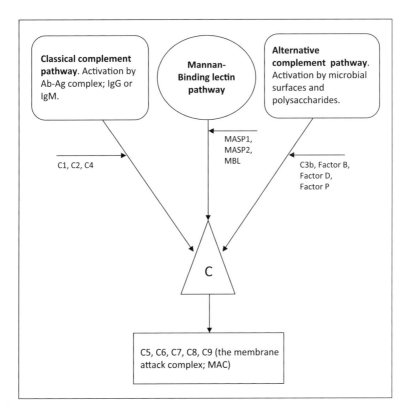

Complement system. This system can be activated by three pathways. The end result of each is the formation of the membrane attack complex (MAC). The lectin pathway is activated by the binding of a lectin to a sugar. MASP-1 and MASP-2 are proteases (similar to C1r and C1s, respectively) which cleave C2 and C4. MASP, mannan-binding lectin-associated serine protease; MBL, mannan-binding lectin; Ag, antigen; Ab, antibody.

2) c.
Deficiency of the early complement components (C1–4) predisposes to the development of autoimmune diseases (SLE and rheumatoid arthritis), while deficiencies of the late complement components are associated with susceptibility to disseminated *Neisseria* infections. Deficiency of the alternative pathway's regulatory proteins carries a risk for *Neisseria meningitides* infections. The majority of these complement deficiencies are inherited in an autosomal co-dominant pattern, except properdin and factor-D deficiencies which are inherited in an X-linked pattern, and C_1 inhibitor deficiency which is inherited in an autosomal dominant pattern. Therefore, properdin deficiency fits the clinical scenario.

3) c.
Mannan-binding lectin, which is part of the complement lectin pathway, attaches repeating mannoses to the surface of microbes. This serum protein resembles C1q; both are oligomers which have a globular domain at one end and a collagenous domain at the other end.

4) c.
CD55 (decay accelerating factor, DAF) and CD59 are abnormal in paroxysmal nocturnal haemoglobinuria. CD55 is a regulatory cell surface protein for C_3 and C_5 convertases; it disintegrates these convertases and prevents cell lysis. CD59 is a glycolipid-anchored protein and a complement system regulator that binds to C_8 and C_9; it blocks the attachment of membrane attach complex and hence cell lysis. CD25 is an interleukin-2 receptor. Basiliximab and daclizumab are antibodies against CD25. Rituxumab is a monoclonal antibody against CD20.

5) c.
Serum levels of C_3, C_4 and CH_{50} (total haemolytic complement) are low during SLE flare-ups and indicate activation of classical and alternative complement pathways. Low serum levels of C_3 and CH_{50} with normal serum C_4 indicate classical pathway activation, while low serum C_4 and CH_{50} with normal C_3 indicate activation of the alternative pathway. Elevation of these serum complements is a reflection of the acute phase response. Very low (or even zero) CH_{50} with normal C_3 and C_4 indicates inherited deficiency of other complement system proteins or in vitro activation.

6) d.
Cystic fibrosis has a carrier rate of 23% while that of hereditary haemochromatosis is 10%. Three per cent is the usual carrier rate of α1-antitrypsin deficiency. Cystic fibrosis is an autosomal recessive disease which usually results from mutation in the *CFTR* gene. The *HFE* gene is mutated in 85% of cases of hereditary haemochromatosis.

7) b.
Myotonia dystrophica has a *non-coding* repeat expansion involving CTG in the *DMPK* 3′UTR gene on chromosome 19, while GAA repeat is

abnormally expanded in the non-coding sequence of the frataxin gene on chromosome 9. Friedreich's ataxia is an autosomal recessive disorder, while other hereditary spinocerebellar ataxias (e.g. type 1 and 2) are autosomal dominant.

8) d.

Kearns–Sayre syndrome is a mitochondrial cytopathic disease which presents with progressive external ophthalmoplegia, heart block, raised CSF protein and sensorineural deafness. Li–Fraumeni is an autosomal dominant disease due to mutation in the tumour suppressor gene *p53*, resulting in increased risk of developing tumours of the brain, breast, adrenal gland, leukaemia and sarcomas. Renal cell carcinoma (which may be bilateral), phaeochromocytoma and intracranial haemangioblastoma are seen in patients with von Hippel–Lindau. Apart from gastrointestinal tumours, cancers of the endometrium, ovary and breast may occur with Peutz–Jeghers syndrome. Patients with hereditary retinoblastoma may develop osteosarcoma.

9) c.

Microdeletion syndromes are syndromes caused by a chromosomal deletion spanning several (contiguous) genes that is too small to be detected under the microscope using conventional cytogenetic methods. Depending on the size of the deletion, other techniques, such as FISH or other methods of DNA analysis, can sometimes be employed to identify the deletion. These are monosomy 1p36 syndrome, Williams' syndrome, WAGR syndrome, Angelman's and Prader–Willi syndromes, Miller–Dieker syndrome, Smith–Magenis syndrome, neurofibromatosis type 1 (only 5%), Alagille's syndrome and DiGeorge syndrome. Machado–Joseph disease is hereditary spinocerebellar ataxia type 3. Wilms' tumour aniridia, genitourinary abnormalities and mental retardation constitute WAGR syndrome which is due to a microdeletion involving chromosome 11. DiGeorge syndrome is the commonest microdeletion syndrome with hypoparathyroidism (absent parathyroids), facial dysmorphism, congenital heart disease, cleft palate and thymic aplasia with low circulating T cells and impaired T-cell function.

10) e.

Common variable immune deficiency syndrome is a sporadic non-inherited disease; there is no risk of inheritance by offspring. Although the number of circulating B cells is normal, these cells fail to differentiate into antibody-secreting plasma cells. Relatives of individuals with this disease might have selective IgA deficiency. Patients may develop repeated sinopulmonary infections, malabsorption, pseudo-lymphoma, lymphoid interstitial pneumonia, amyloidosis and non-caseating sarcoid-like granulomata of the liver, spleen, lung and skin.

11) b.

S-100 is not an oncogene and is seen in tumours of neural crest origin. *Her-2/neu* over-expression is seen in 20% of cases of breast cancer.

CA-125 is a fetal antigen that is present in blood in very small quantities; high levels are encountered in epithelial cancers of the ovaries. α-fetoprotein is produced by the fetal yolk sac and its serum level is very low in normal individuals. Tissues with malignant degeneration have the ability to synthesize and secrete this protein and a serum level >10 000 mg/ml is almost always seen in non-seminoma germ cell tumours. Its half life is 5 days (β hCG's half life is 1 day); therefore, it needs time to achieve a lower level following successful treatment of these tumours. False elevation in alpha-fetoprotein can be encountered in hepatocellular carcinoma and other hepatic pathologies (e.g. hepatitis and cirrhosis).

12) a.

At least 90% of Burkitt's patients have a translocation between *c-myc* (long arm of chromosome 8) and at least one of the following: immunoglobulin heavy chain locus on chromosome 14, kappa light chain locus on chromosome 2, or lambda light chain locus on chromosome 22.

13) d.

Her-2 receptor is one of the epidermal growth factor receptors which are important in the cellular transduction activation pathways controlling epithelial cell growth, differentiation and angiogenesis. There is over-expression of these cell surface receptors in 20% of breast cancer patients; a target for trastuzumab (Herceptin®). *BRCA1* and *BRCA2* mutations increase the risk of hereditary breast (and ovarian) cancers. Mutations in the *p53* tumour suppressor gene are seen in many cancers (like lung and colon).

14) b.

Selective IgA deficiency has a prevalence of 1:700 population and 1:333 blood donors. Up to 45% of these have antibodies against IgA; a situation that may result in severe anaphylactic reaction upon receiving blood or blood product. Usually other immunoglobulins are normal; however, serum IgG_2 subtype may be low and low molecular weight IgM may be raised. There has no curative therapy and regular immunoglobulin replacement has not been successful. The only management is proper treatment and prevention of infections.

15) b.

This is the classical scenario of INF-γR1 mutation on chromosome 22. Asplenic patients or patients with hypogammaglobulinaemia are predisposed to infection by encapsulated organisms. Deficiencies of the late complement components (C_{5-9}) carries a risk of disseminated *Neisseria* infections. CMV retinitis is especially seen in advanced HIV infection (CD4$^+$ count <50/ml^3).

16) a.

The CD40 ligand (CD154) is present on the surface of B cells and activated CD4$^+$ T cells; the interaction between CD154 and CD40 results in antibody isotype switching from IgM to IgA and IgG. Failure of this process will result in low serum IgA and IgG with increased number of IgM (which are polyclonal and sometimes of low molecular weight). The DNA-dependent kinase is mutated in ataxia telangiectasia which shows a combined selective IgA deficiency and defective T-cell function. Janus kinase (JAK) III mutations on chromosome 19 and adenosine deaminase mutations are parts of the abnormal targets in severe combined immune deficiency syndrome with abnormalities in B, T and natural killer cells. Mutated CD18 affects leucocyte adhesion molecule type I. The mutated IL-2Rα in lymphoproliferative syndrome results in poor T-cell responses, impaired apoptosis, increased bcl-2 and autoimmunity.

17) d.

Hepatic nuclear factor Iα mutation is responsible for two-thirds of cases of MODY in the UK. Hyperglycaemia in these cases is mainly seen in adolescents and is usually progressive, requiring antidiabetic medication. Mutations in the glucokinase gene cause 10% of cases of MODY, and usually mild hyperglycaemia is present at birth and can be controlled with diet alone. All MODY types are inherited in an autosomal dominant pattern.

18) c.

The clinical scenario only fits Wiscott–Aldrich syndrome. Survival beyond adolescence is rare and most patients die from overwhelming infections, haemorrhagic complications and Epstein–Barr virus-associated malignancies. Serum IgG may be normal or low. It is one of the diseases that impairs both humeral and cell-mediated immunities; other diseases are purine nucleoside phosphorylase deficiency, cartilage-hair hypoplasia, ataxia telangiectasia and MHC class I and II deficiencies.

19) a.

Serum levels of IgA, IgM and IgG are *normal* as is the peripheral count of B, T and NK cells. In spite of blood and sputum eosinophilia, chest allergic symptoms are usually absent. Histopathological examination of lymph nodes and spleen reveals striking eosinophilia. The eczematous skin rash is not atopic and is usually not persistent (unlike that of Wiskott–Aldrich). Residual pneumatoceles usually follow recurrent chest staphylococcal infections. Low serum levels of IgG are seen in, for example, common variable immune deficiency syndrome and X-linked agammaglobulinaemia.

20) b.

These episodic brawny non-pitting oedemas usually involve the extremities, but external genitalia and mucosal surfaces (especially the upper aerodigestive system) can also be involved. Many attacks have no clear-cut precipitants, but some form of trauma (usually pressure) is usually implicated. Many patients notice increased attack frequency when they are emotionally upset. Between attacks, serum levels of C_2 and C_4 are low and they further decrease during attacks; serum C_3 is characteristically normal during and between attacks. Fresh frozen plasma infusion usually terminates these episodes and long-term danazol therapy is useful to elevate the endogenous level of C_1 inhibitor. About 85% of hereditary angioedema cases are associated with *quantitatively* abnormal C_1 inhibitor; the rest (15%) have abnormal function of that enzyme.

21) d.

The T cells form about 75% of the lymphatic cell pool, and $CD4^+$ cells constitute around 65% of the T-cell population, and the remainder are $CD8^+$ cells. CD3 is part of the T-cell receptor complex and is present virtually on all T-cells (not B-cells). T_H1 $CD4^+$ cells recognize antigen on the surface of macrophages and are the maestro of cell-mediated immunity by secreting interleukin-2 and interferon-γ. T_H2 $CD4^+$ cells recognize antigens on the surface of B cells, and when activated they enhance humoral immunity by secreting interleukin-4, -5, -6 and -10. $CD4^+$ cells interact with antigen on antigen-presenting cells in association with MHC class II, while $CD8+$ cells recognize antigen on the surface of macrophages in association with MHC class I.

22) b.

TNF-α is secreted by macrophages and activates T and B cells. This cytokine enhances angiogenesis, potentiates acute phase responses and stimulates the secretion of interleukin-6 and GM-CSF. Note that TNF-β is secreted by activated T-lymphocytes. T_H1 cell responses enhance the synthesis and secretion of TNF-α.

23) c.

Questions about NNT (number needed to treat), absolute risk reduction and relative risk reduction are very common in the MRCP examinations. Absolute risk reduction (ARR) is calculated as ARR = treated group − control group; this study produced an ARR of 4%. Relative risk reduction (RRD) is measured as RRR = (treated group − control group)/treated group; this study demonstrates an RRR of 36%. NNT is obtained by dividing 1 by the ARR; 25 patients need to be treated to prevent one cerebral vasospasm.

24) e.
The positive and negative predictive values of various tests for the screening/diagnosis of disease can be calculated from:

	Disease present	Disease not present
Positive testing	A	B
Negative testing	C	D

Positive predictive value reflects the percentage of individuals who test positive and who actually have the disease, while the negative predictive value reflects the true percentage of individuals who are negative for the test and who do not have the disease. Positive predictive value = A/(A + B); it is 86% in this question [95/(95 + 15)]. Negative predictive value = D/(C + D).

25) b.
The sensitivity and specificity of various tests for the screening/diagnosis of diseases can be calculated from:

	Disease present	No disease present
Positive testing	A	B
Negative testing	C	D

Sensitivity = A/(A + C); it is 98% in this question [98(98 + 2)].
Specificity = D/(B + D).

26) c.
At the end of a research project, the question needs to be asked 'is there any difference between the two samples studied?'. The null hypothesis always states that there is *no* difference between the studied groups, e.g. there is no difference between disability scores in patients taking a novel medication and those taking conventional therapy for multiple sclerosis. A type I error is said to be present when the null hypothesis is rejected when it is in fact true. A type II error occurs when the alternative hypothesis (fails to reject the null hypothesis) is rejected when it is in fact true. Note that clinical significance does not correspond to statistical significance.

27) e.
Parametric tests use normally distributed data; these tests are the Student's *t*-test and the Pearson's coefficient of linear regression. As well as the first four options, Kandall's and Sign tests are non-parametric tests which are based on 'ranks'.

28) b.
Cross-sectional studies are ideal for detecting the prevalence of a disease in a given population, while the incidence of a disease in that population is better studied using a cohort study.

29) e.

Note the data given are not normally distributed and have been provided with a contingency 2×2 table. This makes the chi-square test the test of choice.

30) d.

Note that the data can be assumed to be normally distributed and the use of a parametric test, like the Student t-test, is reasonable. However, as two groups are being compared for one variable, a 'paired' Student t-test is the correct answer. Anderson–Darling and Kuiper's tests are non-parametric tests.

31) d.

The activity of leucocyte alkaline phosphatase reflects an increased intracellular metabolic activity. Its main use is to differentiate between leukaemoid reaction and the chronic phase of chronic myeloid leukaemia (CML). The LAP score is decreased in the chronic phase of CML (while the blastic crisis has an increased activity and score), paroxysmal nocturnal haemoglobinuria and some cases of myelodysplastic syndromes. Apart from paroxysmal nocturnal haemoglobinuria, the other options are associated with increased LAP score.

32) c.

The supravital stains (methylene blue and brilliant cresyl blue) are used to demonstrate the presence of RNA aggregates in reticulocytes; Howell–Jolly bodies, Pappenheimer bodies and Heinz bodies also take the stain. This stain is used clinically to demonstrate polychromasia, denatured haemoglobin (as in G6PD deficiency) and haemoglobin-H disease.

33) d.

The impaired respiratory burst in chronic granulomatous disease of childhood renders the nitroblue tetrazolium reduction test negative. In this test, the peripheral blood neutrophils are incubated with an activating agent and nitroblue tetrazolium; the neutrophils release superoxide upon activation and this would *normally* reduce the dye into insoluble dark blue formazan (practically seen as granular precipitate within neutrophils). The routine haematoxylin/eosin staining in these patients is unremarkable. Non-specific esterase is positive within blasts of acute lymphoblastic leukaemia and acute myeloblastic leukaemia M_4 and M_5 subtypes. Bone marrow Prussian blue stain is used for iron stores.

34) c.

The myeloid antigens are CD33, CD34, CD117 and HLD-DR. The lymphoid antigens are CD3, CD5, CD10, CD19, CD20 and CD22. Monocytic antigenic markers are CD4, CD11b, CD11c, CD64 and CD36.

35) d.

p53 is a tumour suppressor gene that plays a central role in the control of apoptosis during cellular division. It is mutated in many cancers of the breast and colon, and is the fundamental defect of Li–Fraumeni syndrome. Other options are proto-oncogenes.

36) c.

The hepatocytes form only about 60% of the total liver cellular mass. Kupffer cells are fixed macrophages that sit in the space of Disse. Ito (stellate) cells are fat-storing mesenchymal cells that are very important in the storage of vitamin A; in liver cirrhosis, Ito cells transform themselves into collagen-forming myofibroblasts. In normal conditions, liver portal tracts have a few scattered lymphocytes and an even smaller number of other inflammatory cells; however, in inflammatory diseases of the liver and chronic liver disease, these cells increase prominently in number and arrange themselves into lymphoid follicles. About two-thirds of the liver blood supply comes from the portal vein; the remainder is from the hepatic artery. This dual blood supply is responsible for the red colour of liver infarctions.

37) c.

The apex is formed by the *left* ventricle. The free wall of the right ventricle is usually 4 mm thick while that of the left ventricle may reach 15 mm. The normal pericardial fluid is <20–30 ml. The AV node lies in the interatrial septum just above the orifice of the coronary sinus. The Z-lines separate the myocyte sarcomeres; this is seen with the aid of electron microscopy.

38) e.

The vertebral arteries unite to form the basilar artery which runs in a groove on the ventral (anterior) surface of the pons. The anterior communicating artery connects the proximal portions of both anterior cerebral arteries. The inferiomedial temporal lobe is supplied by the posterior cerebral artery; posterior cerebral arteries are the cephalic continuation of the basilar artery. The internal carotid artery gives rise to the anterior choroidal artery, ophthalmic artery and anterior cerebral artery, and continues as the main stem of the middle cerebral artery.

39) a.

Woven bone is not normally found in the adult skeleton; it is seen in areas of bone fractures, bone restructuring diseases (e.g. renal osteodystrophy) and chronic osteomyelitis. The newly formed bone is not solid and is composed mainly of haphazardly arranged collagen fibres.

40) c.
The size and structure of melanosomes together with the type of melanin determine the skin colour; the number of melanocytes has no effect on skin colour. The upper dermis is the papillary dermis while the reticular dermis forms the *lower* part. Melanocytes are found in the basal layer of the epidermis. The epidermis is clearly demarcated from the dermis by the dermo-epidermal junction.

41) e.
The vasa recta supply the inner and outer medulla and participate in the counter-current exchange system of fluids and minerals. Although 170 L of fluids are filtered by the kidneys each day, the tubular reabsorption of that filtrate lessens it to only 1 L. Both kidneys receive about 20–25% of the cardiac output. The juxtaglomerular apparatus is composed of macula densa (of the distal convoluted tubules), juxtaglomerular cells (of the afferent arterioles) and Lacis non-granular cells.

42) c.
Insulin cell surface receptors have an intracellular domain with tyrosine kinase activity. G-protein-coupled receptors are beta-adrenoceptors and acetylcholine (muscarinic) receptors. Acetylcholine (nicotinic) and glutamate receptors are examples of ligand-gated ion channels. Steroid receptors are nuclear.

43) b.
Albumin has the largest *capacity* to bind T_4 while thyroid-binding globulin has the highest *affinity* to bind that hormone. Under normal conditions, about 99.98% of T_4 is bound and the remainder is the free fraction. The half-life of T_4 is about 7 days. Many medications and drugs can raise the serum concentration of T_4-binding proteins, resulting in an increase in the serum levels of total T_4 while leaving the free fraction constant and the TSH unchanged; oestrogen, heroin, methadone and clofibrate are the usual culprits, as well as pregnancy. In contrast, glucocorticoids, L-asparginase, androgens and danazole decrease the serum levels of T_4-binding proteins; the net result is a reduction in the serum concentration of total T_4, but again this does not affect the free T_4 fraction and TSH.

44) e.
A cardiac ectopic beat or an unsynchronized DC shock that coincides with the vulnerable period might easily precipitate ventricular fibrillation. This vulnerable period lies in the mid-portion of the T wave, i.e. when part of the myocardium is depolarized, part is partially repolarized and part is completely repolarized. This constellation produces a highly favourable environment for establishing a re-entry and circus movement.

45) b.

The adrenal cortical enzyme 21β-hydroxylase catalyses the formation of 11-deoxycorticosterone and 11-deoxycortisol from progesterone and 17-hydroxyprogesterone, respectively. The latter two products will enter the cell mitochondria to undergo hydroxylation resulting in the formation of corticosterone and cortisol by the action of the cytochrome enzyme 11β-hydroxylase. These hormones are present in the zona reticularis and fasciculata from where they diffuse into the systemic circulation.

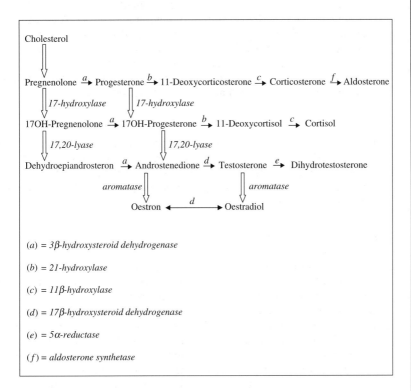

Diagram illustrating the major steroid biosynthetic pathways in the adrenal cortex. Note that many enzymes catalyse these reactions; therefore, congenital adrenal hyperplasias have diverse manifestations due to the accumulation of certain metabolites and deficiency in others.

46) d.

Fibres from the olfactory mucosa high up in the nasal cavity enter the anterior cranial fossa through the cribriform plate of ethmoid bone to terminate in the mitral cells of the olfactory bulb. The amygdala are involved in the emotional reflexes and responses towards olfactory stimuli while the entorhinal cortex is probably involved with olfactory memories. The calcarine cortex is concerned with vision.

47) c.
Cholecystokinin-pancreozymin (CCK-PZ) is a gut hormone that is secreted by the I-cells of the upper small bowel. However, it is also found in the brain (mainly in the cerebral cortex) and in the peripheral nerves in the body. It has a multitude of effects: contraction of the gallbladder, stimulation of the pancreas to secrete its juices rich in enzymes, inhibition of gastric secretion and emptying (and perhaps contraction of the pylorus), stimulation of the release of enterokinase (and enhancing the motility of the small and large bowels) and (together with gastrin) stimulation of the secretion of glucagon (i.e. control of blood glucose).

48) a.
The first step is the combining of acetyl-CoA with oxaloacetate to form citrate. This is followed by a series of reactions ending in the formation of oxaloacetate which forms pyruvate thereafter. The Krebs cycle is the major oxidation pathway for carbohydrates and fats (and some amino acids as well). Aerobic metabolism of 1 mol of blood glucose via the Krebs and Embden–Meyerhof pathways yields 38 mol of ATP.

49) b.
The fear reaction can be reproduced consciously in animals by stimulating the amygdala and hypothalamus. Damage to the amygdaloid nuclei will prominently abolish the fear reaction and its autonomic manifestations. Frontal eye field 8 is concerned with saccadic eye movements.

50) c.
Factors that shift the oxyhaemoglobin dissociation curve to the right (and hence facilitate O_2 delivery to tissues) are: rise in body temperature (fever and hyperthermia), increased concentration of red cell 2,3-DGP (this is low in banked blood; its synthesis is increased by anaemia) and reduction in blood pH (acidosis; chronic renal failure would produce systemic acidosis). Fetal haemoglobin has low affinity for 2,3-DGP; consequently, red cells rich in fetal haemoglobin have greater affinity for O_2 and this facilitates the movement of O_2 from the maternal blood to the fetal blood.

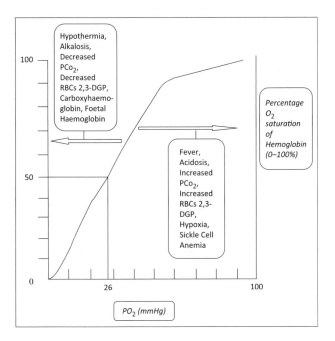

Oxyhaemoglobin dissociation curve illustrating factors that 'shift' the curve to the right or left. Note that at 26 mmHg partial pressure of O_2, 50% of the haemoglobin is saturated (the so-called P_{50}).